Lena Kroeker

In between Life and Death

Beiträge zur Afrikaforschung

ISSN 0938–7285

Herausgegeben vom Institut für Afrikastudien

in Verbindung mit der
Bayreuth International Graduate School of African Studies, BIGSAS
der Universität Bayreuth

Band

61

LIT

Lena Kroeker

In between Life and Death

Decision-making of HIV+ Mothers in Lesotho

LIT

Lena Kroekers's study was awarded with the Young Researcher's Prize for Excellence in Applied Development Research 2013 of the Verein für Socialpolitik with support of KfW Entwicklungsbank.

Published with the support of the German Research Foundation (Deutsche Forschungsgemeinschaft, DFG)

Bibliographic information published by the Deutsche Nationalbibliothek
The Deutsche Nationalbibliothek lists this publication in the Deutsche Nationalbibliografie; detailed bibliographic data are available in the Internet at http://dnb.d-nb.de.

ISBN 978-3-643-90640-3
Zugl.: Bayreuth, Univ., BIGSAS, Diss., 2013

A catalogue record for this book is available from the British Library

Fresnostr. 2
D-48159 Münster
Tel. +49 (0) 2 51-62 03 20
Fax +49 (0) 2 51-23 19 72
E-Mail: lit@lit-verlag.de
http://www.lit-verlag.de

LIT VERLAG GmbH & Co. KG Wien,
Zweigniederlassung Zürich 2015
Klosbachstr. 107
CH-8032 Zürich
Tel. +41 (0) 44-251 75 05
Fax +41 (0) 44-251 75 06
E-Mail: zuerich@lit-verlag.ch
http://www.lit-verlag.ch

Distribution:
In the UK: Global Book Marketing, e-mail: mo@centralbooks.com
In North America: International Specialized Book Services, e-mail: orders@isbs.com
In Germany: LIT Verlag Fresnostr. 2, D-48159 Münster
Tel. +49 (0) 2 51-620 32 22, Fax +49 (0) 2 51-922 60 99, E-mail: vertrieb@lit-verlag.de
In Austria: Medienlogistik Pichler-ÖBZ, e-mail: mlo@medien-logistik.at
e-books are available at www.litwebshop.de

For Mathakane and her daughter Tlhohonolofatso

Acknowledgements

This project started in 2007 with an initial visit to Lesotho during which I made contacts that continue to be of great importance for this publication. From this time onwards numerous people and institutions have been supporting me in the course of this endeavour for which I am truly indebted and whom I would like to acknowledge here.

The Bayreuth International Graduate School of African Studies (BIGSAS) accepted me as a Junior Fellow and provided me with the necessary funding for conducting my research, visiting conferences, and reviewing my findings later on. Moreover, BIGSAS awarded me with a grant for the printing costs of this book.

Aside from the financial assistance, BIGSAS has provided an inspiring platform for intellectual exchange. First and foremost my supervisor, Prof. Dr. Erdmute Alber, and the mentoring team, including Prof. Dr. Martina Drescher and Prof. Dr. Hansjörg Dilger, dedicated their time and intellect to my project. We spent numerous hours discussing interview material and comparing the literature on medical anthropology as well as on family anthropology. Prof. Dr. Drescher introduced debates on linguistics and communication and organised an interdisciplinary workshop for researchers in Bayreuth working on the subject of HIV and AIDS. My project, hence, benefitted greatly from these exchanges. No less important were all the conversations with my fellow Junior Fellows. These are the people who make BIGSAS the nurturing environment it is. Daily interaction with my peers and having a place to work jointly on related topics certainly impacted on the way I see and think about Africa in general, and about my work as a European-socialised researcher.

I would like to thank the Ministry of Health and Social Welfare in Lesotho for giving me clearance for my research. My study was initially under the clinical partnership between the Karabong Clinic at Mafeteng Government Hospital and the HIVCENTER at the Johann Wolfgang v. Goethe University Hospital in Frankfurt/M. After other planned studies were cancelled and I transferred from Johann Wolfgang v. Goethe University to Bayreuth University, I was still allowed to follow my project despite alterations. I am grateful that these organisational changes did not affect the course of research, quite the contrary, the Ministry of Health and Social Welfare was always very supportive.

Despite having studied a similar topic prior to starting this project on HIV positive mothers in antenatal care, I was not able to estimate how far-reaching my findings would be. The project may well not have gone ahead had I known. I greatly admire the work undertaken by the counsellors in Mafeteng Government Hospital and the non-governmental organisation Mothers2Mothers who are doing a tremendous job. Mathakane Metsing, the site coordinator of Mothers2Mothers at Mafeteng Government Hospital has an incredible gift in that she is able to empathetically counsel young mothers who have just found out that they are carrying a communicable virus which may harm their baby. Mathakane always ensured that mothers left the counselling sessions with all the information they needed and a positive attitude. She likewise helped me when the study became overwhelming and I felt that I could no longer continue with my chosen topic. Indeed, she became my counsellor and dear friend. In the course of the counselling sessions, Mathakane reminded me and her clients that we were dealing with the living and not with dead, and this greatly spurred us on when some of us were about to give up. Therefore I dedicate this book to Mathakane and her daughter, Tlhonolofatso.

Moreover, I would like to thank the thirty women who were the key informants for my study. Without them this project would not have been possible. Many of them welcomed me into their families and invited me again after our interviews. When I started the project I thought it would be difficult to find people who would be willing to talk to me about the intimate details of their family life, their medical history, their fears, doubts and sorrows. It turned out to be quite the opposite. Many seemed content with having someone to talk to especially when close family members were not aware of their infection with HIV and the potential harm to a sexual partner and the baby. As a result, initiating interviews and informal talks was straightforward while the topics became more and more taxing. I respect the candidness and openness of these women, some of whom became close friends.

Many of these talks would not have taken place without the help of Relebohile Molapo and Mapoone Lepeletsane who accompanied me as interpreters. Relebohile had a flair for introducing us in a very agreeable way and always found the right words when we became overwhelmed by the narratives. I am extremely grateful to her for this very sensitive approach which included prayers, jokes and drawing on her own experiences as a *bakhachane*, a pregnant woman, at that time.

My host family, the family of 'Me Maletsie, welcomed me as one of their own. After 'Me Maletsie's only daughter left for her marital home I was the only girl left in the house and took over the cooking the way Khobotso had shown me. By that stage I was treated as a family member and not as a guest. In times of happiness, sadness and conflict, I was part of the Letsie family and learned a lot about family interaction. At the same time, 'Me Maletsie and her sons were always ready to discuss with me as a researcher and reflect on Basotho-people social interaction as a female head of household and prospective village chief. I could not have chosen a better place to stay and visits continued for several years after the study had ended.

Dawn Dickson helped me to proofread the thesis and the manuscript for publication. In many cases she added comments from the perspective of an interested reader, which I appreciated. Carsten Mildner looked over the document and posed countless questions and added comments. Moreover, he was always ready to assist with the formatting. Jessica Bier helped to format graphs and tables in the earlier manuscript.

Lastly, I have to admit that it has taken a considerable amount of time to get the thesis to publication. From my current standpoint I feel that it was worth waiting. Becoming a mother in the meantime has enabled me to test some of my theoretical findings personally. Like most women in Lesotho I also relied on my family's support in an uncertain time of change. I would like to thank my parents, Marga and Uli Kroeker, my dear Mark, and our son Thato, for their love and unwavering support. I am grateful to Mark for many things but most importantly for his patience with me and this publication.

Bayreuth, 26 February 2015

Table of Contents

Prologue

Women in precarious situations, such as pregnancy and child-bearing, are in particular need of special care and support from the family network as a whole, a difficult task for families in Lesotho, which is among the poorest countries in Africa. In spite of financial poverty, Basotho people are not at all short of ideas when it comes to mitigating consequences of an insecure livelihood by means of coherence and care.

> The story of Nne[1], aged 22, from a very low income background, who was found pregnant and HIV-positive. After she had dropped out of school she had found work as a maid in a neighbouring village. She fell pregnant by a boy from that neighbourhood, however, he had no intention of being a father figure. Nne, who is a shy person anyway and avoids all kinds of conflicts, was ashamed and sorry about her haphazard situation. Instead of supporting her grandmother, aunt and little niece financially, she now had to leave her job in addition to being responsible for another mouth to feed. Moreover, although invisible to others, Nne also learned in antenatal care that she carried a virus which is said to taint a person's identity[2]. Humiliated and sad, she neither found the right situation nor the words to disclose this piece of bad news to her grandmother, who was only aware of Nne's pregnancy. Nne was now left wondering what steps she could take in order to protect the child from getting infected during pregnancy, delivery or breastfeeding, and how to manage her precarious situation and that of her family while keeping face at the same time (Fieldnotes Kroeker 4: 28/10/2008-21/05/2009).

In addition to social causes for uncertain living conditions, such as poverty, familial disruption and limited opportunities, pregnancy, birth and the immediate post-partum period are a time of increased vulnerability for both mother and child. Jordan and Davis-Floyd (1993), the 'midwives' of anthropological birth studies, summarise:

> In most societies, birth and the immediate post-partum period are considered a time of vulnerability for mother and child – indeed, frequent-

---

[1] Names of all informants have been changed. For further detail, a list can be found in the Annex.

[2] cf. Goffman, E. (1963): Stigma - Notes on the Management of Spoiled Identity, Prentice-Hall.

> ly a time of ritual danger for the entire family or community (Jordan & Davis-Floyd 1993: 3-4).

The transition of mother and child entails dangers, which differ from one culture to another; yet, medical and non-medical solutions are found to make this life-changing event as successful as possible. The advent of HIV/AIDS had added a new component to the already uncertain situation of pregnant women.

In Lesotho, with the third highest HIV prevalence worldwide, medication is available to prevent transmission of the virus from mother to child. However, health practitioners do not recognise the precarious social situation young mothers find themselves in when adapting to a new social role. In Lesotho, just as with everywhere else, they depend on important tips, loving care, and support at home from experienced women, which are not easily combined with medical guidelines.

> Nne chose to change households time and again to avoid confrontations. When the delivery approached and she still did not dare to speak with her family members about her dilemma, she suddenly found a solution: A counsellor from the hospital would help her to talk to her elders and counsel them like she was counselled. Nne would not need to enter an uncomfortable discussion, her grandmother, with whom she was staying, would receive the information on her medical condition and advise her as it is her role as an experienced female family elder.
> Six months later Nne's baby tested HIV-negative but had at the same time developed a sickness of witchcraft affliction: The child was "touched by a rich person", which resulted in an undernourished child. Would it have been "safer" to prioritise the prevention of spiritual harm over biomedical safety precautions? (Fieldnotes Kroeker 4: 28/10/2008-21/05/2009)

This book recounts the stories of thirty expectant mothers with HIV and how they made their way during an uncertain time.

Introduction

Safety precautions and preventive considerations for mother, child and the community already start during pregnancy and last for some time after the birth. Particularly elderly female family members, who know what it is to become a mother both in a biological as well as in a social sense, assist the new mother. It is their task to ensure the well-being of the mother-child pair as well as to manage the network of support which includes considerations about natural and supernatural causes of disorders, ritual and medical practices, allocating financial and logistic resources, among other aspects, in order to prevent harm and facilitate a successful transition to becoming a mother. In addition to offering preventive means, elderly female family members also serve as a great source of knowledge on curative therapies for various disorders. In any case, female household members will easily assist the mother both throughout the pregnancy and upon the birth of the baby, a state of *being and becoming* (Vigh 2009: 419-438).

Furthermore, over 90% of the expectant mothers in Lesotho also seek antenatal care and counselling[1] within a biomedical health facility (MoHSW et al. 2010: 103). Just as at home, expectant mothers are also informed here about dangers and means of prevention. The examinations, counselling and care follow the National Guidelines for the Prevention of Mother-to-Child Transmission of HIV (in short: PMTCT) which mention safety in the form of

- Safe obstetrical practices (...)
- Safe delivery practices to decrease the risk[2] of infant exposure to HIV.

---

[1] In this book, *counselling* shall be defined as an institutionalised talk with a professional counsellor, whereas *advice* indicates all kind of verbal and non-verbal directive. More precisely, my notion of counselling follows the description of Silverman (1997: 5-7). A counsellor enables a client to cope with life in a professional way and within an institutional framework. The professional has some acquired body of knowledge and interpersonal skills. A client often has different options, which are discussed with the counsellor, who may in the course of counselling give advice on one or the other option. Counselling, however, is not biased per se but rather an interactional information exchange on the client's personal situation and his or her respective options.

[2] Risk is mostly defined by calculable factors, such as the probability of an accident and the expected loss in case of an accident. In my study these figures are neither known nor relevant. I am more interested in the subjective feeling of uncertainty, beyond rational calculations, which nevertheless governs human behaviour. Thus, I do not find the term risk applicable here and avoid it except in quotations. Having said that, a whole sociological debate revolves

- Infant feeding information, counselling and support for safer practices (MoHSW et al. 2009: 4-5).

Both domains of knowledge, the knowledge of family elders and that of biomedical health professionals, follow the mission of assuring the well-being of mother and child, yet recommendations derive from differing perspectives, positions and follow differing interpretations. A hospital delivery, as recommended in the national medical guidelines (GoL 2009), foresees hygiene, attendance by trained staff and medical equipment which is at hand in the event of any adverse incidents. However, with respect to individual assistance by well-known and trustworthy birth attendants and loving care in the bosom of one's family, a home delivery may well be preferable. It is also the case that family elders may recommend traditional medication to prevent harm caused by malevolent powers, while hospital staff members prohibit traditional medication due to drug interaction and unpredictable side effects.

Thus, in this book I assess the advice given by family members and biomedical practitioners who propose expectations on "safe" and therefore "correct" behaviour to my study informants. Both forms of advice postulate ideas on the prevention of harm that may happen to pregnant and HIV-positive women. However, it remains uncertain how "safety" is actually conceptualised and what type of harm shall be prevented. Moreover, in the absence of a concrete definition and concurrence, conflicting advice is very often given to expectant mothers. Nne, for instance, also visited the health facility, where she learned about her HIV-positive status and received advice on how to prevent HIVtransmission from mother to child. She was also told to come back to the health facility for monthly check-ups for which she did not have the financial resources. In addition to her already insecure marital and financial situation, Nne learned that she also had to confront an unstable medical condition, which could also affect her child's well-being and her reputation. With normal pregnancy-related conditions she would have approached her aunt who was a traditional healer and could have treated her at no cost. But her diagnosis with HIV added to an already difficult situation. What care was now needed? Expectations of "good" and "safe" conduct thus differ creating a dilemma for pregnant and child-bearing women on how to

---

around risk as part of modern societies; how risk is perceived, evaluated and contextualised. For example, see Beck, 1986, on the "Risk Society", Macamo, 2008, on "Taming of Fate", Bloemertz et al. (Eds.), 2012, on "Risk and Africa", and others.

position themselves and justify their decisions. Speaking to expectant mothers Jordan concludes:

> In order to deal with this danger and the existential uncertainty associated with birth, people tend to produce a set of internally consistent and mutually dependent practices and beliefs that are designed to manage the physiologically and socially problematic aspects of parturition in a way that makes sense in that particular cultural context (Jordan 1993: 3-4).

Here, the cultural contexts can refer to familial care on the one hand and the biomedical setting on the other, to which I will refer as *frames of reference*[3]. A frame of reference stands for groups of actors who share particular norms and values, such as standards of evaluation and orientation, which mark "fundamental statements about the actual and ideal nature of the world. (...) Frames of reference are thus a form of supra-individual orientation and they apply to groups of people" (Loimeier et al. 2005: 17). Comparing the notion of a pregnant lady in Basotho society and in a biomedical care unit one finds a very basic difference between the two frames: community members in Lesotho usually see the mother as well as her child as social beings within a larger network of supporters, while a patient[4] in western-based biomedicine is often seen as an individual, who acts and decides on the basis of an informed decision of the potential outcome and possible dangers of a procedure. In contrast, family care is embedded in intergenerational relationships on a long-term basis whereas medical staff shifts and changes, which makes

---

[3] The application of the term "frame of reference" has previously been suggested by Loimeier, Neubert and Weißköppel (2005). These authors approach internationally diffused assets in various local "frames of reference" in which they are embedded. In the field of medical anthropology, Dilger and Hadolt encourage the study of constellations, or "contexts", in which health practices make sense (2010: 25-26). The term "context" describes a relation between a social practice and its situation. Communities, which are not bound to state borders, build social units that mobilise social and political constellations rather than mirroring them. A performative act (including the researcher's performance) therefore forms the context (Dilger & Hadolt 2010: 23-24).

Despite the active, performative connotation of "making" a context, I will use the term "frame of reference", which seems to adequately express social interaction, technical innovations, economic and political constellations, as well as changing power relations in a certain locality.

[4] Different terms apply for those who visit health facilities: medical staff members speak of *patients*, while non-governmental organisations (NGO) speak of *clients*. I will also refer to *clients* which highlights their agency, whereas *patient* conversely carries a connotation of sickness and a need for help.

a trusting relationship between client and staff impossible and little desirable. The relationship in a health facility will be merely professional and short-term. HIV, being a chronic disease, however, requires long-term commitments, on-going care, and trust. The situation can thus be characterised as ambiguous.

In the meantime expectant mothers find themselves in a volatile situation of rapid social change. At the same time, in biomedical facilities not only human resources, but also medical practices, undergo frequent changes, too, which affect the clients as well as staff. The guidelines for clinical management of HIV in pregnant women were revised four times during the study period (in 2004, 2007, 2009, and 2011). Some recommendations became the opposite of earlier guidelines and both counsellors and patients found it difficult to know what was "correct", "false", "safe" or "dangerous" and to keep abreast of any changes.

A third opinion-building domain (although not a frame of reference) needs to be mentioned as well: the client's individual situation including her marital status, lifestyle, historic and future aspirations. Her previous contact with medical practitioners, and here I mean those within the traditional as well as the biomedical school, impacts upon her personal confidence. A history of disease and pain, in short her embodied knowledge, may also influence her decisions in pregnancy, delivery and infant feeding, too. Of course, psychological pain, loss, anxiety but also happiness, comfort and self-confidence must not be ignored. In short, biography, the socially immediate and the socially imagined (Vigh 2009: 419-38) build a valuable orientation for a person. A lack of financial and social resources, however, such as in Nne's case, limits her livelihood not only materially but also the options she has when making her daily decisions.

External advice and personal feelings cannot always be easily reconciled. Indeed, it is more often the case that there is a conflict of behavioural expectations. Although complex power relations within a political-economic hegemony of biomedical AIDS care as well as a no less restrictive system of kinship, familial interdependence and bio-moral explanations of affliction undoubtedly affect individuals, these structures do not render individuals powerless. Quite the opposite in fact, and I strongly refute a notion of these women as passive victims who are trapped between structural forces (cf. Farmer 2005). Instead of presenting solely restrictive conditions I intend to discuss urban Basotho women's responses. In spite of this, I found active decision-making agents while facing conflicts of interests, which include considerations of etiquette, keeping face, receiving love, support, care and the stability of a social security network. Sets of practices and beliefs, yet, underwent adoption, appropriation, modification, aspects may be neglected, distorted, delayed or exercised openly or surreptitiously in an attempt to make ends meet – that is, to navigate between conflicting demands towards a notion of well-being.

Consequently, this book tackles the following questions:

1. What is the social framework in which, and with which, HIV-positive pregnant women in urban Lesotho interact?
2. What conflicts do these women face while aiming for the well-being of mother, child, and the family as a whole? Which arguments influence women's behaviour in the health facility, at home and towards their social environment?
3. How do they navigate between conflicting demands and therewith put the most crucial aspects into a feasible practice? What methods and tools are utilised to bridge the gap?

I do not intend to criticise structural forces of biomedical technology or traditional medical systems *per se*. Instead, I intend to describe and discuss their anchorage within the cultural setting and in view of social challenges presented by HIV/AIDS. My intention is to document decisive aspects and highlight the individual manoeuvres, and very often detours which these women make (I am, however, well aware that they sometimes merely deviate rather than gliding through, although this is nevertheless part of the tour).

Secondly, this book contains factors that appear crucial in decision-making and thus describe the grammar of health-related interaction. We can hopefully learn from how people act under changing living conditions and in uncertain times.

Thirdly, I need to add here that schools of medicine are not monolithic by any means. Both traditional medicine and biomedicine appropriate new aspects and are prone to change. Moreover, the terms "traditional" and "modern" found throughout this book are used merely to distinguish one from another[5]. I am aware that with this book I am drawing a situational

[5] I will use the term medicine as an umbrella for all kinds of schools of health care. Biomedicine refers to a medical school based on human biology and physiology, which is the predominant school of medicine in Euro-American societies. Other schools of medicine are referred to as local or traditional medicine in this book. I will stick to these terms wherever they match policy-makers' terminology, despite criticism of the terms "modern" and "traditional" in the

picture, much like a photograph which becomes part of history as soon as it is taken. Nevertheless, it needs to be taken in order to document change.

The way today's HIV-positive mothers deal with conflicting demands may become a key characteristic for their generation, especially since the women who are currently becoming mothers grew up with prevention campaigns, HIV-positive acquaintances and the consequences of the pandemic. Despite numerous attempts, the scourge of HIV/AIDS does not seem to be abating in the foreseeable future and neither are its devastating effects on Southern Africa. Looking at the past thirty years, the era of HIV/AIDS in Lesotho is also an era of constant social and economic change. In an environment of male redundancies from South African mines, female family bread-winners, domestic labour migration, and land degradation which increasingly hampers subsistence agriculture, rapid social change seems to be the only constant feature (Kroeker 2011).

In the course of examining this complex situation, I will draw upon the biographies of thirty expectant women with HIV in the Mafeteng District of Lesotho. The mothers allowed me to follow up and document their concepts, notions, decisions and impacting factors, for which I am greatly indebted to them. During numerous home visits as well as biomedical counselling sessions we discussed their challenging life trajectories. Following the abovementioned questions, I am particularly interested in their agency, motivations and justifications.

In the scope of this study, I intend to discover *uncertainty, innovation and the quest for order*. In the course of doing so, I wish to raise a debate on the household decision-making of people living with HIV/AIDS. In addition, my study engages with debates on *social navigation* (Utas 2005; Christiansen et al. 2006; Vigh 2009), uncertainty (Evans-Pritchard & Gillies 1978; Douglas 1994, Whyte 1997; Jenkins et al. 2005), and some aspects of conflict avoidance (Goffman 1959, 1963; Hirschman 1974; Scott 1985, 1990).

---

scientific community (cf. Wolf & Hörbst 2003; Greifeld 2003). The terms are criticised as being too dichotomous; moreover, "traditional" implies a monolithic, derogative or out-dated notion, whereas "modern" apparently means the opposite. While "modern health system" is easily avoided by calling it biomedical, cosmopolitan, western, evidence-based and the like, I lack an appropriate term for describing the variety of local institutions and people. I will therefore use *traditional* healer or *traditional* notions which shall be read as a system in flux and by no means monolithic. Just as in many African countries, "traditional healers" in Lesotho, i.e. sangoma, ngaka or mathuela, are part and parcel of the contemporary health system, just as much as biomedical practitioners. Clients visit traditional practitioners as a complementary or alternative treatment option to biomedicine.

1.1 Aim and Outline of the Book

Since about 2006 studies on HIV and infant feeding choices have increased significantly, most of which have concerned East or West African countries. So far, however, I have not found any anthropological study on pregnancy, delivery and the infant feeding choices made by HIV-positive women. Various studies describe clients' difficulties when complying with globally valid biomedical health protocols, but omit to mention local reasons behind these conflicts. Therefore, it is my intention to address this gap in knowledge. In accordance with Hazam, I see biomedical care as an "additive" to a local health care system:

> It is perhaps inevitable that the research posture rooted in an appreciation of the established cultural context in which Lesotho's medical system finds expression invites the study of cosmopolitan medicine largely as a kind of "additive" to the indigenous system. Like the cream in one's coffee, it alters but does not change the underlying nature of the brew, a dimension not to be ignored but as much an alien in an enhancing additive (Hazam 1983: 3).

Due to plurality in the medical field clients opt to use biomedical and local traditional health facilities in a complementary way. I therefore intend to describe why they appropriate information to their current situation and what their arguments were for doing it in one way or the other.

Secondly, I would like to position this study in relation to a debate on *Social Navigation*[6] under uncertain living conditions. Social Navigation is often studied within the context of violent conflicts and situations of war, although Chistiansen et al. (2005) provided examples on how young people navigated when entering adult life. In either case social navigation concerns the direction people take within this insecure and uncertain field. However, after Whyte (1997), as well as Jenkins et al. (2005), defined health hazards as an existential cause of an uncertain situation, my study contributes to an analysis of how in times of disease one struggles to achieve a more certain and stable situation. These ideas are accompanied by observations on the political realm of anthropology, namely avoidance of conflicts.

---

[6] "Strategy is the process of demarcating and constituting space and tactics in the process of navigating them" (Vigh 2003: 136), "the way agents guide their lives through troublesome social and political circumstances" (Utas 2005: 10-11).

Thirdly, this analysis connects studies in the field of political anthropology and medical anthropology. My study describes subordinates' behaviour towards dominant parties in decision-making processes and counteracts the notion that subordinates, here females living with HIV, are passive or victims. Instead I emphasise their active role as decision-makers within the social hierarchy. However, the women in my study in no way intended to invert the social hierarchy. By way of contribution to the theoretical body of knowledge in political anthropology, I would like to present ways of dealing with conflicts by avoiding them. Under situations of uncertainty I found five ways that were used in close long-term relations of dependency with unequal power distribution, namely: feigning agreement, physical absence, finding excuses, disturbing the normal procedure, and involving a mediator.

This book comprises eight chapters. Following on from these introductory remarks (Chapter 1, Introduction), Chapter 2 (Research at the Intersection of Debates) will relate this study to on-going anthropological debates. Chapter 3 (In Sickness and in Health) discusses the value of a biographical approach for this work. I will thereafter introduce the reader to the geography and social structure of Lesotho, with a focus on women and their living conditions in urban Mafeteng (Chapter 4, Shifts and Changes in Uncertain Times). Three subsequent empirical chapters (Chapter 5, Pregnancy: Navigating between Conflicting Demands; Chapter 6, Delivery: "*In between life and death*"; and Chapter 7, Options for Safe Infant Feeding) should be read as one entity, although I decided to organise them as three subsequent events. Organisationally, the triad of pregnancy, delivery and infant care follows the structure of *rites of passage*. Van Gennep (2005) and Turner (2005) suggested that rites generally follow a threefold structure comprising *rites of separation*, *rites of liminality* and *rites of incorporation,* which corresponds with the three chapters I present here.

Chapter 8 concerns the use of contraceptives and to what extent the prevention of HIV transmission to a child impedes on the desire for children. In particular HIV-positive women are counselled to refrain from having offspring. Due to the inductive approach to the topic, a subsequent chapter (Chapter 9, Uncertainty, Innovation and a Quest for Order) concerns strategies of "muddling through" as well as hidden agendas of resistance.

Finally, in the last section (Chapter 10, "*This thing of HIV makes childbearing difficult*") I summarise empirical and theoretical findings and conclude how means of *social navigation* help to create "something like order". HIV-positive pregnant and child-bearing women present pragmatic and flexible ways of reconciling their life in a framework of uncertainty, innovation and a quest for order.

Research at the Intersection of Debates

In recent years, particularly researchers from two South African research centres have published on the social context in which the programme for Prevention of Mother-to-Child Transmission of HIV (PMTCT) was applied. One of these is the interdisciplinary African Centre for Health and Population Studies at the University of KwaZulu Natal in South Africa which published extensively on Preventing Mother-to-Child-Transmission in South Africa. Authors such as Bland et al. (2007, 2008), Coovadia et al. (2007), Coutsoudis et al. (1999, 2001), among others, published on mother-child health and HIV. At the second of these centres, the Human Science Research Council (HSRC), particularly Peltzer et al. (2007, 2009, 2009a, 2010) and Phaswana-Mafuya (2008), who also heads the Social Aspects of HIV/AIDS Research Alliance (SAHARA), wrote extensively on PMTCT in South Africa. The papers mention difficulties faced by women when complying with biomedical treatment and PMTCT advice, and list a number of factors which interfere with treatment compliance. However, their studies rather contribute to the discipline of public health and behavioural science and speak from a staunchly biomedical standpoint. In fact, many studies describe how patients are "failing their treatment" or are "non-compliant" but neglect to describe their interests, motives and arguments for doing so. Nevertheless, the authors list aspects that are worthy of being studied in more detail and with ethnographic depth. In contrast, medical anthropologists looked into health-related behaviour beyond a natural scientific perspective and rejected making a judgement on right and wrong behaviour, which at times makes collaboration difficult, since anthropologists do not necessarily have an interest in improving the situation or listing policy implications but tend to document the status quo.

Recent anthropological studies on HIV/AIDS in Africa were predominantly concerned with what Janzen (1978) called the *treatment management group*, that is, the group of people caring for the sick. Furthermore, various anthropological studies approached HIV/AIDS from a clinical, political as well as a pharmaceutical perspective. A detailed analysis on expectant mothers with HIV is still lacking. My study not only intends to fill this gap, but aims to connect debates.

This book hinges on several research visits to the town of Mafeteng, the second largest town in Lesotho. Mafeteng town, like nine other district capitals, provides a governmental referral hospital. Mafeteng Government Hospital includes Karabong Clinic, which caters solely for HIV-positive clients who receive antiretroviral therapy. Despite the fact that part of my study took place in a hospital, the study is *on* health care systems rather than *within* health care facilities. Here, I distance my study from those in clinical anthropology even though the place of study is within a clinic. This study on mother and child care in the HIV era rather hovers at the intersection of diverse scientific disciplines, global guidelines, governmental interpretations and local practices.

By and large, a clinic is a place saturated with hierarchies, laws and orders. Consequently, while describing the interaction of health personnel and their clients, much can be inferred about asymmetric power relations and how people act as dominants and subordinates in such social processes. Here, the study leans towards political anthropology. Secondly, people approach a health facility solely because an unusual physical condition forces them to do so. Thus, they are uncertain whether "normal" life can be re-established and if their discomfort will be brought under control. Themes of this kind and how people act to bring an unusual situation under control are currently discussed among anthropologists under the heading of "uncertainty". Uncertainty is debated beyond disciplinary boundaries and not necessarily with a focus on health. I, however, intend to make a statement on uncertainty when speaking about HIV-positive expectant women too. I only found out about these connections to political anthropology and the interdisciplinary debate on uncertainty while carrying out research on mothers and children in Lesotho. Due to the inductive approach of my study, the lion's share of the theory will be discussed and summarised in Chapters 9 and 10 following the empirical chapters. In the next chapter, however, I will briefly outline these debates to orient the reader. Therewith, I would like to draw attention to the framework in which this research is embedded. This includes: medicalisation, childbirth as a medical event, sickness and uncertainty.

2.1 Medicine of the North, Medicine of the South

A basic disagreement exists between the social and natural sciences on to what extent health and, thus, normal life, can be manufactured by means of medical technology[1]. Social scientists (by now) deny that there are universal

[1] Technology means the science of techniques and includes the tools, crafts, methods, knowledge systems and personnel that surround a technical solution. Technique solely means

laws and point to the social interpretations of normality and abnormality whereas, in contrast, in the natural sciences it is assumed that universal laws exist which lead to certain consequences. In short, natural scientists seek justification from natural scientific laws which build a formalised analytical frame for explaining the world (Loimeier et al. 2005: 18). Respective research, built on such universally valid laws, produces models demonstrating functions and malfunctions.

Academically studied medicine originated in humanist philosophy and advancements in European scientific work in the 19th century. It follows the assumption that natural science can explain what causes disorders in the human body based on the symptoms the body presents. Treatment mechanisms are likewise based on natural-scientific laws and medical practices are legitimised if they evidently do more good than harm to the afflicted human body. That being so, medical technology relies on evidence-based, rational, reliable and globally applicable principles (Borck 2003: 139-141). For these reasons, western-based biomedicine is considered to be superior to other locally prevalent medical systems, which are not supported by scientific evidence. Having said that, health technology is a product of the cultural setting. Despite the assumption of biomedical researchers that natural sciences work globally, they are nevertheless imbued with the norms and values of the researchers and their technological standards. The scientific concepts on which biomedicine is based are themselves products of a particular research background, as well as political and social interests associated with particular biomedical products[2]. Moreover, the history of moral norms and values is inscribed into the social institutions produced by society. In the end it is the scientific community which accepts or rejects a study and its outcomes. In the social sciences the tools, methods, knowledge systems, the institutions, health personnel and political economy are part of the research object. This context is relevant for functionality and representation of a health care system and needs to be taken into account. Institution, material

---

the device or practice as such. Medical technology includes devices (instruments, machines and pharmaceuticals), information on their functions and applications, and services offered in biomedical health facilities, hence, everything and everyone involved with diagnosis, monitoring or improvement of human conditions (Paslack 1999: 837-856).

[2] With regard to the history of medicine, I am reminded here of the endeavours of microbiologist Robert Koch (1843-1910) which, without doubt, led to significant medical advancements. Notwithstanding this, his inhuman clinical trials with African populations would not have been possible without the encouragement of the British and German colonial administrations, and thus the backing of the contemporary political and social culture.

and personnel have a major impact on biomedical processes. This impact cannot be underestimated.

Religious notions disappeared from medical explanations and were replaced by secularisation. Individualisation and natural scientific patterns of explaining the world took the place of religious interpretations. Social deviance, which was previously judged according to religious norms, became a matter of criminalisation and, subsequently, of medicalisation, and deviant behaviour had to be corrected in social institutions. The religious, judicial and later medical treatment of people in a physically or mentally disordered state was dealt with by professionals from the health sector, who therefore became gatekeepers. Foucault argued in the 1970s that people in social institutions are there solely because of their social deviance. Patients of a health facility thereby serve as the medium of sickness; organs are afflicted body parts in a merely technical sense and a hospital is the place where disease carriers are gathered. In the "Birth of the Clinic" (1973) and "Discipline and Punishment: The Birth of the Prison" (1991) he illustrates how governmental institutions characterise inmates as deviant and in need of correction. All material and immaterial goods in the realm of the institution including the architecture are intended to observe the clients' progress in becoming a "normal" member of society (again).

Since the 1970s social scientists have gone on to analyse the health sector and its social representation. Hospitals are places where the norm is established given that patients are basically people who cannot physically function according to their normal capacity. In his book on the "Limits to Medicine: Medical Nemesis" (1977), Ivan Illich argues that the normality of human life is increasingly judged from a medical point of view. Illich provocatively criticises the way health care institutions have gained control over the lives of humans to a degree which perhaps does more harm than good. Dysfunctions of the human body became the sole medical concern and thus the medical sector gained ground as a moral institution that defines and treats what is considered abnormal, deviant and prone to being treated using medical technology and institutions. He therewith points out that the public health sector has implications in the social sphere beyond the individual patients' well-being. Illich concludes by determining this institutional framework of health care as being a pandemic in itself. Physicians have gained access and authority over human bodies, while the patients have forfeited this right. Resulting from this notion, Illich objects to a quasi industrialised production of health whereby humans are merely objectified carriers of disease within a rampant health care system.

Conrad and Schneider (1983), Zola (1972) and Conrad (1975, 1992) develop this argument further by determining that medicalisation implies conceptional, organisational and interactional aspects. Conrad elaborated upon his definition of medicalisation by saying:

> Medicalization consists of defining a problem in medical terms, using medical language to describe a problem, adopting a medical framework to understand a problem, or using a medical intervention to "treat" it. This is a sociocultural process that may or may not involve the medical profession, lead to medical social control or medical treatment, or be the result of intentional expansion by the medical profession (Conrad 1992: 211; cf. Conrad 1975).

The medical sector works on various levels, which are nevertheless intertwined, namely medical technology, collaboration of medical and non-medical institutions, ideology legalising and supporting certain practices, and monitoring of sick humans. Examples of medicalisation include the reproductive system (menstruation, pregnancy, delivery, breastfeeding, menopause as well as sexual deviance), development of children and the elderly, as well as addictions, learning disabilities, eating disorders, violent and criminal behaviour to name just a few. In all kinds of medicalised conditions physicians are pivotal in the access to treatment. Medical staff decide whether a person fulfils the "role of the sick" (Parsons 1964) or not and if a person needs to be referred to (social) institutions for further treatment and care. In the process of re-establishing order medical staff, as executors of health policies, legitimise and pre-define the steps needed to arrive at normality. Thus treatment and debate are no longer the concern of the public domain but are the realm of professional caretakers who are part of a strong backbone: the health sector. Due to high societal acceptance, if justification comes from a professional physician then various institutions and their employees in the judicial and education sector collaborate with medical facilities. The sector appears reliable and strong as the hegemony is built on natural science which suggests objectivity and reliability as well as political independence, which doctors shall guarantee.[3] A whole health sector is instrumental to the representation of biomedical approaches to minimise or eliminate disorders or to

---

[3] For a critique and elaboration on the different levels where medicalisation comes into effect, see, for example, Halfman (2011).

make them a normal part of life. These social, economical and political implications are attached to the health facility and all associated social institutions as immaterial characteristics. These immaterial implications surround the institution whenever they are transferred out of their context of origin, for instance, if a western-based biomedical health care system is set up outside the scope of western countries. This is discussed in a debate on travelling models or travelling ideas, which I will outline here in connection to health[4].

Biomedicine is the dominant medical system in industrialised countries and since most globally acting institutions of health and healing are dominated by westerners[5], biomedicine was transferred to other world regions. Missionaries, and later international agencies such as the World Health Organization (WHO), international development agencies and many more, spread biomedical technology all over the world. It was assumed that this generally applicable school of medicine would cure pathologies independently of local interpretations, and hence, in the global arena, biomedical approaches were promoted as the predominant school despite a large variety of other therapeutic systems worldwide[6].

International agencies such as the WHO, and institutions of the United Nations, have named malaria, tuberculosis and HIV/AIDS as global scourges that are the focus of biomedical research. HIV/AIDS received overwhelming attention in the West as well as the rest of the world. Despite the fact that biomedicine claims to be the only school of medicine which can detect and treat (but not yet cure) infections with the HI-virus, the largest population of those infected can be found in developing countries, namely Southern African countries. In order to control the HIV pandemic, blood screening methods, biomedical treatment and prevention techniques were developed in the global North and promoted by international agents in the global South, where the immunodeficiency syndrome is most prevalent. Thus, biomedicine

---

[4] Travelling models or travelling ideas are discussed in development sociology and sociology of knowledge, respectively, as well as in development anthropology. Its foundation was laid by Latour (1986), Loimeier et al. (2005) and Rottenburg (1996, 2009). It concerns the diffusion of material and immaterial goods which are produced in one social and cultural context and applied in another. Examples stem from development agencies, globally acting companies and the international distribution of pharmaceuticals.

[5] The UNICEF and WHO International Conference on Primary Health Care held in Alma Ata in 1978, or the UN Millennium Development Goals of 2000, reflect this global spread.

[6] For a discussion on globalisation and medicine, see Wolf & Dilger 2003; Wolf & Hörbst 2003; Dilger & Hadolt 2010.

is part and parcel of international health politics and a health economy driven by western stakeholders. For instance, antiretroviral treatment, received by HIV-positive people, has its own social life due to the highly politicised and global markets, sparked by debates on availability, economic interests and the high demand in resource-constrained areas (Comaroff 2010). The biomedical health sector undoubtedly claims a monopoly over the treatment and care of people living with HIV and AIDS, meanwhile, the institutional sector and political-economic backing supports and shapes this hegemonic representation. Manifold hybrid organisations build a framework around biomedical HIV/AIDS testing and treatment sites in which people living with HIV/AIDS are taught how to live "positiHIVly" (see, for instance, www.AIDShilfe.de).

Besides biomedical ideas, material goods such as pharmaceuticals are also transported from the laboratories to the patients. Only in recent years have anthropologists started studying "biographies" of biomedical products. A debate arose on the immaterial values of pharmaceutical goods, their institutional backgrounds and their social texture. As commodities that travel the world, from the place of manufacture to the consumer, pharmaceuticals have a *social life* of their own and through the people who are handling them (v.d.Geest et al. 1996; Whyte et al. 2002; Whyte 2002; cf. Appadurai 1986). Medical technology, such as commercial pharmaceutical products, is exported globally, and also to developing countries where social and cultural conditions, available expertise and the supporting infrastructure differ from the place where the product was developed, produced and marketed. With this global export, a technology is disconnected from its source context and is applied as new technology in its target context. Here, humans are more than mere recipients of technology. Antiretroviral medication, for instance, changes not only in its geographical setting, but also its social context beyond its mere pharmacological function. Effects and side effects ("unintended consequences") must be evaluated afresh in a global-local setting (Rottenburg 2002). Developers of technological assets, nevertheless, often assume effects and functions to follow the laws of natural science, irrespective of the time, place and social setting which are lost to the technology through the global transfer. Determinants are hence the technology which functions by itself (Technikdeterminismus) rather than the human supported by social institutions (Sozialdeterminismus). In summary, a geographical shift includes the construction of knowledge which surrounds antiretroviral therapy as it is produced and transferred within health institutions and at the patient's home.

In the context of my study of HIV-positive women in Lesotho, medicalisation plays a major role. Pregnancy, delivery and early infant care were not considered in most non-western societies as pathological events which required medical attention. In contrast, the western-based biomedical school foresees medical attention during pregnancy, delivery and the post-partum period. These days, most pregnant women in Lesotho attend antenatal care in a biomedical health facility at least once and consent to being screened for HIV in the course of their examination. With these antenatal check-ups medical professionals gain access and authority over two human bodies in their care: the mother's and the child's. A HIV-positive test in pregnancy alerts health personnel to a severe obstetric disorder. Even if the expectant mother does not have any feelings of sickness, she will be advised to enrol in medical care following national and international guidelines for the prevention of HIV transmission from mother to child. From now on a whole machinery of health technology will control the mother's compliance with treatment protocols to keep her and her child fully functional, "normal" members of society. In any event, normality and abnormality is defined by biomedical, mostly western, policy makers.

2.2 Medicalisation of Life

Many functions of the body have undergone a paradigm shift through medicalisation. Particularly women's bodily functions are under medical scrutiny whereby normal process adopted some pathological aura and became a matter of medical technology (Binder-Fritz 2003; Kneuper 2003). Pregnancies, for instance, receive overwhelming biomedical attention and mothers are advised to attend antenatal care in medical facilities. Jordan & Davis-Floyd described births in four cultures and contrasted the degree of medical technological intervention and social interaction between a mother and her birth attendant in the US, Sweden, the Netherlands and Mexico. Care for mother and child in confinement in a non-medicalised setting differed significantly from a "medicalised" delivery in a biomedical setting (Jordan & Davis-Floyd 1993; Davis-Floyd 1997; Teijlingen 2000). In all four cultures confinement was associated with risks for mother and child and the need for the special expertise of birth attendants to assist during this crucial time. However, the definitions of the risks, the tools and expertise needed to contain it and the time when the risky period starts and ends is a matter of debate. The authors illustrate how the standard protocol of care relates to different perceptions of the harm that parturition entails. Notwithstanding this, supervision of pregnancies and deliveries with biomedical methods did not give better results per se than a non-biomedically attended one.

On the whole, having children is a normal part of women's biography and one of the most crucial experiences in a woman's life, in both a social and biological sense. Even though pregnancy, delivery and early child care is not a pathology, biomedical policy makers claim authority over supervising confinement. International agencies promote biomedical antenatal care as well as delivery services worldwide to reduce maternal and infant mortality. In fact, maternal and infant mortality rates shall determine the development of a country. However, Jordan & Davis-Floyd do not consider hospital births to be safer in their examples from the US and Sweden, as they praise training and practices of birth attendants in Mexican and Dutch home births who deliver children with equally good results.

In many regions, women awaiting the delivery of their child have a choice between places to give birth and between different schools of thought. Sargent (1982, 1989) studied obstetric choices of women in urban Benin and found a correlation between women's educational attainment and the place of delivery. Women with little formal education, living in rural areas and from a peasant background delivered at home, whereas elites with formal education and employment opted in favour of a hospital delivery. However, not only the mother's but predominantly the father's and husband's achievements correlated with the place of birth, as Sargent argues. In spite of this, fears of witchcraft affliction of the child leading to infanticide were shared among all social strata. Besides proverbial virtues, as well as religious, economic and medical aspects play a part together with status aspirations, although proverbial and religious factors are less influential when women have greater access to education and opportunities of social mobility (1989: 205). In conclusion, not only rational arguments based on hard facts are decisive, but emotional and spiritual arguments.

In addition to the birth, the post-partum phase has been a matter of interest in biomedicine as well as in anthropology due to biological, nutritional as well as sub-social processes. Authors from both natural and social sciences agree on the benefits of breastfeeding for mother and child but focus on different aspects. Basically, authors disagree on the question of to what extent breastfeeding is a natural law or a social construct.

In anthropology, breastfeeding has been researched in relation to duration, fertility and post-partum sex taboo, and mother-and-child interaction (Dettwyler 1988; Guz & Hobcraft 1991; Yovsi 2003). Studies in bio-anthropology provided information about the interrelatedness of biology and social-interactional aspects of breastfeeding. Stuart-Macadam and Dettwyler (1995) as well as Maher (1992) combine biomedical and nutritional considerations with social and religious notions of infant feeding. Maher, on the one hand, focuses on the historical development of ideas surrounding breastfeeding in the Western World, whereas Stuart-Macadam and Dettwyler, on the other hand, describe breastfeeding from a cross-cultural perspective and look into associated social relations. Ethnographic examples, in summary, categorise breastfeeding as neither a solely biological nor a social matter, yet, psychological, cultural and biological processes interrelate and, consequently, breastfeeding signifies much more than nutrition. Moreover, breastfeeding can have spiritual implications when it is embedded into a whole ritual process of reproduction. Yovsi (2003) compares the infant feeding practices of sedentary Nso farmers and Fulani pastorals in Cameroon and embeds the feeding practice into a spiritual understanding of child development. In this context, mother-child-interaction in general and breastfeeding in particular bridges the development of a foetus from its ancestral stage into a social human being. In contrast to the other authors, she connects breastfeeding with the whole ritual cycle of human being and becoming. Therefore, some rites which commence with conception and terminate with weaning only become comprehensible in their broader social context. In conclusion, pregnancy, delivery and infant feeding affect the community as a whole and become a matter of family well-being. Biomedical notions of pregnancy, delivery and infant feeding cannot grasp these aspects. Biomedicine usually focuses on individual patients and not on their social background. For the same reason, international guidelines for early infant feeding do not take social factors into consideration.

Of course, the above mentioned implications affect people's behaviour. Changes in the medical recommendations are not easily accepted due to the far reaching consequences in the social realm. The medical finding that HIV can be transferred from mother to child during breastfeeding additionally poses some difficult decisions for the infected mothers. Moland analysed the dilemma faced by HIV-positive mothers in the Tanzanian Kilimanjaro Region when having to decide on infant feeding practices. On the one hand, they risk transmitting a potentially fatal disease, on the other, breastfeeding is seen as an integral part of "good motherhood". This causes uncertainties due to choices brought about by the medicalisation of breastfeeding (Moland 2004). Further studies on the Kilimanjaro Region were offered by Leshabari, Blystad and Moland (Leshabari et al. 2007, 2007 (a)). They arrive at the conclusion that rural economically and socially vulnerable women with HIV prefer breastfeeding as it would further stigmatise their situation not to do so (Blystad & Moland 2009). They argue that the irreconcilability of notions of new life (of the child) and death (of mother or child through AIDS), as well as social versus economic costs, contribute to mothers' choices. Desclaux and Alfieri (2009) arrive at the conclusion that the choices HIV-positive mothers make are not solely based on either local or biomedical knowledge. They need to balance economic availability and social obligations.

A good overview on Southern African practices of HIV-positive breastfeeding mothers is offered by the Centre of Health and Population Studies at the University of KwaZulu-Natal from a Public Health perspective. Bland et al. (2007, 2008), Coovadia et al. (2007), Coutsoudis et al. (1999, 2001), among others, published on mother-child health and adherence to biomedical advice in South Africa between 1999 and 2007. As with the interdisciplinary group which studied Tanzanian breastfeeding practices, the South African group also recognised the difficulties in reconciling local medical and biomedical recommendations, resulting in the low compliance of HIV-positive mothers. However, researchers take a predominantly medical view when looking into factors which inhibit medical success.

Even though expectant mothers do not usually have any symptoms of carrying the virus breastfeeding shifted from a mere social sphere into a pathological, medicalised one. Since interventions to prevent HIV transmission from mother to child differ due to economic reasons between industrialised and developing countries, Desclaux and Taverne speak of "AIDS of the North" and "AIDS of the South" (Desclaux & Taverne 2000).

It is unfortunate that medication which can prevent the transmission of HIV from mother to child is available in western countries where only a few patients are in need of it, whereas in developing countries with high HIV prevalence medication has limited availability due to economic reasons. In industrialised countries patients can expect to be treated with medication which is combined depending on their individually assessed health conditions and treatment history. In poorer countries a standard therapy is available which is not tailored to individuals. Subsequently, therapy outcomes are worse because there is no choice for physicians and their patients. For instance, in industrial countries, where most medical technology is developed and tested, various diagnostic methods and treatment schemes are available. As a result, HIV-positive pregnant women will be on lifelong treatment with close monitoring of changes in their immune status.

Pharmaceutical interventions are expected to reduce vertical HIV transmissions from mother to child to around 1% (Cooper et al. 2002). A combination of preventive measures includes highly active antiretroviral therapy (HAART) for the mother, close monitoring of the viral load, caesarean section, post-exposure prophylaxis for the child and replacing breast milk with formula milk. In contrast, in developing countries such as Lesotho, the Ministry of Health and Social Welfare (MoHSW) published PMTCT guidelines which follow the WHO guidelines for resource-constrained countries. These guidelines recommend a choice of two options depending on the maternal immunological condition. Either mothers in a fairly good condition receive a short course treatment over 14 weeks before confinement, or, if the immunological condition is fairly low, the mother will be offered life-long treatment. Delivery takes place as a normal vaginal delivery. HIV-exposed infants shall receive a short course exposure prophylaxis for seven days post partum and mothers will breastfeed the child for six months exclusively or use replacement exclusively for the same time span. Looking at the transmission rates four weeks after delivery, a study from Abijan, Ivory Coast, showed that 2.2% of the children were infected (Tonwe-Gold et al. 2007). Thus, the rates are more than double those witnessed in industrialised countries. The aforementioned feeding assumption proves greatly difficult in practice as breastfeeding significantly depends on cultural norms, as noted by the aforementioned anthropologists. For instance, familial systems also impose hierarchies of age, respect and decision-making power over young and somewhat inexperienced family members (Jordan & Davis-Floyd 1993). Despite criticism by anthropologists, public health approaches do not integrate local obstetric practices. If at all, rites and practices were merely considered as outdated and hampering the effectiveness of biomedical care. In a rather ethnocentric way, patients shall be persuaded to abandon "harmful cultural practices" and accept biomedical care instead.

Earlier anthropological studies from the 1970s to 1990s discussed pregnancy, delivery and early infant care with respect to the debate on medicalisation. Starting from the 1990s and 2000s, anthropological studies have shed light on obstetric practices and breastfeeding with respect to HIV/AIDS. With the present study I intend to follow up on both debates.

2.3 Managing Sickness, Managing Uncertainty

The anthropological literature on uncertainty is predominantly based on Evans-Pritchard's "Witchcraft, Oracles and Magic among the Azande" (Evans-Pritchard & Gillies 1978), Mary Douglas' "Purity and Danger" (1994) and Whyte's "Questioning Misfortune" (1997).

Neither the society Whyte studied in Uganda, nor the Azande studied by Evans-Pritchard, doubted that misfortune was an unavoidable experience in human life. However, all societies provide material or immaterial tools for dealing with and preventing mishap, or to explain unfortunate and therefore uncertain situations. However, the cause often needs to be defined by knowledgeable people or by means of oracles so as to find the right way of handling the situation. Uncertainty basically means unease or discontent with the present and/or future and engagement does not intend to eliminate misfortune as such, which would also not be possible. Usually, individuals are advised to perform rites properly and regularly to prevent unfortunate occurrences. Yet, witchcraft or improper fulfilment of rites can do harm in any case. Well-being is, in contrast, defined as the absence of misfortune in a physical, spiritual and social sense according to Whyte (1997).

Whyte highlights four groups of causes for misfortune, which she categorised according to traditional healer's records. Cases fell into the categories: absence of physical or mental health, lack of prosperity (i.e. job, money, livestock), failure in conjugal relations (finding a partner, reproductive disorders, absence of marital harmony, etc.), and absence of safety (accidents, unfavourable environmental circumstances, seeing signs of death) (Whyte 1997: 16-18). In order to tackle the unfortunate and uncertain situation sustainably, the agents need to be determined and, hence, the necessary steps to be taken. In general, the search merely aims at a quest for order in a time of crisis (Whyte 1997). The strategies societies had developed rather helped to control, minimise or eliminate the cause of an uncertain situation.

A person found in the uncertain state of unwell-being, usually in a first attempt to find assurance, compares their own experiences, embodied knowledge and a history of what had helped when dealing with similar situations previously. Secondly, household members, close acquaintances, or a representative of the family, may offer help to reinstate confidence at the household level. In a third attempt to bring a situation under control, knowledgeable people, such as traditional healers, may be approached. Whyte concludes that

> there is the issue of the sociality of uncertainty and control: the means of dealing with uncertainty are accessible through social relations. Differentials in power and influence are relevant to people's experience of uncertainty and attempts to steer through it (Whyte 1997: 247).

Evans-Pritchard explains that the Azande blame witches and sorcerers for evil, antisocial practices which bring harm upon fellow men. If any kind of misfortune such as disease, or any other mishap such as the collapse of a building, occurs, the collective of affected people will need to investigate in order to uncover the agent. An oracle shall often indicate the cause of an impaired condition or unfortunate occurrence, which may nevertheless be found in a biological realm. Whyte warns against underestimating these profane causes of misfortune (Whyte 1997: 27), whereas Evans-Pritchard stresses that even if a biological cause is known, the agent still needs to be identified (Evans-Pritchard & Gillies 1978: 66-68).

In the aftermath, ways of containing uncertainty need to be found. Some problems are solved by buying (material or immaterial) medicine (Whyte 1997: 204-205, 229) or the performance of a ritual to re-establish well-being is jointly needed to mitigate the problem.

A more holistic approach of traditional healers entails social interaction and a close inter-linkage of cure and healing in a religious sense. African therapeutic systems do not distinguish between spiritual and physical dysfunction, but rather categories of causes for the absence of well-being. Among the Azande, for instance, approaching diviners, interrogation of oracles and medication alleviate and disarm the consequences of witchcraft and sorcery (Evans-Pritchard & Gillies 1978: 39). Hence, health practitioners combine medical and magical interventions in order to recover health, prevent spiritual harm and keep social order. Dealing with the consequences of misfortune equals dealing with the uncertainty for which medicine as well as rituality can be tools for achieving control (Whyte 1997: 204-205).

Rituals can, on the other hand, guarantee a regular order in a preventive way. Douglas argues that hygiene, for instance, and thereby health, depends on certain rituals. In a quasi religious way norms are manifest and followed in a regular behavioural way. In many cases it cannot be explained what the rationality behind a taboo, law or moral standard was originally, but the behavioural norm is shared by the community and remained in place over generations. In the end, it does not matter whether certain rules are followed due to rational, scientific explanations or due to religious laws as long as they are followed and, hence, sickness is prevented (Douglas 1994: 48-49). In the reverse conclusion, the cause of sickness and other unfortunate events, and thus uncertainty, can be found in an improper or irregular performance of a ritual. Crossing moral lines entails a risk for the individual, the family, or the society overall (Douglas 1994: 182).

Haram and Yamba speak of agency rather than rituals. The authors agree, nevertheless, that everyday actions of individuals can be seen as the counterpart of uncertainty:

> It is through agency that a person makes choices (rational or irrational, depending on the particular type of logic we apply to others' choices) in order to minimise uncertainties in everyday life (Haram & Yamba 2004: 4).

Steffen, Jenkins and Jessen presented a volume on the management of health crises in which they (Jenkins et al. 2005) determine that dealing with uncertainty is a quest for control which may, however, lead to a new uncertain situation. Their introduction entitled "Matters of Life and Death" draws attention to "social and symbolic aspects of life and death. These are aspects of well-being that are no less real than the body and its frailties" (Jenkins et al. 2005: 9). Treatment translates into care for the purpose of resurrection or relief, which spans far wider than a biomedical notion of health and health care. Hence, this study contributes to discussions on the management of uncertainty displayed in a health crisis.

> there is a (...) sense in which matters of life and death are necessarily bound up with uncertainty, in that *attempts to control, reduce or remove uncertainty may actually lead to the generation of further uncertainty, or the accentuation of existing uncertainty*. [Matters of life and death are] concerned with *the control of uncertainty, the uncertainty of control,* and *the creation of uncertainty* (Jenkins et al. 2005: 17-18; emphasis in the original).

Whyte (1997) also concludes that there is no guarantee of success, but alternative strategies may be tried out to identify sources of uncertainty. Depending on the cause of the affliction, a health professional will advise on how to eliminate, minimise or normalise uncertainty. If the cure does not provide relief and the cause of affliction is assumed beyond this realm, another treatment needs to be tried until a satisfactorily solution is found. Approaching biomedical facilities may be one of the alternatives. Notwithstanding this, alternative options again represent uncertainty due to a choice and a dearth of reliability. A pluralism of medical facilities (and medical shall here be read in a more holistic definition) contributes to the confusion of clients. It should be noted, moreover, that institutions and people within these frames of reference are not hermetically separated. Quite the contrary, institutions are interlinked and patients approach health professionals and relatives in a complementary way. Likewise, explanatory models of a person's affliction are intertwined. In the search for the cause of an illness certain aspects can be traced back to biomedical notions as well as to local philosophy forming a unique local explanatory attempt.

Carrying a symptomless disease (Helman 2007: 150), as well as symptoms without disease, conflicts with local *explanatory models* (Kleinman 1980). Thus, HIV mostly falls under the western disease aetiology, while others stress that the cause, which is related to a sick person's individual fault, weak morals and negligence of sexual taboos, is what leads to HIV (Gausset & Mogensen 1996). Others argue that HIV is transmitted through witchcraft from one person to another. Intentional or accidental transmission from one person to another resembles the western medical category of communicable diseases. HIV-positive support groups, however, particularly promote the idea of HIV as merely a chronic disease and therefore of divine origin. Following this notion, social intervention, which would sanction a sick person, for example, through the application of a stigma, must not be applied since the sickness is not the person's responsibility[7]. In Lesotho, people consider HIV/AIDS a biomedical disease which needs to be treated by a biomedical doctor, whereas diseases which appear in relation to HIV (opportunistic infections in biomedical terminology) may however be interpreted according to emic classifications and treated by a traditional healer (Field notes Kroeker: 06/2008). If the cause of a disease lies in the spiritual realm or was due to witchcraft, a healer may be consulted along with biomedical attention. While interpretations on the cause of the sickness and the subsequent treatment are not consistent, either notion may provide guidance in interpreting the situation as well as organising the way forward through an uncertain situation. Traditional and biomedical facilities are therefore approached alternatively or complementarily with an uncertain outcome.

---

[7] I discuss this in my M.A. Thesis (Kroeker, (forthcoming a), M.A. Thesis, 2007, Johann Wolfgang v. Goethe University, Frankfurt/M.). Support groups for people living with HIV/AIDS try to destigmatise their disease by arguing that it was of divine origin. Thus, people living with HIV must not experience exclusion but support.

In Southern African countries the HIV/AIDS pandemic poses a scourge of public health. Moreover, consequences affect conjugal relations and due to the fact that HIV/AIDS mostly affects people in their productive years many families suffer from the absence of prosperity. HIV/AIDS is, in conclusion, the cause for the general absence of well-being. Devoid of a cure, HIV/AIDS provokes high levels of uncertainty and fear for those infected and affected by the pandemic. Lesotho is a country with an extremely high HIV/AIDS prevalence. Therefore, it is an interesting field to study in terms of health and the management of uncertainty.

2.4 Inductive Approach to Authority and Resistance

Rompel (2003), Dilger (2005, 2010), Whyte (2005), Nyanguru (2005), and Wolf (2006), to name just a few, have linked social interaction in health facilities concerning treatment management for people living with HIV with their *treatment management group* (Janzen 1978), thus, the social environment of the sick. In many cases HIV-positive people experienced stigma and feared rejection from their next-of-kin, although many also needed support to get on with their lives. Studies, thus, tend to focus on those who are already in an advanced stage of AIDS and are dependent on others either at home or within treatment support groups. Besides, there has been a focus on care networks for the sick and AIDS orphans (Foster 1998; Foster et al. 2005; Rompel 2003; Wolf 2010).

In many studies the patients appear as minors, weak and helpless. For instance, in Paul Farmer's book, "Pathologies of Power" (2005), HIV-positive people also appear as victims of human rights violations due to political structures and structural violence. Females in particular are prone to fall victim and be deprived of health care because of the social pressures under which they live. In contrast, there are studies which emphasise the rights and duties patients receive and their active involvement. Reference is made to studies on *therapeutic citizenship*, based on Nguyen and Peschard from 2003, Nguyen 2005, and 2010. Nguyen describes how being HIV-positive binds people together in an international network. Organisations which cater for people living with HIV build a platform of norms, thus, a biosocial environment. National and international bodies select those people who are well positioned within the network and choose "dynamic" members who are therewith eligible to undertake treatment campaigns. Politics within the network, known as biopolitics in this case, determine who represents people living with HIV, their medication and their needs. The debate centres on the extent to which people living with HIV/AIDS perceive rights to health care and antiretroviral treatment merely through a medical test result. This debate rather concerns a political discourse on "biopower", often in correlation with debates about the neoliberal order and national health management.

> Therapeutic citizenship is a biopolitical citizenship, a system of claims and ethical projects that arise out of the conjugation of techniques used to govern populations and manage individual bodies (Nguyen 2005: 126).

Health group participants became advocates in a global political sphere of antiretroviral treatment provision (Comaroff 2010; Dilger 2010). Zachie Achmad, for instance, a treatment activist in South Africa, used his popularity gained from and through negotiations on antiretroviral treatment provision on a national political level (Nolen et al. 2007).

Meanwhile, I am more concerned with people living with HIV who are not necessarily on life-long therapy, but on a short-course treatment regime. My study participants were actively involved in decision-making, which offered them opportunities to avoid conflicts and structural violence. Interpretations of causalities, treatment advice and applicability, however, affected their course of action.

In this study, the female patients' (or rather clients') active role in the whole biomedical, traditional medical realm, as well as interaction with the social embedding, shall therefore not be underestimated. The analysis of the data I collected in Lesotho showed that the decision-making pathways of women with HIV entailed resistance against the hegemony of medicalisation, strict treatment protocols and other behavioural expectations which do not fit their life situation. The manoeuvres somewhat resembled Scott's description of the "Arts of Resistance" (1985) and "Weapons of the Weak" (1990), and what Scott calls "forms of everyday resistance"[8] which will be discussed in Chapters 4.6 and 4.7. HIV-positive women in Lesotho tended to avoid conflicts with those assumed to be dominant parties in social interaction, i.e. those who represented biomedical institutional structures and those holding authoritative knowledge. Methods of putting decisions into practice

---

[8] While Scott speaks about peasants, slaves, beggars, and likewise politically underrepresented groups or individuals, he describes their way of muddling through when interacting with authorities in a similar way.

showed that women had agency in decision-making but opted to use concealed or indirect strategies to get by. Although uncertainty nevertheless forced them to accept a social hierarchy overall, they were allowed some variation in everyday manoeuvres.

Since these ideas of interpreting HIV-positive women's behaviour resulted from the analysis of the empirical material, I will refrain here from explaining my take on authority and resistance. A further debate on these matters, usually discussed in political anthropology, will follow the presentation of the empirical material in Chapter 9 of this book.

In Sickness and in Health: Biographical Studies

This chapter will illustrate how I gathered biographical information on sensitive topics such as HIV/AIDS, sexuality and family affairs. Clients of a hospital comprised the target population of the study, whereas health professionals and family members formed the social framework. With the selection of expectant women who attended antenatal care at least once, I intended to find those who were literate on the prevention of mother-to-child transmission of HIV. In order to follow their ways of manoeuvring through an uncertain situation, I needed to learn about earlier experiences, attitudes and interests, which I did by applying a biographical approach. This chapter contains a discussion on the process of selecting informants and provides information on the possibilities as well as the challenges of reconstructing biographical data on the basis of interviews.

3.1 Background of Selecting Informants

The anthropological research grew out of a clinic partnership between the HIVCENTER of Frankfurt University Hospital and the Karabong Clinic at Mafeteng Government Hospital. Between 2007 and 2009 I spent eleven months in Mafeteng at the hospital, at family homes and with non-governmental organisations which work in the field of interest[1]. Several shorter visits followed until 2012. Formal interviews as well as informal conversations with various stakeholders in the broader field of research built the corpus of data[2]. Formal interviews were prepared in advance and followed a half-structured, open-ended questionnaire. Some conversations cannot be clearly determined as formal or informal interviews. In fact, informal conversations accompanied the whole course of the study whenever specific questions came up. Due to the fact that meetings between interviewees and interviewers were mostly on a daily basis and conversations continued during subsequent meetings, I refer to these conversations as informal and to the advantages outlined by Ochs and Capps:

---

[1] Approval and ethical clearance for the study was sought and granted by the Ethics Committee of Johann Wolfgang von Goethe University Hospital Frankfurt/M., the Medical Association of Lesotho and the Ethics and Research Committee of the Ministry of Health and Social Welfare in Lesotho.

[2] For more detail, a list of interview partners can be found in the Annex.

> Informal conversation is the communicative glue that establishes and maintains close relationships in many communities. This does not mean that close relationships require continuous talk, but rather that commiserating, gossiping, philosophizing, exchanging advice, and other informal discourse interlaces lives and builds common ways of acting, thinking, feeling and otherwise being in the world (Ochs & Capps, 2001: 8).

The data collection was accompanied by *individual* and *interactional* participant observation[3] (see also Morgan, 1997: 8-10)[4].

Due to a general lack of data on the topic, a triangulation of quantitative and qualitative tools proved valuable[5]. In conjunction with the District Health Management Team[6] I designed a questionnaire called "Attitudes Towards Child Birth in Mafeteng" (ATCBM). It assessed factors that influence the choice of the place of delivery for the expectant mothers and the general attitudes towards antenatal care in hospitals, health centres and with traditional birth attendants. In total, the questionnaire was administered to 161 pregnant women in twelve health centres in the Mafeteng District. This questionnaire built the foundation for the qualitative data collection in the next phase of the research.

---

[3] By that I mean participant observation of one individual or of more than one individual who interacts. For instance, in a support group my observation concentrates on particular key informants and their interaction with others who are not part of the study. Although I would not call this a focus group, as I did not assemble participants or direct the discussion (Morgan, 1997: 8).

[4] Expert interviews followed an open-ended half-guided questionnaire. The interviews were conducted in English and recorded, transcribed and analysed by myself. Several interviews were not recorded either because of practical reasons, as we had to move through the health facility during the course of the conversation, or due to noise interference.

[5] I refer to field notes that relate to personal interviews with study participants with the following reference, "Field notes Kroeker: *Date of conversation*", whereas formal and informal conversations will follow this diction, "Field notes Kroeker *Indication of Interviewee*: *Date of conversation*"). For notes which are based on the qualitative/quantitative study it is likewise indicated in the reference: "Field notes Kroeker ATCBM: *Date of conversation*".

[6] The District Health Management Team (DHMT) for the Mafeteng District, which consists of a Public Health Nurse, Health Information Officer and Statistician, and an Information Officer. In total, the questionnaire was administered to 161 expectant mothers in twelve health centres in the Mafeteng District between 1st and 17th of July, 2008. The study was funded by the HIVCENTER of Frankfurt University within the Clinical Partnership on HIV. Unfortunately, the results have not been published to date.

This phase included thirty expectant women who attended antenatal care at Mafeteng Government Hospital and were found to be HIV-positive during their first visit. Pregnant women who tested positive remained in the health facility and waited for further counselling with psychosocial supporters of the international NGO Mothers2Mothers[7]. Mothers2Mothers counsellors - all women who had previously received PMTCT with their own children – function as intermediaries between medical staff and clients. During their counselling sessions I was able to select women for my qualitative study. Following a methodology of *focused sampling* I intended to identify clients who

- tested HIV-positive in antenatal care or earlier,
- expected to give birth between November, 2008, and May, 2009,
- consented to my presence at their health counselling sessions,
- consented to visits either at home, or elsewhere if preferred, and therefore remaining within the proximity of the urban area of Mafeteng,
- no more than 25 in total.

To my surprise, more women were interested than I could have reasonably dealt with within the proposed time frame. Within one week 25 women volunteered to take part in the study and only two women refused to be questioned when the counsellor introduced the study, due to the fact that they had tested positive on the same day and found themselves in a state of shock.

In order to cover more contrasting social groups, I included five further study participants. Therewith I attempted to meet Elwert's *cross-perspective approach* (2003: 31) which basically looks for contrasting elements in informants, perspectives and research methods. I therefore also included:

[7] The roll-out of psychosocial support for HIV-positive women in Lesotho resulted in the introduction of Mothers2Mothers in Mafeteng. This international NGO provides counselling and care for pregnant and breastfeeding HIV-positive women. Due to their position, Mothers2Mothers facilitated my taking part in medical as well as social activities within the hospital, and the site coordinator guided me through the procedures. Moreover, the counsellors allowed me to take part in sessions, provided the clients agreed, as part of my interactional participant observations. Both the district manager and the district coordinator of the NGO were also based at Mafeteng Hospital. Both were a constant source of information as formal and informal informants, and we exchanged ideas on a daily basis. Hence, the contact with Mothers2Mothers and their activities shaped the outline of my further study and longitudinal study significantly, since our field of interest is interlinked.

- MaHlano, a pharmacist and former employee of the hospital. Her background suggested a unique view on health and health care from a private and professional perspective.
- MaMararo was a traditional healer by profession and I included her for the same reasons as MaHlano.
- MaSupa was employed by a funeral home, which suggested a professional and private perspective on AIDS.
- MaRobeli had already been staying in the hospital's shelters for expectant mothers for several weeks and preferred it due to conflicts with her in-laws.
- MaRobong's did not meet my criteria due to her expected due date in June, 2009. However, we kept in touch and I approached her later as she qualified as a research assistant. Since I learned a lot about MaRobong's experiences during our work, I later considered her as a participant as well.

MaSupa and MaRobong were known to me before and during the course of the study. With both women I had discussed issues of my study informally before they were integrated as key informants. Our informal conversations broadened my outlook on the topic.

With those thirty women I conducted open-ended guideline interviews, informal conversations and participant observations and was given access to their medical records. Between four and twelve visits followed our first meeting in the hospital, during which I assessed their biography, family and medical history as well as future prospects and the decisions that needed to be made for these.

Every meeting was prepared by myself and discussed with MaKhotso, my interpreter[8], in advance in order to agree upon the guiding questions. Thematic fields that applied to all interviewees included:

---

[8] Most of the conversations in the second phase of the field work were conducted in Sesotho unless the interviewees were able to express themselves fluently in English. Conversations in Sesotho were initiated by a research assistant; a graduate in Social Work from the National University of Lesotho to whom I will refer as MaKhotso in this book. She had previously worked as a voluntary counsellor in HIV/AIDS Clinic and had been trained on voluntary HIV testing and counselling. However, she was not known to the study participants. In addition to MaKhotso's professional expertise she was also pregnant at the time the study took place and study participants accepted her easily as *mokhachane*. This coincidence proved of great value since discussions about pregnancy developed almost automatically when we met with other expectant women.

- pregnancy (retrospectively, present, prospectively),
- delivery (retrospectively, present, prospectively),
- infant feeding (retrospectively, present, prospectively),
- matrimonial situation (current and desired situation),
- education and employment (current and desired situation),
- housing conditions and close social environment,
- HIV test,
- disclosure of the test result (current and desired situation),
- reactions and support of family members (retrospectively, present, prospectively),
- use of biomedicine and traditional medicine (retrospectively, present, prospectively).

When agreed with the study participants, the same thematic fields were discussed with their family members either individually or jointly. Study participants and their relatives gave exhaustive accounts of their biographies including sensitive, personal information. While some informants talked freely and narrated earlier experiences boldly, others were rather quiet or insecure, which often spoke volumes. Due to the fact that MaKhotso was local and pregnant at the same time, interviewees generally felt at ease. Moreover, MaKhotso managed to create a sensitive and trustful atmosphere, which enabled interviewees to talk about bad experiences but also allowed us to ask critical questions. This had a great impact on the situation and on the information we were able to obtain, such as in the following example of feeling frustrated and insecure, as illustrated by LeTharo:

> During our first meeting in the counselling session LeTharo had just received the test result of her immunological status. While it was still high with a CD4 of 900 in the last test, three months later the test showed 204. Confused and crying she refuses medical care when the counsellor suggested she shall start lifelong ARV-treatment immediately. She argues that she still does not feel ready and needs time as well as further counselling.
>
> MaKhotso and I go on a first home visit shortly thereafter. LeTharo instantly starts to ask questions about HIV and the ARV-treatment, she obviously considers the home visit as an individual counselling session to persuade her to enrol on the treatment scheme. I explained again that she must not confuse us with counsellors; nor do we intend to persuade her to do anything. We changed the topic and started talk-

> ing about her biographic background. LeTharo is an evangelic pastor and therefore feared losing face in front of her parish if members learned about her HIV-status. Apparently, her husband did not know about her status either, since he worked in Maseru and was not around most of the time. Adding to her own problem, eight weeks before her husband was beaten up by *tsotsi*[9] at night and subsequently had to be admitted into hospital time and time again. He still had not fully recovered. MaKhotso interrupts the conversation and suggests that we pray together for LeTharo's husband and that her health shall improve so that she does not need to start HIV-therapy at this stressful time (Field notes Kroeker 13: 14/11/2008-17/11/2008).

LeTharo obviously found herself in a stressful and uncertain situation. Worries about her husband, her own health, the child's well-being and her reputation as a role model in her parish added to that. Thus, Makhotso's suggestion brought about sympathy and trust which impacted on the elaborate nature of further narrations. As time went by, we experienced greater candidness and confidentiality during interviews than we had previously expected. Concluding from this short meeting, I have to admit that the interview situation significantly affected further collaboration and the information I took into account. In short, creating a comfortable atmosphere was essential when talking about sensitive issues. However, this was a precondition we could not plan but hope for.

When analysing a situation and information, we constantly needed to bear in mind that experiences are not recounted in the same way they took place, narrations rather depend on the current state of mind, situation in which they are told, and memories also develop over time[10]. As memories fade, gaps are filled in by the narrator and expressions are adjusted to the recipient's comprehension.

Autobiographical narratives can only state the informant's present view on a past occurrence. The interviews already imply an analysis of the past in the way they were narrated, which might not have been the case when the situation took place. Therefore, a narration always implies the situation as experienced (*erzählte Zeit*) and the situation of now (*Erzählzeit*) from which

---

[9] Tsotsi: (South African urban Slang): Thug, gangster, thief.
A glossary of Sesotho terms can be found in the Annex.

[10] Riemann mentions here processes of orientation, conversion, interpretation, self-definition, legitimation, fading out and blanking out in the narration of a biography (Riemann 2006: 45-48).

perspective occurrences are interpreted (Lucius-Hoene & Deppermann, 2002: 24-29).

The reality of narration thus merely gives information about the present situation someone finds him or herself in. For my study the current situation was the most important part and I therefore did not view this as a disadvantage but as a strength for the study. In contrast, a narrative may be embedded retrospectively into a context. In many cases a narrator might not even be aware of social enmeshments[11]. Subjective strategies of coping with conflicts, for instance, depend largely on earlier experiences, social relations and cultural frameworks. Perceived reactions of others to a particular piece of information, such as the disclosure of a HIV-positive test result, may be instead attributable to the interpretation of the narrator. As Lipp (1975) explains, individuals with a tainted identity tend to assume discrimination and behave accordingly. Therewith, a stigmatised person may have adopted deviant behaviour irrespective or not of whether others had actually enforced it. For my study, though, it is irrelevant whether discrimination was enacted or not as long as an informant felt stigmatised or discriminated. The 'felt' rather than the 'enacted' stigma shaped identity, biographical narratives and personal relations (Jacoby, 1994).

3.2 Three Observers and Four Stories

A sociological debate concerns the *Biographical Illusion* (Apitzsch & Jansen, 2003: 95-110), which discusses whether a "good story" is necessarily based on a "true story". I will now include a story told by different actors to illustrate my point:

MaMeli's first baby passed away the day after she gave birth in the hospital. Her mother-in-law explained the situation in the presence of MaMeli, MaKhotso, and myself, as follows:

> After the delivery the baby had dropped out of the nurse's hands while the midwife was sewing the episiotomy. The head of the child was fractured and, generally, the whole staff did not treat MaMeli, the baby and the mother-in-law nicely. The nurse spoke in rather a rude way to her and she and MaMeli overheard them complaining that the in-laws came too often and interrupted the nurses' duties. When the

---

[11] See also Erdheim, M.: Die gesellschaftliche Produktion von Unbewusstheit, Frankfurt/M. 1984.

> midwife discharged MaMeli from the hospital after the delivery MaMeli was told to come back for a check-up after only two days.
> The mother-in-law at that point of the narration turns to MaKhotso and I to ask if it is usual for a baby to be brought in for a check-up after two days. I answer "No, usually after one week", which indicated to the mother-in-law that something was wrong with the baby, but the nurse had kept her in the dark. She proceeds: When MaMeli brought the baby the next day the mother-in-law mentioned again that the deformed head of the baby seems to be the cause of the baby's nose bleeding. The doctor examined the baby and wrote something in a book, tore out the page and sent it to maternity ward, the mother-in-law recalls. He also immediately sent a call to the midwife who had delivered MaMeli's baby and who was still on duty. When the doctor asked the midwife about what had happened with the child she did not say anything and just kept quiet.

The mother-in-law spoke negatively about the nurse and made it clear that staff behaved in a careless and rude manner in front of the mother, child and mother-in-law. At odds with the statement that MaMeli was asked to come back after two days, her medical book indicates that she was asked to come back after seven days. MaMeli tells a slightly different version in the absence of her mother-in-law and in the presence of a counsellor called MaThloni:

> MaMeli states that she had already realised in the post-natal room that her baby was unwell. I asked her what symptoms made her think that the baby was unwell. She answers first of all the deformed head, which her mother-in-law had interpreted as a fracture. The nurse however had told her that "the baby won't have a problem with the head". Secondly, it worried her that the baby was crying a lot. Other babies in the post-natal room were quiet and their mothers told her that she must have lived in a noisy place all the way throughout her pregnancy so that the baby is now crying so much. MaMeli recalls that she thought, "the baby may calm down at home, but it got even worse".
> MaMeli spent the night at her mother's house. The baby cried and had hot flashes like high fever, she explains. Moreover, it was not breathing well and she rushed back to the hospital the same night. The mother-in-law also went to the hospital. The baby had severe nose bleeding and when they arrived at the maternity ward and undressed

> the baby, they realised that the inside of the clothes was all bloody. They were then referred to casualty, where they found a doctor.
> MaThloni asks if she had applied anything on the umbilical cord or whether she had dressed the child rather tightly. MaMeli denies this.

Later, I approach the doctor who had attended MaMeli, her sister-in-law, her mother-in-law and the baby that night. The doctor recalls the story in my presence like this:

> MaMeli and her sister-in-law arrived only after 7 p.m. when he was on call for the night shift. The mother-in-law dropped in later and immediately started to talk furiously. She blamed the nurse for having dropped the child which had resulted in the baby's malformed head. The bleeding was, as she understood, a consequence of the head fracture the nurse is responsible for.
> The doctor then checked the baby and noticed the baby's bleeding nose but it was not severe. He asked when the baby's condition started, but the mother-in-law was not able to answer. He figured that the mother-in-law was not with the child during the night and asked her: "Who is the mother of this baby?" and the mother-in-law pointed at MaMeli. The doctor interrogated MaMeli and she explains that the baby had been crying all day starting from 8 a.m. He therefore told them that they had come too late. The baby had a neonatal sepsis, which he could have treated if they had come earlier.
> Directed towards me, he adds that traditional people often apply Vaseline or cow dung on the umbilical cord, which causes infections of the blood cycle[12] (Field notes Kroeker 22: 25/11/2008-09/03/2009).

This case narrated from three perspectives shows some overlaps in the story, but also varying interpretations. The speaker re-interpreted an occurrence and re-staged the plot. While the mother-in-law places the emphasis on the bad medical and social behaviour, the doctor blamed the mother's ignorance and the local culture. In all cases I was the recipient of the narrative. While the basic story became clear, all the narrators added details which embellished their presentation of the self and blamed the other party. Ochs & Capps note:

---

[12] I did not find any further indication of such traditional practices either in the literature or in my empirical data. The doctor is also not of local origin and does not have children himself.

> All narratives exhibit tension between the desire to construct an overarching storyline that ties events together in a seamless explanatory framework and the desire to capture the complexities of the events experienced, including haphazard details, uncertainties, and conflicting sensibilities among protagonists (Ochs & Capps, 2001: 4).

The narratives already entailed foreshadowing and back-shadowing which gave hints as to what the narrators aimed to convey (Ochs & Capps, 2001: 5). The narrator already forecasts his/her point or, in contrast, justifies and interprets a situation retrospectively. Therewith stories are put into a context.

In summary, autobiographical narratives may not necessarily match an objective description (Apitzsch & Jansen, 2003: 95-110) by a long way. In fact, in MaMeli's description as well as in the descriptions of others, Basotho narrators presented it like they were present, although it seems to be a stylistic means of letting someone in authority recount what happens, despite their being absent at the time of the event. A narrator may, with or without the intention of fabricating a story, consider certain parts and explanations more important than the listener.

> Narratives of personal experience do not present objective, comprehensive accounts of events but rather perspectives on events. (…) [they must be considered] as selections rather than as reflections of reality (Ochs & Capps, 2001: 45).

Occurrences that would be important for explaining the self of that past time might not be considered relevant by the speaker and he/she therefore fails to explain a situation completely. This information may have blurred over time or is not worth telling due to different assumptions of the topic under study by the informant and myself, as recipient. Details will be generalised, selected or completely neglected, since they did not seem a crucial part of the story. However, despite the inaccuracy and disadvantages of biographical narrative interviews, the absence of a more accurate method makes this procedure nevertheless a suitable method.

Due to the long period of interaction with the mothers in Lesotho and the repetition of questions, I was able to revise topics after a length of time. Inconsistent narratives were cross-examined and either interpreted by me as unclear memorisation, re-staging due to the current situation, seeking to conceal information or masking a lie. I assume that accounts exaggerated the situation in some cases to make the speaker look like a victim or a hero(ine). Gestures and facial expression while speaking and reactions of others in the room said a lot about the feelings a person encountered while talking about earlier experiences. Hence, observation was an important part of the interviews besides the semantic value. Some matters, however, were merely reconstructed by myself, in particular those concerning disclosure of the HIV status to the partner. If a story failed to become clear even after questioning someone for a second time and comparing statements with other people's interpretation of events, I decided to believe the informant's version for the sake of our further collaboration. Notwithstanding this, my interpretation may yet be the fourth version of MaMeli's, her mother-in-law's, and the doctor's narrative.

When taking limits and challenges into account, biographical interviews along with cross-examining the narratives of related informants, medical records, several study visits, and repetition of questions worked surprisingly well.

3.3 Researcher's Dilemma: Mediating in Conflict Situations

Working in a cross-disciplinary field and exchanging research approaches initiates reflections on methodology. The intersection of my study in medicine and anthropology, and my close collaboration with medical practitioners from Frankfurt/M. University clinic, facilitated an exchange on good research practice. While I basically intended to document the information flow, uncertainties, authoritative structures and life trajectories, I became aware that this is impossible. The target group, women in an uncertain situation of pregnancy and sickness, actively sought assistance from me in mutual exchange for giving their story and I was accepted as one of the insiders (cf. Goffman, 1963: 28, 31).

Biomedical research envisages the improvement of the patient's physical condition or looks to facilitate procedures which are measured by natural scientific "objective" indicators. Anthropological research works quite the opposite. A documentation of social norms may suffice. An active interference in the situation, which is the aim of medical research, may be undesirable for anthropologists. Some authors stress that ethnographic fieldwork shall merely document situations in their cultural context with little or no bias.

> The method of participant observation builds the core of the field research, which attempts to observe all-day life in a possibly unadulterated way; with as little as possible interference through the investiga-

> tion (Friebertshäuser, 1996: 75, Translation Kroeker; cf. Girtler 2001: 116).[13]

While physicians intend to create an unbiased research setting, anthropologists argue that there is nothing like objective research and their presence has already created an artificial situation. Without doubt both contrasting pre-assumptions, interference vs. no interference, affect the outcome of the study. Yet, I try to analyse my role as researcher within the process and therewith evaluate my results in relation to it, since it would be impossible to deny it completely.

Interference in medical anthropological studies must be discussed from an ethical point of view. Can a researcher leave an informant to suffer physically, spiritually or psychologically after obstacles come to light? Do conventions on confidentiality between doctor and patient also apply for researcher-patient relations in a medical field? Should a researcher be answerable to medical staff, relatives or merely the key informant? Should the researcher help to secure collective or individual well-being if they are mutually exclusive or neither of the two?

The situation of expectant mothers in the study was particularly complex since they were worried about their personal situation and that of their child and family. Would it have been ethically defensible for a medical anthropologist to interfere in the situation? Would it have been ethically defensible not to interfere? Of course, my notion of good ethical practice largely depends on my western socialisation and personal norms and values.

In the course of the qualitative study I became aware that my person and the content of the study influenced study participants more than I expected. The discussions with the women during home visits raised issues they avoided thinking about or did not find problematic until a topic was openly addressed.

> Familiar conversational partners (…) provoke further thinking about an incident. Such sustained collaborative reflection can destabilize a person's prevailing interpretation of the self and others, leading the way for alternative ways of remembering the past and inhabiting the present (Ochs & Capps, 2001: 17).

---

[13] "Die Methode der teilnehmenden Beobachtung bildet das Kernstück der Feldforschung, der es darauf ankommt, das alltägliche Leben möglichst unverändert zu beobachten, und -soweit es geht- möglichst wenig einzugreifen oder mit der Untersuchung zu verändern" (Friebertshäuser, 1996: 75).

Yet they suddenly had to confront something they may not have reflected upon. While answering a question, thoughts were organised and arguments evaluated. However, it is not possible to answer a "what would have been without" question.

I am of the conclusion that in situations where my study participants open up and include me in their concerns, worries, discussions and dilemma, I have already gained influence. It would moreover be naïve to believe that study participants do not have their own agenda when agreeing to the study and interaction. Study participants may have intended added value for their own benefit when they agreed to participate and spoke surprisingly openly about conflicts and debates within their household community. Contrasting with my pre-assumption, most women saw a need to exchange ideas on the topic I was researching. Informants took our conversations as a chance to air unresolved life events, particularly conflicts (cf. Ochs & Capps, 2001: 7). Indeed, some approached me directly to act as their mediator, given that I had researched their stories and could therefore speak to third parties on their behalf[14]. This social function incorporated me into a local structure of conflict management, as I found out much later. I served as a messenger between generations, while not knowing that this position existed locally, and I was involved in local methods of conflict resolution. The role of a messenger between generations includes some rights and duties, which I subsequently undertook despite my earlier hesitation. In the beginning I did not consider this role as an opportunity for participant observation; in fact, I did not like this position and avoided it as much as possible. I initially viewed the role of mediator in a conflict situation as a hindrance and interference in the study, although it later provided the possibility to gain valuable insights while acting as a messenger between parties. Hence, my involvement at the request of the informant can be characterised as *active participant observation* (Girtler, 2001: 63) as I was given a role within the local social texture, or as *thick participation*, which Spittler described (2001). This methodology allowed me to analyse a situation from experience and not only from observation.

I eventually decided that my interference in the study must be part of the mutual immaterial exchange. I would not feel comfortable letting mother

---

[14] I would prefer to use the term ambassador for this function in relation to the missionaries who assisted the Basotho in talks with the Cape Government throughout the 19th century. In the cases I observed, the social status of a diplomat was more relevant than the accurate knowledge of (medical) information. However, ambassador is not an established term in anthropological and sociological literature. I will revisit this point later.

or child, who had become friends, suffer while I knew about an easy solution to the problem. In several cases I was asked to bring along HIV testing kits to test a reluctant partner at his home in a fake testing campaign. I refused to do so. First of all, I am not authorised to use the kits, but more importantly, I am not trained to counsel people. I agreed, however, to be present when the mother disclosed her HIV status to a relative, since it gave her confidence to have someone with her. Moreover, sometimes I arranged a professional counsellor to be present, if the mother so wished. This was as far as I was willing to interfere as a participant observer.

Respect for the informants meant that these kinds of interferences would be discussed and agreed upon with the study participant. I had no intention of damaging the relationship between the mother and me and, quite the opposite, the aim at all times was to strengthen the possibility of mutual exchange.

With regard to these considerations my interference entailed the following:

- Assistance in disclosing the HIV-positive test result at the mother's request. In those cases a Mothers2Mothers counsellor was made aware of the situation. The participant had to be present when the counsellor initiated the talk with the relative and the counsellor prepared the ground for the participant to disclose her HIV status. Thereafter, the individual and family member received a counselling session on what this situation meant for mother and child and where they could receive further information.
- Help with transportation, if there was no other option. Due to the fact that I had access to a car, small favours of transporting things and people from time to time strengthened the relationship and provided opportunities for informal talks.
- Due to my network with other representatives of the NGO which assisted people living with HIV, I referred needy participants to those facilities for aid. In some cases my interpreter kept them company to assist in the process.
- I refrained from giving financial assistance under any circumstances. However, one family whose situation I assessed received financial support indirectly. The family did not have sufficient income to pay for a hospital delivery or transport and asked me for help. My interpreter and I discussed the situation and decided to buy vegetables

and fruit from the head of the household and handicrafts from the participant's husband to facilitate income generation.
- Aside from the impact on the participants' lives, the study significantly impacted on the counsellors and their training. Through my close contact with the Mothers2Mothers counsellors, particularly the trainer and supervisor, opportunities and challenges were discussed with them and obviously influenced the training, supervision and programme policy. A presentation with their regional manager also included suggestions and challenges based on my findings which I again consider part of a mutual exchange of knowledge. Furthermore, the study had already impacted on the employment of study participants as counsellors, since they were already known to staff.

I assumed that my visits strengthened the women's resolve to adhere to PMTCT and the counselling they received, which definitely biased my study in this aspect. Would that bias be avoidable and would it be desirable to avoid it? Yes and no. The study affected the outcome, although in a situation where a researcher learns about life and death conditions, mothers infecting their children, partners getting infected with a deadly disease, research results may have to bear the brunt of this influence.

I strongly believe that the aim of my anthropological study should not be limited to data collection but to provide findings to those who may benefit from it. Eventually the data collected was discussed with the counsellors' supervisor, MaThloni, without any reference being made to participants' identities. Therewith, comments and criticism improved the comprehension and performance of counsellors in the hospital. Likewise, these discussions brought about interesting insights into the counsellors' understanding of their work and their interpretation of clients' situations.

Shifts and Changes in Uncertain Times

The following chapter provides a deeper insight into the history of Lesotho. It contains notes on social, military and economic developments with a focus on the past three decades which have led to major changes in society. Secondly, the chapter illustrates the factors which contributed to women obtaining powerful positions, which they have held up to the present date, and which affect their agency in household decision-making. Moreover, as I will argue, these changes impacted on reproductive decision-making and fertility. Female decision-making is, however, somewhat limited in terms of gender and generational affairs, as I will show in the conclusion of this chapter.

4.1 Historical Overview: Resistance and Resilience

Landlocked within the Republic of South Africa, Lesotho is situated at the heart of Southern Africa. The small mountain kingdom was founded in the 1820s during a period of constant trouble in the Southern African region. The Kingdom of Lesotho, with a population of 2.1 million in 2012, is inhabited predominantly by the Basotho people. The population is often described as ethnically homogeneous (Rosenberg et al. 2004: IX), even though composed of various tribes united under King Moshoeshoe I. Today, the Basotho define themselves as one ethnic group, even though some cultural differences are still apparent, such as in clan-related practices during rites of passage. The fight against the Boers, settlers of Dutch origin, united the clansmen as one nation which draws its identity largely in contrast to the white South Africans. The Basotho people withstood the Boers in the 19th century and again in the 20th century: while other ethnic groups were incorporated into the Republic of South Africa, Lesotho opposed the Cape Colony under white rule and apartheid. Although other homelands later became part of the Republic of South Africa, Lesotho has remained an independent constitutional monarchy to the present day. At the time of Apartheid in the Republic of South Africa, Lesotho's geographical and political position as an independent kingdom made the country a stronghold of opposition with support from western countries. Lesotho therefore acted as a safe haven for refugees and foreign agencies acting against the racial segregation.

Rosenberg (2004: ix) characterises Lesotho as "very different from the rest of Africa. It's (…) a rare place that has retained much of its pre-colonial form and has stubbornly gone its own way". Since some of the clan-related practices are still visible in the rites of passage, i.e. during marriage ceremonies, in preparation for birth, under confinement and in death rituals, the social structure needs to be highlighted. It is impossible to understand the importance of these practices without looking back in time.

In the late 18th and early 19th century, a large number of Sotho-Tswana and Nguni clans dwelled in the area which is currently known as the Transvaal and the Orange Free State in the Republic of South Africa (Gill 1993: 16). These two Bantu sub-tribes occupied a large portion of land in today's South Africa, which they used as cattle keeping agriculturalists[1]. The large and powerful *Koena* clan occupied the Transvaal region between the Caledon River and the Vaal River from around 1550 AD, however,

> the enviably fertile and well-watered *Mohokare* (Caledon) River valley, (...) attracted a series of powerful predatory enemies, first Bantu-speaking (Hlubi, Ngwane, Tlokwa, Ndebele) then Khoi/'*Coloured*' (Koranna, Bastard, Griqua), then white settler colonial (the Afrikaner *voortrekkers*) and finally both colonial and imperial British (Coplan 2003: 978).

Moshoeshoe I (1783 or 1786-1870), descendant of a minor *Koena* subclan, presided over a growing chiefdom during the period of unrest called *Lifaqane*. He managed to incorporate various clans into his kingdom when invasions of Nguni-traders from the East, Khoi-raiders from the West, the military rise of Shaka Zulu in Natal, and Voortrekkers enforced territorial dislocation (Gill 1993: 24, 66). The white settlers of Dutch descendants subsequently created the independent Boer Republics of the Transvaal, the Orange Free State and Natalia.

> It was the Afrikaners and other white settlers of the Orange Free State who proved the most rapacious and relentless. The period 1840-1870 was one of almost constant conflict between Basotho and Boers, with other Bantu, Griqua and even San ('Bushmen'/*Baroa*) doing their part to keep the pot boiling, and the British getting their fingers burnt while clumsily trying to put out the fires on their colonial borders (Coplan 2003: 978).

---

[1] Stock farming Iron Age people may have settled in the region which was also vastly occupied by nomadic hunter-gatherers around 200 AD. Cattle-keeping Bantu arrived around 900 and 1400 AD and, despite contact zones and inter-marriage between the ethnic groups of Sotho and Nguni, we find distinctions in language, settlement patterns and kinship system (Gill 1993: 15, 21).

As part of a shrewd strategy of government, Moshoeshoe I offered fields and welcome presents in the form of livestock to impoverished clans in exchange for their loyalty. In times of insecurity, famine and cattle diseases, he managed to unify scattered groups of different ethnic origin as one folks-people. Their struggle was predominantly oriented against the Boers who fenced off the land and marked it as belonging to them, an idea still disputed by Basotho people today, as land can only be used but not possessed by individuals[2]. In addition to holding alliances with several tribes, Moshoeshoe I also invited French missionaries from the Paris Evangelic Mission Society (PEMS) in 1833 and the Roman Catholics in 1862. The Boer authority of the Orange Free State had also deprived several missions of their land in 1858 and missionaries also found refuge in Basutoland. Eugène Casalis (1812-1891) became a close friend and political advisor of Moshoeshoe I and assisted by writing letters to the Orange River Sovereignty. With the missionaries' knowledge of European languages and political structures they also worked as influential ambassadors for the Basotho with the British Cape Government (Rosenberg et al. 2004: 49, 351).

> In 1868, after three years during which the Basotho took very much the worst of it, Britain stepped in to save the Basotho kingdom from complete conquest. But the resulting treaty, arranged between the British High Commissioner and the Free State government without the participation of the Basotho nobility or their trusted French missionary advisers, deprived the resulting Basutoland reserve of the better part of its cultivable lands and, perhaps as importantly, the abodes of many chiefs and the graves of their ancestors that constituted Basotho notions of home and connection to the land (Coplan 2003: 978).

Basotho ambassadors were nevertheless heard and Émile Rolland (1836-1915), a second generation missionary, suggested to the Cape Administration that they leave Basotho chiefs in power in the form of a *parallel rule* whereas many African countries in the Commonwealth experienced *indirect rule*.

---

[2] Land right is somewhat different in Lesotho than in other African countries: land is generally owned by the ancestors of a totemic clan (Coplan 2003), which means that Moshoeshoe I's direct descendant is the current King of Lesotho and solely his next-of-kin is responsible for land allocation. Hence, conflicts occur over land use not land possession and merely the right to use the land is transferred from one person to another person through the patriarchal line. In recent times, however, unmarried women and widows can likewise be beneficiaries of land inheritance or tenure since laws changed as recently as 2006.

Lesotho became an autonomous protectorate (1868-1966) under the British Crown rather than a colony. Thus, Moeshoeshoe I had experienced missionary education as a politically powerful resource for his people. Girls were explicitly included in the primary schools run by the French missionaries and a secondary school for girls was opened in Lesotho as early as 1871, although it was attended mostly by King Moshoeshoe's royal clan members (Silase et al. n.d.: 34). Even today local politics relies on the royal clan members and women are actively involved as acting chiefs. However, privileges for female *Koena* clan members did not generally undermine women's subordinated position in the patriarchal social structure.

As a consequence of the continuous promotion of education for girls, present-day Lesotho has a high literacy rate. Over 80% of the Basotho people are literate and more girls attend school[3] than boys, which is unique in Africa's educational landscape (Unesco 2005: 257). Particularly at the time when large numbers of men migrated to the mines, young boys had to take over male chores at an early age and therefore dropped out of school. Some herded livestock during the day while others left their village for several months a year to work at cattle posts. In any case, few young herders had access to education and health facilities and lived far away from their families, exposed to harsh climatic conditions[4]. Girls' education in contrast was more easily combined with female chores including caring for small livestock, working fields and jobs around the family home. I will come back to the effects that the education and economic participation of women have on fertility trends later on in this chapter.

4.2 Basotho Cosmology and Societal Structure

Southern Sotho tribes enjoyed an economy, consisting of extensive cultivation, pastoralism, hunting, gathering, pillaging and cattle raiding. The duties in and around the settlement were divided between men and women presided by a chiefly family of the *Koena* tribe. The gendered division of labour can be illustrated when looking at rural housing arrangements. Villages provide

[3] Enrolment in primary education comprises 74% of girls and 71% of boys, secondary school: 31% girls versus 20% boys; further education: 4% of females and 3% of males (Hausmann et al. 2010: 192).

[4] UNICEF estimated that 15, 000 boys were herders in 2007, many of them aged 12-18 years, others up to the age of around forty (UNICEF 2007).

two geographical and cosmological spheres, which divide male and female work places spatially[5].

The male-dominated most inner part of the settlement forms the core of politics and control. Decisions which concern the community as a whole are made by male family elders who meet at the court *[khotla]*, which serves as the spiritual, juridical and political centre of the settlement (cf. Comaroff & Comaroff 2012: 45-50). The male-dominated sphere of politics also hosts the *kraals* where livestock, capital and household resources are kept. Male capital such as livestock provides safety for the members of the compound and any income generated is allocated through the household head, which is the eldest female member. Male ancestors inhabit the cattle enclosure, the *kraal* (Rosenberg et al. 2004: 349). Lineage members were laid to rest (in Sesotho, "to sleep for the living") close to their animals and are thus controlling and protecting the wealth and well-being of the community.

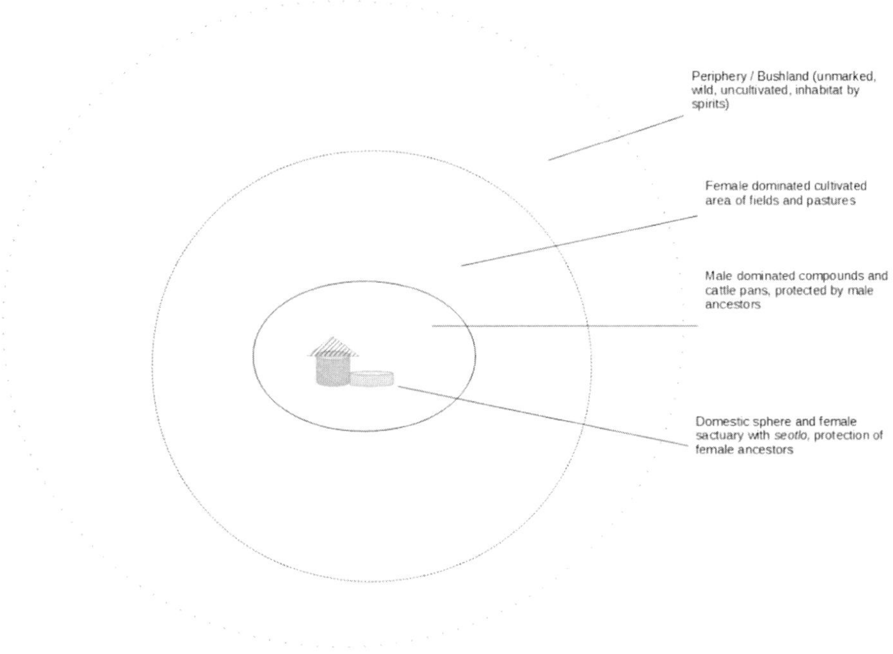

Basotho settlement and cosmology (cf. Comaroff 1980)

---

[5] I will refer to Comaroff (1980) and Comaroff & Comaroff (2012) who have been working on the Southern Tswana subgroup of *Barolong*, who are closely related to the Basotho.

Conversely, the female sphere comprises the private room and the periphery and women in pre-colonial Southern Africa were valued for their traditional chores of family management (productive activities) and family enlargement (reproductive activities) (Gay 1980; Gill 1993; Rosenberg et al. 2004: 44). When labour organisation in the household was organised within homologous tasks between male and female family members, obedience to the head of household's demands had an immediate effect on the productivity. The bride wealth the groom's father had to pay to the bride's family was given as a pledge in exchange for a bride's fertility and obedience, and if she did not fulfil these demands, cattle and thereby wealth could be claimed back by the husband's family.

> 'obedience' meant that the wife had to fulfil her function as an agricultural producer within her husband's homestead; 'fertility' meant that she had to produce children whose labour would, in time, be used for the benefit of the homestead (Walker 1990: 39).

While sexuality was controlled by men, obedience was judged by female family elders, both acting as traditional authorities in the house for their respective sphere. These terms were not controlled by young women until they were older and supervised a household. Until then, they were under the auspices of the eldest female in the compound who thereby made sure productive as well as reproductive activities were fulfilled for the family's benefit.

Female productive chores included the production and processing of consumables originating in the wild to serve the household's daily needs. Thus, women also handled small animals and the agricultural production, while large livestock was firmly part of the male domain. It could also be said that while women produced and domesticated every-day consumables, men held the resources with their livestock, also known as "banks with legs" (Rosenberg et al. 2004: 50) or "God with wet nose" (Comaroff 1985: 68).

Similar to the male *khotla*, female elders held meetings with the chief's senior wife, who negotiated women's issues in their court *[thakaneng]* (Rosenberg et al. 2004: 399). Depending on the case, either the elder women in the court would summon quarrelling community members, for instance, an abusive spouse and a further family member or chief to speak on behalf of the woman (Gay 1980: 270). Women were, however, not without means of protest in a patriarchal society. In domestic conflicts for example, women had the right to withhold from conjugal duties or return to their maternal home, which would set up a process of mediation (Gay 1980: 268, 274; Rosenberg et al. 2004: 400; cf. Alber 2004). In severe cases of the wife being mistreated, the mediation results in an annulment of the marriage without return of the bride wealth (Rosenberg et al. 2004: 45).

The core of the female sphere, however, was not the *thakaneng* but the home as the most intimate place of family affairs. The doorway opened into a vestibule, *seotlo*, a sanctuary protected by female ancestors (cf. Comaroff 1985: 56-57, Tswana: *seghotlo*). Female household members utilised this area, shielded from wind and gazing eyes, to prepare foods and kindle the fire. It was here that all activities took place to domesticate goods before they entered the household and before returning to the wild once more. Everything that left the core of the family residence carried personal applications and hence needed to be handled with special care. Therefore, women were also responsible for safeguarding everything that left the house afterwards such as ashes from cooking the family meal and all other kind of waste material from the inner sanctum of the homestead. *Thothobolo,* the waste place, was therefore established where the female living dead were laid to rest and protected such refuse, since substances which related to intimate family issues may be misused by strangers for witchcraft if they had access. Moral norms and sanctions attributed some order to the male and female realms as well as to the public and private sphere (cf. Comaroff 1980). Rites and taboos protected the family from affliction whereas neglecting such rites may result in misfortune, loss of resources, and render family members sick. The eldest woman in the house therefore not only coordinated household chores but instilled correct behaviour in younger family members in order to maintain family well-being.

The public sphere was situated at a further distance from the core of the settlement. While the male sphere is associated with politics and control, the female sphere is associated with production, reproduction and fertility. Even further away, the periphery opens out into the bush and even further into the unknown areal, which is associated with spiritual danger and rank environment. The wild does not relate to any gender or political sphere but to an undifferentiated and socio-morally unmarked nature. Therewith, it relates to wild fecundity and disorder (Comaroff 1980).

4.3 Shifts and Changes in Production

Dealings with the missionaries throughout a period of rapid change facilitated acceptance of a new economy and brought along significant societal changes. Capitalist production and Christian values added notions of female subordination to men to a "separate but equal" social structure (Walker 1990: 29). This whole process started with the land pressure which consequently led to a sedentary economy on, for the most part, infertile land.

The territory which the Basotho had defended against the pressures of dislocation was predominantly mountainous and resources of all sorts except water were extremely scarce. New border formations had deprived the Basotho of both fertile areal as well as the land of their ancestors and the mountainous territory left people struggling to find resources. Droughts, lack of farming land to support families, increased trade of cash crops and wool in South Africa and the opening of trading stores in Lesotho, subsequently resulted in high levels of economic insecurity. The soil did not allow for the same strategies of subsistence and the Basotho had to mitigate shortages by means of large social networks. Eventually, the introduction of ploughs by missionaries in around 1850 brought changes to both the economy and gender relations:

> Prior to the 19th century, women's main economic contribution centered on the gathering of fruits and wild vegetables in addition to agricultural work. The introduction of the plow in the 1850s led to a dramatic increase in agricultural labour performed by women. Because women were forbidden from handling cattle, plowing became the domain of men, yet most of the other responsibilities were left to women. Although some men helped with harvesting and threshing, in general the plow increased women's work while men controlled the profits as surpluses were used to buy cattle and European manufactures (Rosenberg et al. 2004: 398-399).

In addition to shifts and changes in the local agricultural production, the discovery of diamonds and gold led to major changes in household economy. In 1867, diamonds were found in Kimberley and shortly thereafter gold mines sprang up around Johannesburg in South Africa. Instantly, an increasing number of Basotho labourers began to migrate to South Africa to supplement their families' arduous agricultural production with income they could send home from the mines. With their cash remittances their wives and mothers defrayed costs for basic family expenditures such as food, clothing, livestock, bride wealth, housing, furniture, agriculture, and savings (Gay 1980: 139).[6] Besides, labour migrants also facilitated good exchange as mine

---

[6] List according to value in descending order (Van der Wiel 1977: 80 in: Gay 1980: 139).

workers returning from South Africa brought along farming assets and monetary resources to the families in Lesotho which helped to mitigate the consequences of insecure resources (Walker 1990: 172-175; Muzvidizwa 2003; Silase et al. n.d.: 45, 52). Meanwhile women who stayed behind in Lesotho spent their time grinding corn, cooking, fetching water and fuel, making clothes, weaving, making pottery, maintaining homes, and raising children. Petty cash was generated by raising and selling small livestock, such as chickens and pigs and from brewing beer for sale, which was particularly a pastime for elderly women.

The number of Basotho migrant labourers increased constantly and one decade later mine work was the most important labour market for Basotho men. Migrants from Lesotho were recruited and quite often stayed for ten months or more (Silase et al. n.d.: 42; Gay 1980: 74). Thus, by the 1960s and 70s almost half of Lesotho's adult male labour force worked for months at a time in South Africa's gold and diamond mines. Until recently, Lesotho had the highest percentage of its labour force working outside the country than any other nation in the world (Cobbe 2004; Rosenberg et al. 2004: 84) which left women to become *de facto* heads of household. Walker notes:

> By drawing off the able-bodied men, the system put more and more strain on the rural homestead as a productive unit. This heightened tensions between the sexes and between the generations, which in turn brought further pressure to bear on the homestead as a social and economic unit (1990: 19).

Due to the absence of men, women were substantially involved in building the country following Lesotho's independence in 1966. Female workers dominated many areas of local infrastructural development such as construction, water supply, and in the tertiary sector (Matete-Lieb 1997). Women were better qualified for administrative jobs due to their higher educational attainment, while boys left school at an early age to herd the cattle or engage in migrant labour. However, despite the strong presence of women involved in community development, major decisions were often made by men on their short visits home from South Africa or upon retirement when they returned to their marital homes for good (Rosenberg et al. 2004: 399; Gay 1980: 135).

4.4 Empowerment of Women

The extended family pattern was in crisis from at least the early 19th century which manifested itself in a lack of stability of gender and generational arrangements on which the smallest units of the society were built. Male absence and marital breakdown led to female-centred families. Nevertheless, traditional bodies tried, as far as possible, to consolidate the residual structures.

Family law was amended under Griffith Lerotholi, the paramount chief from 1913-1939, and the Basotholand National Council in 1903. Lerotholi ruled as a fairly conservative leader who disagreed with any changes that would jeopardise the power of traditional men and family elders. Despite the absence of men due to labour migration, this did not change the position of women as minors under male custodianship[7]. However, since the 1920s women have taken on political positions as village and ward chiefs in place of their fathers, husbands or sons. Ironically, Lerotholi's daughter-in-law, 'Mantsebo, took over as first queen regent from 1941-1960 after her husband had ruled for only one year (Silase et al. n.d.: 61) and until her son, Seeiso, was old enough to succeed her as King Moshoeshoe II and head of parliament.

During her reign, 'Mantsebo restructured the powers and hierarchies of the chiefs and integrated them into a constitutional monarchy with a parliament (Silase et al. n.d.: 58). In the middle of the 20th century four of the 22 principal chiefs, who must be affiliated to the royal clan, were female and to date it is estimated that 35% of the villages are represented by women (Gay 1980: 41; Rosenberg et al. 2004: 403-404).[8] Despite female chiefs and women's agency in many aspects of social life, when it comes to large household expenses, such as land tenure and house ownership, women's participation remains marginal. Regardless of women's agency in traditional bodies, the parallel colonial administration and the colonial civil law subordinated women perpetually.

---

[7] The 1927 Native Administration Act in South Africa regarded women as perpetual minors under the auspices of their father, their husband or their son (Walker 1990: 185). Hence, it was the colonial administration that put an end to an "equal but separate" system and installed a gender hierarchy instead of an age hierarchy.

[8] The Global Gender Gap Index does not recognise female participation in traditional bodies but recognised a gender gap in parliament and ministerial positions. 24% of the MPs are female, while 32% of the ministerial posts are held by women (Hausmann et al. 2010: 193; cf. Kroeker 2011).

Despite 'Mantsebo's reign, "Lerotholi Law" has remained in force, although *realpolitik* would suggest otherwise. De Jure, the Land Act as of 1979, for instance, allows every Basotho individual, despite their marital status, to hold land titles, while the Marriage Act prescribes community of property under male custodianship. However, particularly unmarried, separated and widowed pro-active women have defied this practice by holding land titles allocated by traditional chiefs, opening bank accounts and by speaking for themselves. The extent of this was such that in 2006 laws were eventually passed that entitled women to do all of the above, although this fact does not seem to have been widely publicised (Women Thrive Worldwide 2010).

4.5 Young Women's Lives in Urban Lesotho

In the 1980s and 90s the economic landscape changed again dramatically and the Basotho had to adjust once more to new conditions which affected the generation of household income. Technological developments in the mines, declining global prices for gold and diamonds, and shifts in South African labour policy, aggravated the situation of male migrant labourers from Lesotho. After the end of Apartheid in the Republic of South Africa in 1994, South Africa's policy had additionally changed with the result that domestic employees were favoured over international labour migrants. Many labourers were dismissed and returned home as the opportunities for men in South African mines decreased. Curtailing labour migrants in South Africa severely affected the Basotho people by cutting down their foreign income. Remittances still accounted for almost half of Lesotho's Gross Domestic Product in 1987, while in 2005 it shrank to 20.4% (United Nations - INSTRAW)[9]. Redundancies as well as the down-scaled agrarian production and health situation resulted in less family income, a reduced ability to produce cheaply (e.g. agricultural products, food, handicrafts), and higher costs for goods that could not be produced (e.g. medication, clothing, building material, school equipment). The rate of unemployment rose to about 45% (2002), however, 86% of the resident population were engaged in subsistence agriculture to supplement other sources of income (CIA World Fact Book: Leso-

[9] However, about 60% of the mine workers are still foreign. In 2000, labour migrants in South African mines came from Lesotho (58,000), Mozambique (57,000), Swaziland (9,400) and Botswana (6,500). (Crush et al. 2005: 8). This number went down to 46,000 Basotho labour migrants in 2006 (UN-INSTRAW & UNDP 2010: 15).

tho, numbers as of 2003). Lower unemployment and agricultural production figures were indicated for 2009 by the Demographic and Health Survey. Unemployment was at 22% and agricultural occupation at 50% (MoHSW 2010: 35-41).

While men perceive rights of property and status through their citizenship and patrifiliation, women solely receive recognition through marriage, unless they have the opportunity to join the urban working class[10] by their own means (Gay 1980: 45). Gay, who carried out research in the 1970s stated:

> Since most rural Basotho women have no hope of joining the employed urban elite, early marriage is regarded as essential to provide cash and productive resources and the rights to utilize such resources. It is only through legal marriage that a girl can break from childhood dependence, be respected as a woman, and obtain lifelong rights to a homestead and a house of her own, to the labour and cash support of a man, to fields and livestock, and be assured the legitimate right to the labour and earning of her children (Gay 1980: 45).

From the 1980s onwards employment prospects for women rose in the formal sector. The opening of Chinese textile factories in Lesotho offered new opportunities. Textile companies were predominately situated in the lowland belt which stretches from Butha-Buthe in the north to Mohale's Hoek in the south. Employment as seamstresses enabled women to supplement or compensate for the loss of family income, and to gain recognition at the same time. Many women additionally combined formal and informal[11] occupations to generate income and took on the role of migrant breadwinners when men were no longer able to sufficiently provide for their family networks (Gay 1980: 295; Kimane & Ntimo-Makara 1998: 119). However, women did not only become *de facto* heads of household in lieu of their fathers, hus-

[10] Gay speaks of the urban elite. I doubt, however, that there is an urban elite in Lesotho. Traditional elites are rather found in the rural areas where their political power and social rank plays out. Here, I rather speak of those people relying on money from non-agricultural production and in formal employment and assume that Gay meant the same when speaking of urban elites.

[11] Formal employment in Lesotho consists of skilled manual labour in offices as well as unskilled labour such as in textile factories and shops. Informal occupation includes the aforementioned traditional female income generating activities, which migrant labourer wives practised, in addition to jobs as domestic helpers, selling from door-to-door, vegetable and pastry vendors, telephone kiosks, etc.

bands or sons, but also *de jure* as they entered labour migration. In the late 1970s, around 70% of the rural households had been managed by women, but major decisions were often made by men (Rosenberg et al. 2004: 401; cf. Walker 1990: 184). Yet male migrants in their brief visits home rarely managed to reassert their authority or continue to generate sufficient family income. Marital breakdowns, excessive drinking, and domestic violence became common (Rosenberg et al. 2004: 399; Gay 1980: 135; Gill 1993: 195). Women's negotiating position was marginal when a male custodian was in charge despite having primary responsibility for the household. Now, as household heads, women were in an inevitable position as agents in economy and household autonomy, which also impacted on gender relations: while the economic situation for men deteriorated and intensive agricultural production made the land more and more infertile, women's agency rose manifoldly in line with their labour participation. In 2003, the number of female workers in the textile industry alone peaked at around 60,000 (Rosenberg et al. 2004: 384; ILO [n.d.]: 10).

Unlike in other African countries, female workers in Lesotho usually work in towns, away from their family home, for several years (Walker 1990: 188-189), while in many cases elsewhere (cf. Ungruhe 2011: 58-79) girls come to town for a short period, for example, to gather their trousseau and personal assets. In his study on Nigeria, Caldwell (1982) recognises that predominantly young, unmarried and childless women left the villages for Nigeria's urban centres to seek employment. In Lesotho, however, in addition to numerous unmarried women, married mothers and wives also migrated as a means of escaping from abusive relationships or abandonment by migrant husbands (Rosenberg et al. 2004: 400; Walker 1990: 189). Basotho women move due to an increased demand for financial resources such as additions to the family, school fees, medical fees or in place of a (male) breadwinner (Field notes Kroeker: 17/11/2008; 30/10/2008; 18/11/2008). In Lesotho, most women moved from rural areas to bustling town centres. The repercussions of this included changes in livelihood, family relations, household decision-making, and eventually a change in the demographic.

Urban female-headed households tended to be smaller and/or more decentralised. As in many urban areas around the world, leased urban dwellings are characterised by changing neighbours, a more anonymous lifestyle and small families of one to five household members. Social and financial ties nonetheless continued to bind female employees in urban areas to the households of their extended family; this structure differs from the rural female-headed households, which still depended on male migrants' wages.

Men who migrated did so to provide their dependent extended family with security and status. An employed husband is expected to spend the generated income on the family and provide his wife and children with resources for their daily needs. Marriage used to promise a lifelong right to a homestead, which the husband would have to build, access to resources such as financial support, social standing as a mature member of society, and a familial network of security for wife and children (Gay 1980: 45). In practice, family income such as remittances from the husband and unmarried brothers were handed to the eldest female family member, who then allocated it on request to the younger household members. With the advent of high unemployment rates among men due to redundancies, marriage no longer fully assured a family's livelihood. Women, on the other hand, were not obliged to support their partner financially and once they left the village it was more likely to be a permanent break and more difficult to return to the female work sphere they had left (Walker 1990: 188).

In contrast to male income, female income was never managed by family elders. Migrant labourer wives, for instance, who generated their own petty income, even when living with agnatic or consanguine family members, were not expected to hand money over to their elders. Earnings belong to the woman and can therefore be used for her children, personal needs, or the family as she wishes (Field notes Kroeker: 03/02/2009). Both heading a household and generating independent income can be said to increase the independence and self-confidence of Basotho women (Gay 1980: 293; Griffiths 1990: 13-16) regarding life decisions and power in negotiations as the following case reveals:

> MaRobong, 22 and recently married, lived with her in-laws when she was offered a job as interpreter. Her husband requested that she must hand over her salary to the mother-in-law to support the family in the same way he, as a taxi driver, does. He requested her to help buy formula milk for his baby nephew who lived in their household. MaRobong refused, arguing that a wife's salary is supposed to be her own and must not be considered as family income. She thus decided to give half of the salary to her mother in order to save up for a mobile phone and bought groceries for the in-law's household with the other half. While mother and mother-in-law accepted her decision, the hus-

> band became angry since she disobeyed his decisions for the first time (Field notes Kroeker 29: 02/02/2009).

Many employed women who did not live with their family but who rented were, in addition to their income, interested in more independence and access to consumer goods. Solvent women mostly decided to use money on rent, groceries, sending money home, children's school needs and to save a little (Mapetla 2005).

More importantly than their financial independence, the situation raised their self-consciousness (Gay 1980: 293; Griffiths 1990: 13-16) regarding life decisions as one of my informants illustrates:

> LeRobong comes from a rather well-off household and dropped out of school when she got pregnant and married aged 17. She intended to further her studies after weaning her child, however, her husband forbade it[12]. He was not comfortable with the idea of her eventually becoming financially independent from him due to her being better educated and having a better job than him. His job as a contractor in South Africa did not suffice to provide for the family when their second child was born. LeRobong took up employment in the textile factory and moved into rental accommodation in town on her own. After having forbidden her to go back to school once she now says: "I suffered so much, I don't want him to block me again" (Field notes Kroeker 19: 23/11/2008).

Anthropologists such as Haram (2004) and Silberschmidt and Rasch (2001), who have studied female employees' reproductive life in East Africa's urban centres, show how conjugal life can be affected by women's financial independence. Men were afraid that their wife's financial independence would lead to disobedience and marital discord (cf. Bourdieu 2002). Silberschmidt (2004) highlights that men in Kenya and Tanzania lost their 'biologically given' status of household heads since they ceased to be able to provide bride wealth and cater for their family's daily needs. With respect to sexuality being key to masculinity, however, men have tried to keep traditional role models even if this has meant by force.

---

[12] "Girls who have had some education are considered more eligible for matrimony than the uneducated, but this must not be taken too far; highly educated girls are the object of awed and envious admiration but are also considered too advanced for the ordinary male to control or be happy with" (Ashton 1952: 60).

Apparently, sexual violence of men against women is a serious challenge in present-day Lesotho. Aggressive sexual behaviour with high rates of rape has been increasingly reported in recent years. It remains, however, unclear, whether the rates are actually rising or simply more women are willing to report such offences to the Child and Gender Protection Unit of the Police, which would, in contrast to the first assumption, prove women's self-consciousness when speaking up against men (cf. Motsoeli 2009). Brown et al. (2005) do not give any indication of the change in gender perception but report solely on the magnitude of sexual violence. The authors conclude that:

> Sexual violence is common with 61% of the sample reported having experienced sexual violence at some point in their lives of which 22% reported being physically forced to have sexual intercourse. Women with lower economic status and limited education were more likely to report sexual violence. Young women are at great risk of sexual assault with 33% of respondents reported having experienced forced sex by 18. Boyfriends were the most common perpetrators of forced sex (66%) (Brown et al. 2005).

The Demographic and Health Survey of Lesotho reported accordingly that not only sexual but also domestic violence against women happens at a high rate in Lesotho. The Survey reports that "many women and men find wife beating to be justified in certain circumstances", such as arguing with the husband, neglecting the children, going out without informing the husband, or refusing to have sex with the husband (MoHSW, 2010: 228).

Silberschmidt concludes that in East Africa while women were empowered by socio-economic changes, the role of men remains neglected. In her analysis, as men became more and more disempowered by socio-economic change, there was not only a breakdown of masculine roles, reduced male self-esteem, and a general lack of social value associated with men; men attempted to compensate for this loss by dominating sexual relationships, domestic violence and 'escalating gender antagonism'. In the face of poverty, unemployment, and a lack of access to education, masculinity has turned to a show of irresponsible, promiscuous and aggressive sexual behaviour towards women (Silberschmidt 2004: 234, 242). In Lesotho the situation seems comparable.

Due to disputes over power, resources and traditional roles, solvent employed Basotho women would rather live away from their husband or family. Due to the family economy, spouses and their children may therefore live in more than one household and members may oscillate between various urban and rural residences. As a result, female labour migrants often rented a room in town in order to avoid conflicts and to enjoy independent decision-making without having to consult the head of the household on day-to-day decisions. In short, women who moved to town on their own gained a great degree of autonomy while at the same time losing material and social security, both of which marriage into an extended family network would provide. Consequently, young urban mothers are quite conscious that the circumstances of female labour migration and separation of spouses are not the ideal type of family life.

Many female migrants try to keep in touch with their extended family by providing them with goods and paying visits, if their budget allows, and sending children to stay with them. Migrant women generally live in rented terraced houses with one or two rooms, so called *malaene,* which are modelled after the male migrant houses near the mines or large construction sites. Those dwellings were not designed to house families but single men and the accommodation women rent close to the textile factories, for instance, is also not suitable for family life. The architecture of the *malaene* settlements often does not allow for separate sleeping arrangements according to gender or age. Families are, thus, separated because of the available housing in town[13]. For this reason, child fosterage arrangements with rural family members gain weight (Field notes Kroeker: 29/05/2008; 03/06/2008; cf. Chipeta 2005; Gay 1980: 78, 295, 308; Griffiths 1990: 6; Field notes Kroeker: 05/11/2008; 11/11/2008; 23/11/2008). Moreover, shifts in the textile factories can last up to 12 hours and therefore a child minder would be needed. The high cost of raising children in town and the lack of time to care of them forces textile workers to send their children to stay with relatives.

In the rural area children are usually welcomed as helpers in and around the house. Moreover, they connect their mother with a family-based fail-safe network. In fact, all kinds of care arrangements involve the extended family in the absence of private welfare arrangements. Few can afford insurance premiums which require a permanent and regular wage. Therefore care for the elderly, children and the sick is organised by unemployed members of the extended families. Support of the family will moreover be considered as long-term insurance and urban-rural relations as well as cash remittances secure crucial family bonds especially in times of HIV and AIDS, when nu-

---

[13] Chipeta (2005) illustrates the inter-linkage of gender and architecture in urban Malawi.

merous people of a productive and reproductive age fall sick (Mapetla 2005). Sending children home is a common way of keeping close ties with relatives outside the urban area. Migrants mostly visit their family on a monthly basis after payday to deliver money and groceries which Muzvidziwa (2003: 24) describes as "double-rootedness" (Field notes Kroeker: 03/06/2008; 23/11/2008; 12/05/2009). The support system is, thus, far from eroding as it is a pre-condition to combining paid labour with care (Gay 1980: 294-295). Thus, in Lesotho, single female tenants or single-mother households can no longer be considered exceptions[14]. Having a place on one's own also allowed for some sexual freedom and partnerships with or without long-term commitments.

Despite the high value of having children, it does not come as a surprise that the history of family planning is closely connected with women's increasing participation in formal employment (cf. Mapetla & Moultrie 2011). Employed women chose to have fewer children because although children were considered as a valuable gift, having many children was too expensive and therefore female income-generation impacts on family planning (cf. Easterlin & Crimmins 1985; Caldwell 1982; Kaufman et al. 2000: 26). Lesotho's Government advertised family planning and monitored fertility rates from 1970 in order to reduce population growth and employed women in particular accepted contraceptives[15]. Besides, heading a household also allows unmarried as well as married female labour migrants in Lesotho to engage in casual relationships. Due to the use of contraceptives, the majority of these relationships do not result in offspring since the 'use of contraceptive methods allows women to postpone pregnancy, alter the timing between pregnancies, or avoid pregnancy completely' (Tuoane et al. 2003: 105).

Employed women mentioned that they did not expect to get pregnant due to an unfavourable financial situation, signified by a correlation between

---

[14] Accordingly, I distinguish between household and family. With family I mean the extended family, which may be spread over a larger geographical scope and include more than one generation. A household, in contrast, consists of people who are living together in one place. An urban household may include only one person renting a single room, as well as a couple or a single mum with her child(-ren) or an in-house helper, who stays overnight at the employer's house. Household refers instead to one residential unit, whereas family refers to a social, agnatic entity.

[15] A more detailed discussion about Lesotho's fertility rates in connection with women's employment can be found in Kroeker (forthcoming).

the employment of women and contraceptive use[16]. The low land belt shows higher contraceptive use and good access to family planning services. In 1989, the Ministry of Health and Social Welfare estimated that this area had a significantly higher attendance rate of family planning units from 21 to 69 visits per 1,000 people in contrast to 3 to 19 visits per 1,000 in the foothills and mountainous region (Lucas 1992: 151). Contraceptive prevalence rose from around 7% in the mid-1970s to 47% in 2009 throughout the whole of Lesotho (Tuoane et al. 2004).

Due to the fact that many female breadwinners were actually not only responsible for their own offspring but supported their family networks (Mapetla 2005), employed women mentioned that they did not expect to get pregnant in view of their unfavourable financial situation, such as the case of my informant, Leshome:

> Leshome, aged 36, started to migrate between village and town in 2001 when she found employment in Mafeteng's textile sector. Leshome, being the firstborn, committed herself to the family hardships and later generated income to sponsor her younger siblings' education. Now that the last-born was about to graduate she and her long-term boyfriend started planning their own family. However, she still did not intend to marry or move in with him. He, being a widower with children, neither intended to marry into a second family (Field notes Kroeker: 07/11/2008-21/05/2009; cf. Kaufman et al. 2000: 24, 26).

---

[16] The correlation between employment, education and decline in fertility has been most prominently discussed by Easterlin and Crimmins (1985) or Caldwell (1982). The economist, Easterlin, argued that fertility can be directly linked to relative income and a "fertility revolution" will accompany social and economic shifts. He argues: 'The principal changes in reproductive behaviour associated with modernization relate to fertility and fertility control. The change in fertility is from an average of six or more births per woman over the reproductive career to around two' (Easterlin & Crimmins, 1985: 4).
In his theory of fertility transition, Caldwell (1982: 72) argued that economic and social change alters the flow of wealth between generations, making children more expensive, and thence fertility declines. In his quantitative and qualitative study of household economy and fertility decline in Nigeria, he states that the benefits of having many children will be superseded by the costs of upbringing, education and the like. Employed parents in urban centres are therefore more likely to reduce the number of offspring and invest instead in the intensive care and finance of their fewer children. Moreover, contraceptive use correlates with employment and education of women, with their age, and with place of residence (a positive impact of living in an urbanised area) (Caldwell 1982: 18).

4.6 The Dominant Party: The Grammar of Social Interaction

On a practical level, urban women in Lesotho actively switched between productive and reproductive activities which was similarly the case during industrialisation in 19th century Europe. Becker-Schmidt (2003) analyses that gender roles had a reciprocal relation in a historical context, whereas male spheres dominated female spheres. Industrialisation urged women to combine "male" and "female" work chores resulting in a double workload, which is the basis for women's *double socialization* (*"doppelte Vergesellschaftung"*). Productive activities were highly appreciated as these enabled participation in public and social life, but meant that women struggled as time-consuming female household and family chores had to be fulfilled as well. Nowadays, the socialisation of girls rather allows for the blurring of lines between productive and reproductive activities and for them to follow mother or father as a role model, unlike boys solely following the male model. Becker-Schmidt concludes that the homologous social gender arrangements became weak due to women's double socialisation, although not in spheres of political and economical relevance; the spheres of strong male hegemony. These findings of Becker-Schmidt can be compared with the situation I found in Lesotho.

Women were "drawn into the maelstrom of proletarianisation and urbanisation" (Walker 1990: 17) and left the traditional distribution of gender roles as they combined their paid and unpaid activities at their own households and, at the same time, maintained close ties with their family network. At their neolocal home traditional distribution of roles and chores will not apply since females adopted traditionally male chores besides their female activities. Employment increased their autonomy over housing arrangements, in day-to-day decision-making, maintenance of social relations, formal and informal partnership and enhanced self-esteem. Women thus took responsibility for their own, their child's and their family's well-being. Those who were engaged in paid employment and rented rooms in urban areas, or were respectively exposed to this lifestyle and its representatives, were somewhat divorced from gender and generational arrangements. By that, I mean that urban female-headed households were organised on an individual basis, either removed from multigenerational living arrangements or resulting in the geographical separation of spouses.

While there are numerous female-headed households without a male partner, I did not find a single urban household where an employed woman was providing for an unemployed partner. If that were the case they would rather not stay together and separate their spheres. Presumably, a wife in that situation would even protect her husband from rumours ("He is not able to provide for his wife and children") and rather state that he works elsewhere than admit that he depends on female income.

Of course, male employees likewise rent rooms in town, where they, in the absence of females, perform female household chores such as cleaning, cooking and washing. However, if a wife, sister or girlfriend were present she would be expected to take on those chores which had culturally female connotations and as such prevent a deconstruction of gender roles. Thus, the situation has in fact not changed much when different genders and generations found themselves in the same sphere.

Looking at this from the perspective of a political anthropologist, we find some valuable points in Scott's description on the interaction between dominants and subordinates which enable us to elaborate on the complex gender and generational relations among urban Basotho women. While they gained recognition as heads of household, earners and decision-makers on their own, women fell back into old behavioural patterns of patriarchal dependency when men were present. Behavioural patterns entailed domination by males and subordination by females who therefore preferred to live on their own. In Scott's examples on dependent peasant groups, the subordinate party in the social relation did not intend to contest the structure, quite the opposite, subordinates rather accepted the social order and agreed *per se* upon the principle stratification of society. Individuals or groups may consider a certain social strata as basic contours; an assumed environment that may not even be noticed by the subjects. Though lacking ideas on alternative ways of organisation, individuals and groups have "at least a fatalistic acceptance of that social order and perhaps even an active complicity" (1985: 39). Elsewhere he states:

> It is precisely this public domain where the effects of power relations are most manifest, and any analysis based exclusively on the public [norms of behaviour] is likely to conclude that subordinate groups endorse the terms of their subordination and are willing, even enthusiastic, partners in that subordination (Scott 1990: 4).

Superiority, as part of power relations, cannot be described without simultaneously stating who accepts this domination because the social stratification is not solely established by the dominant but in accordance with the subordinate subject, who accepts domination through acts of deference. If no one recognises a superior, superiority is lost, just as in Arendt's definition of *Macht* (Arendt 1996: 45) where subordinates accept it (sometimes, however, they are forced to accept it, which Arendt then calls *Gewalt*). Similarly, Comaroff describes the social relations between a chief and his community among the Batswana with a common proverb: "A chief is a chief because of the nation. If we cannot see you in the court *[kgotla]* we shall draw away from you. And if we do will you still call yourself a chief?" (Comaroff & Comaroff 2012: 119).

The relationship between the dominant party and subordinated party can therefore only be described in relation to each other. Scott calls the interplay of the two parties consequently a "self-fulfilling prophecy":

> If subordinates believe their superior to be powerful, the impression will help him impose himself and, in turn, contribute to his actual power (Scott 1990: 49).

To describe the power relation in more detail we need to look into the characteristics of interaction. Scott suggests that dominants merely control the pathways of participation of subordinates and are thus powerful. Dominants exercise coercion and influence both openly and covertly by means of the media (Scott 1990: 73). Among the Batswana, for instance, dominant forces, in this case males in traditional political positions, made sure to control change-making bodies. The respective bodies would be needed to bring about a change of hierarchy and gender relations respectively, which were therewith somewhat manifest (Comaroff 1985: 48, 60; cf. Preston-Whyte & Zondi 1989). Griffiths notes likewise:

> Women are actively engaged for support, compensation or distribution of property but they have less access to those resources which confer status and power and this makes them more vulnerable in their dealings with men (Griffiths 1990: 8).

Lesotho's patriarchal and gerontocratic family structure demands respect in the form of normative power which is also reflected in the interactive process. During communication between the parties certain norms apply which, in addition to discourse, include body language, non-verbal communication and avoidance of topics. Comparably, young Basotho women accepted the "grammar of social interaction" and in the case of open disputes, though, subsequently in expectation of disagreement, women argued from their "traditionally founded position of weakness" (Mapetla 2005; Ntimo-Makara &

Makara-Khatleli 2005). Mapetla as well as Ntimo-Makara and Makara-Khatleli investigated an awareness of a traditional divide in private and public domains in Lesotho. Seemingly, women were quite aware of traditional gender and generational roles and referred to them when power-holders were involved (Mapetla 2005). Where the "traditional" family stayed together, "traditional" contracts of gender also remained more or less intact despite female participation in the economy. Even if women were better informed and more aware of ongoing debates, they remained disempowered and acted according to societal gender expectations in situations of dispute (Ntimo-Makara & Makara-Khatleli 2005: 195-217).

A fundamental reform of gender roles would require access to religious, political and economic forms of transformation, thus, the core of the male sphere. Consequently, gender roles were not contested, while the livelihood of women changed tremendously owing to economic changes. Urban women, despite geographical distance from their family members, had no intention of challenging the social hierarchy but respected the dominance of males even in cases of violence and abuse.

This argument can be broadened: not only men but also elders, both representatives of "traditional" power holders, had a say in issues that extended beyond the female-headed urban household. Thus, gender arrangements remain manifest where male and female spheres meet, and interaction between people of different ages also remained in place. For instance, wherever daughters (-in-law) and mothers (-in-law) meet, traditional role models determined behavioural expectations in a highly politicised relationship. In the interaction between dominants and subordinates in a family network, women accepted authority, support and their role as such. Young women attempt to keep face and therewith showed respect to elders. An elderly teacher explains to me:

> Younger ones are not allowed to ask questions to elder ones but must adhere to the advice they give. Therefore they may never be told why things are supposed to be like this or that (Field notes Kroeker Malikhoele: 15/03/2009).

Moreover, young people assumed that quarrels would affect the relationship which guaranteed love, care and support from elders and considered it part of a family's heritage. A young teacher in Lesotho agrees with the aforementioned statement and explains from his point of view:

> I respect what our forefathers did because I know it was good. Therefore, I respect our culture. There are certain rules and norms that can't

> be understood by me now, but I know that at a certain age I will understand them and I will adhere to them now and accept the regulations without asking why. (…) They will become comprehensible at a later stage of life. (...) I understand that [the current youngsters] should be told when it is important to educate their own children, before they should just obey to the rules the elders give them without understanding the reasons (Field notes Kroeker Theko: 28/07/2009).

Scott adds that gerontocractic orders are very stable since young people expect to achieve this powerful position for themselves one day. Looking forward to becoming a respected parent eases the acceptance of a subordination and compliance with authoritative orders at present. Gerontocratic dominance and subordination seems merely part of being and becoming:

> The expectation that one will eventually be able to exercise the domination that one endures today is a strong incentive serving to legitimise patterns of domination. It encourages patience and emulation, and, not least, it promises revenge of a kind, even if it must be exercised on someone other than the original target of resentment. If this supposition is correct it would help to explain why so many age-graded systems of domination seem to have such durability. The junior who is exploited by elders will eventually get his chance to be an elder; those who do degrading work for others in an institution – providing they can reasonably expect to move up – will eventually have that work done for them; the traditional Chinese daughter-in-law can look forward, if she has a son (!), to becoming a domineering mother-in-law (Scott 1990: 82-83).

Coming of age may solve the dispute at a later stage in life, when reasons may become clear and decisive power is by-then in an aged person's hands.

One-generational households headed by young women, in contrast, allowed for some geographical distance between them and family authorities. Female household-heads with independent income and decision-making agency enjoyed the opportunity to avoid interaction with men or elder relatives that would subordinate them. Urban living conditions were therewith both a tool and a pre-condition to avoiding gender and generational disputes. One could also surmise that women took on economic duties but did not yet have access to the rights which conferred political and strategic decision-making outside the traditional female chores. Without doubt, women employees manage their life in town and decide how to support the extended family. However, women did not take over in extra-household decisions and the underlying patriarchal system remained intact. On the whole, women who were able to make extra-household decisions did not subvert traditional gender arrangements as the next examples illustrate. All these women took on productive and reproductive activities in and outside the household in a vacuum, since there was no custodian who could fulfil this function.

> LeRobong, MaRobong as well as Hlano had some financial independence and made household decisions on a day-to-day basis. However, none of them made decisions outside the household for long-term investments for the family's well-being, such as building a house, buying sites and registering them in their name. Only women who may not conflict with traditional custodians did so according to my findings. MaThloni, for instance, who was orphaned and unmarried bought a site. Neither a husband nor father or brother could have signed a contract in her stead. MaSupa was widowed. She also bought a plot and wanted to build a house, which her husband had not managed during his lifetime (Field notes Kroeker: 10/2008-05/2009). MaRobong's mother and grandmother, both of whom were widowed, even overtook ritual functions in absence of a male household head (Field notes Kroeker 29: 06/02/2009).

In a national comparison of all districts, women in the Mafeteng District were the most involved in independent decision-making. 66% decided individually on health care, 49% on large purchases, 68% on daily purchases, 67% on family visits, and 81% on nutrition. Agency was particularly high in the textile industry districts (MoHSW 2005: 41-42). However, quite in contrast to these findings, women were hardly ever in charge in extra-household decisions which they only took over temporarily in the absence of men. In general, subordinates, for their part, chose not to provoke conflicts with the dominant party, which makes avoidance of their supervision a rational tool of dispute settlement (various types of avoidance will be outlined in Chapter 9).

4.7 The Subordinate Party: Silent Agents Who Keep Face

The manifestation of social hierarchies and related etiquette did not render the subordinate party, here young women, powerless. Despite an intention to separate spheres of dominants and subordinates and therewith avoid conflicts, empirical data suggested that study participants actively made room for their own preferences while playing the role of subordinate. In fact, young people behaved according to the norm of respect for elders and avoided challenging the existing social order, but developed techniques which they could use for their own benefit. Subordinates may generally not have the power or the intention to overthrow a social system but will attempt to navigate within its limits in order to achieve greater freedom or less inconvenience. Hobsbawm, on whom Scott partly bases his notion of social hierarchy, also realises that a rebellious group intends to cause upheaval but only within the existing social framework as they have neither the means nor the ideology to construct a replacement structure by themselves (Hobsbawm 1962: 74). Without a political mindset these groups seek reform rather than revolution and, thus, the architecture of society remains untouched. In his analysis of power relations, Scott therefore distinguishes between the *hidden* and *public transcript* of either party and the respective normative behaviour within each party and towards the other party. Meanwhile, the hidden transcript implies knowledge about differing behavioural expectations as well as ways to keep face. For instance, talking behind a superior's back implies a hidden agenda, etiquette though prevents openly acknowledged talks.

> Like many female family elders, LeRobong's mother told her not to sleep during the day when pregnant since it will harm the child. LeRobong disagreed with this order she got and complained towards me: "It is only told to scare women!". Though, under close supervision she decided to adhere to it grudgingly. Although she now assumes the consequence of sleeping during the day to be irrational, she does not know what the rationality was to give her that advice. Up to now she was not confronted with the hidden transcript of the taboo since discussions did not take place and she disobeyed instructions when elders were not at home (Field notes Kroeker 19: 01/04/2009)[17].

Of course, LeRobong did not allow her superiors to find out about her disobedience. Neither did she inquire as to the reasons why she must not sleep during the day but accepted the instructions which came from people she considered to be in a dominant position.

The interaction itself, according to Scott, follows a certain set of behavioural norms. Notwithstanding, certain personal preferences will be concealed from the other party as the behavioural etiquette demands. This means that, in spite of somewhat manifest gender and generational hierarchies,

---

[17] The explanation will be given in Chapter 9.4.

young urban women in Lesotho are in no way left without the means and techniques to pursue their interests. Nevertheless, their strategies may not be debated in public and in view of superiors in the social strata. In his study, Scott uses *public transcript* for openly avowed ideas, and *hidden transcript* for ideas that imply everything that is said in addition to non-verbal expression, such as gestures, general behaviour and the like, in fact every representation of verbal and non-verbal communication[18]. Individuals, though, usually use an open interaction "on stage", in the public communication, if speaking across hierarchical frontiers.

> What we have here is a difference between "onstage" and "offstage" behaviour; to the extent that the deference expressed in the public, power-laden situations is negated in the comparative safety of offstage privacy, we can speak unambiguously of false deference (Scott 1985: 25).

The hidden transcript comprises "discourse that takes place off stage", beyond direct observation by power-holders and thus, the hidden transcript is derivative as it confirms, contradicts, or inflects what is performed in public. To describe the hidden transcript in relation to the public transcript one could therefore ask: what are the issues we usually try to hide in public? Of course it will somehow be implicit in the public discourse, yet, etiquette and knowledge of adequate behaviour ensures that discontent with the situation is kept away from the public sphere.

> The analysis of the hidden transcripts of the powerful and of the subordinates offer us, I believe, one path to a social science that uncovers contradictions and possibilities, that looks well beneath the placid surface that the public accommodation of the existing distribution of power, wealth, and status often presents. (...) The analyst in any situation like this has a strategic advantage over even the most sensitive participants precisely because the hidden transcripts of dominant and subordinate are, in most circumstances, *never in direct contact* (Scott 1990:15).

The hidden transcript of LeRobong's mother, in consequence, was not known to LeRobong, while she also tried to shield her hidden transcript – the disagreement and the subsequent disobedience – from her mother. The public transcripts entailed, however, subordination to elders. Nevertheless, there

[18] We will talk about this in 5.2.1.

is criticism and dissatisfaction within the public interaction, which is, however, enrobed in norms and conformity. This corresponds with Lesotho's gerontocratic educative structure, which demands respect in the form of normative power which shows in the communicative process. In linguistic terms we would thus speak of *politeness*, which qualifies social relationships in a positive or a negative sense. Brown and Levinson (2006) argue that we can draw universal strategies, which underlie cultural differences. One of these universals is the rational use of "face" which relates to the planned utilisation of more or less direct confrontation as a means to an end. "Face" refers to Goffmann's notion (1963) which is connected with embarrassment and humiliation. People interacting with one another hence attempt to maintain face, aware of the mutual vulnerability and the risk of negative politeness and face threatening acts. In a constructivist approach, Brown and Levinson's rational bases of conventions are described, which allow one to lose "face" while every person eagerly seeks to be unimpeded and carries a desire that actions of every "competent adult member" be of good intentions (Brown & Levinson 2006: 62). Notwithstanding this, keeping face in public ties in with more extreme ways of making ends meet. Scott mentions the "weapons of the weak", which still appear as if subordinate parties comply with the dominant party's expectation. However, this is only to disguise an actual, hidden interest:

> Here I have in mind the ordinary weapons of relatively powerless groups: foot dragging, dissimulation, false compliance, pilfering, feigned ignorance, slander, arson, sabotage, and so forth (…) They require little or no coordination or planning; they often represent a form of individual self-help; and they typically avoid any direct confrontation with authority or with elite norms (Scott 1985: 29).

Interestingly, some of the strategies Scott describes by analysing the interaction of peasants, slaves, monarchs and dictators[19] can, on a micro-level, be transferred to hierarchical relations within the family. With advanced strategies young women avoided conflicts with men, elders as well as medical staff in the hospital, as we will see later. Nevertheless, they managed, for instance, to

---

[19] While in "Domination and the Arts of Resistance" (1990) Scott emphasises the interaction between subordinates and a collective interest as a key characteristic of a hidden transcript, in "Weapons of the Weak" (1985) he mainly draws examples from individual resistance. Hence, I am talking about individuals and applying Scott's concept to individual women who are HIV-positive as well as pregnant or child-bearing.

participate in crucial family issues and prearranged their preferred outcome of negotiations. Having said that, in the end they made it look like the dominant party made the decision and not them. For instance, young women found ways to force a man's hand in marriage and to make their parents agree to the liaison.

4.8 Marriage Proposal as Individual Decision

In pre-colonial times, a pre-nuptial pregnancy or child among the Swazi and the Zulu would guarantee the fertility of a woman, and thus make it easier for a man to agree to marry her. Even non-biological children would be accepted as his offspring once he agreed to marry the mother (Kuper 1950: 88). The Basotho and Tswana, in contrast, expected a bride not to have had penetrative sex. Both then and now, parents generally discouraged premarital sexual relationships and encouraged early marriage as a means of preventing pre-marital pregnancies (I will elaborate on this in Chapter 5.1.2). The Basotho did not require proof of the bride's virginity (Maqutu 2005: 36) but premarital meetings between boys and girls ought to be modest. Marriage decisions were in the hands of elders who married their daughter off when chances of illegitimate offspring were high due to premarital sexual activity (cf. Preston-White & Zondi 1989) which must have been the norm rather than the exception. Today, in many cases, parents would turn a blind eye to one of their children being in a relationship provided contact was not displayed in public and there were no consequences (cf. Bochow 2007). If a relationship was in the public domain, the parents were blamed for the lax moral upbringing of their offspring. Moreover, having a grandchild out of wedlock would also be the fault of the girl's parents and therefore it was preferred to arrange marriage in a timely manner. Often a child born out of wedlock will receive a bad name and consequently "everybody will know that something is wrong with the mother of this child" (Field notes Kroeker Malikhoele: 15/03/2009). Usually, a child's name was chosen by elder relatives with reference to an ancestor or historical incident, however, this also applies when referring to a disobedient mother. LeSupa's baby, for example, was called "Thuto" (Sesotho: Lecture) by its grandfather. The grandfather explained that she fell pregnant for the second time while she was still at school and he hoped that the child would serve as a lesson to her (Field notes Kroeker 17: 15/01/2009).

Missionaries had encouraged the Basotho to abolish customs such as polygyny, initiation schools and bridewealth *[bohali]* which they considered inimical to Christian values (Walker 1990: 14; Rosenberg et al. 2004: 349), albeit without success. Today, officially, marriages are monogamous (98%) and 95% of women aged 45-49 in Lesotho have been married at some stage (MoHSW 2010: 69, 71) which indicates that marital life is still highly valued. However, informal polygamy – that is extramarital relationships – of both sexes cannot be denied.

While during earlier times familial supervision interfered with unacceptable behaviour, such as illegitimate sexual relations of their youngsters, distant housing arrangements and migration diluted moral norms and values. Initiation schools which teach about morals, norms and behaviour, still exist, attended by some boys and fewer girls. Earlier, at the onset of puberty, young girls and boys were separately enlightened about their marital rights and duties in these schools. Now, a handful of young people are taught by traditional healers on marital life and neither is sexual education a topic between children and their parents. Perhaps this is why sexual morals among adolescents are now lax since neither initiation schools nor alternative structures provide adequate sexual education. Yet, some of the norms still apply.

The boy's maternal uncle, *malome*, still has the role of advisor to a young boy inquiring about marriage. He discusses whether a match is favourable beforehand and negotiates bridewealth *[bohali]* (Ashton 1952: 18-19). The exchange of goods still remains a crucial part of marriage arrangements (Rosenberg et al. 2004: 349, 351), despite Christian wedding ceremonies.

Whenever supervision waned due to weakened networks of neighbourly control and geographical dislocation, and young people became more independent, the initiation of marriages also changed. Nowadays, it is the young couple that initiates marriage negotiations at a specific time when they intend to come out in the open about the liaison. More often the boyfriend decides to take his girlfriend home and let her stay overnight with or without warning his parents and thereby reveals his more serious interest in the girl (Maqutu 2005: 155). From the exhaustive protocol of traditional marriage arrangements which I will discuss in 5.1.3, present-day young couples appropriated an individualised version of elopement *[chobeliso]* and abduction:

> Today most of the Basotho Customary Marriages are irregular and start as elopement. (…) people who wanted to marry for love forced

> the hands of their parents through blackmail. Young people used to elope if their parents were in the way. They ran away and consummated their relationship through cohabitation. Parents to avoid scandal were forced to marry them off. (...) Almost nine out of ten Basotho Customary Marriages are through *chobeliso* (...) Chobeliso has gained a degree of social acceptability that it did not have thirty years ago. This is inevitable because people are becoming poorer and poorer, and yet the custom of *bohali* remains deeply embedded into the culture of the Basotho (Maqutu 2005: 152, 155).

Economic hardships often exclude men from marriage altogether due to the bride wealth payments up until their late 20s. If a man cannot manage to pay his debts to the girl's family, and thereby shows that he is unable to provide for a wife and all her offspring the children resulting from the union will belong to the maternal lineage.

MaRobong told me her story of their elopement:

> MaRobong met her future husband while she was still a student in 2006. They dated for more than a year without her parents' knowledge and his parents were not aware of the relationship either. Even prior to this, MaRobong had been in another relationship although her parents had never found out about her first boyfriend.
>
> Since her husband-to-be worked as a taxi driver the couple usually met in town. One day, when she came from the saloon, he picked her up to give her a ride home like he always did. That day it was late however, when he branched off to his neighbourhood instead of hers without preparing her. He pretended that he only needed to pick up a jacket but asked her in when they reached his place and she stayed over. Later she learned that his mother has already been informed about their due elopement.
>
> MaRobong's mother though was angry and worried all night. The mother called a meeting with family elders and the grandfather decided that MaRobong shall marry the man she had spent the night with (Field notes Kroeker 29: 02/02/2009).

Young people joke that the traditional way of marriage is the best one since no preparation or money is needed and it solely depends on their choice. They assume that parents only need to accept the girl in the morning after the elopement and with that the couple is instantly married (Field notes

Kroeker: 30/06/2008). However, the secrecy of a relationship and insecurity about whether the elders will approve of it or not when a pregnancy becomes apparent as a result of the liaison, affords further steps: many girls get married because they are with child.

Elders may suspect this to be blackmail and doubt the truthfulness of their children. However, to avoid stigma they will usually agree to enter marriage negotiations.

4.9 The Female Way of a Love Proposal

In fact, a more individualised lifestyle also meant a more individualised sex life dissociated from reproduction which is reflected in the high uptake of contraception amongst Basotho women (Gay 1980: 294; Kaufman et al. 2000; Griffiths 1990). Most of the girls manage to get through puberty without falling pregnant[20], and, in fact, the age for having a first child rose in recent years in Lesotho and marriage was likewise delayed. First pregnancy for Basotho women occurs in their early twenties, and teenage pregnancies were recorded less often than in other Southern African countries[21]. The average age for marriage is now at 21 years for women and 26 years for men (MoHSW 2010: 72). First pregnancy is also delayed to approximately 22 years for first mothers in urban areas, and 20 years in rural areas.

The temporal and informal nature of some relationships and male dominance in gender relations, made it difficult for young women to build relationships and to arrange for marriage. Hence, many girls in Lesotho, as well as in South Africa, seemingly chose to show their serious interest in the boy by getting pregnant. Despite the widespread availability of free condoms as a form of male birth control, safe protection against pregnancies seems to be a female responsibility, and this enables girls to use fertility for the purpose of initiating marriage negotiations when they consider the circumstances to be just right (Field notes Kroeker MaMong: 15/04/2009; Field notes Kroeker Theko: 15/04/2009; Field notes Kroeker LeSupa; Field notes Kroeker MaMeli; Field notes Kroeker MaTharo).

---

[20] Mafeteng Government Hospital lies within walking distance of some secondary schools and teenage girls wearing their school uniforms seek family planning advice in their breaks or after school. A big family planning unit, run by an NGO, opened in 2010 on the fields between the hospital and the taxi rank, and is therefore easily accessible for school girls.

[21] Teenage pregnancies (15-19 years): Botswana 21%, Namibia 14%, South Africa 13%, Zimbabwe 4%, Lesotho 3% (Mturi & Moerane 2001).

The secret use of contraceptives by women is most common as this pragmatically avoids awkward discussions on sexuality between partners (Field notes Kroeker: 02/02/2009). Despite open talk about sexuality and procreation in biomedical and educative arenas and despite women's knowledge and agency in family planning, communication between partners on sexual issues remains a taboo. Due to etiquette, explicit discussions on procreation seldom take place between partners and between elders and their children (cf. Horstmann 2006)[22]. Consequently, most women prefer contraceptives which can be used secretly such as three month-injections that suppress ovulation as well as menstrual flow (Field notes Kroeker: 10/02/2009; MoHSW, 2010: 85; Bledsoe 2002: 83-84)[23]. Due to a taboo on menstrual blood, women had to abstain from intercourse during their monthly period anyway (Ngubane 1976; Gausset 2002). Killing two birds with one stone, women avoided pregnancies, their period, and discussions on abstinence with their partner when using hormonal injections.

Thus, women used hidden, but powerful strategies to put their interests into practice. In quite a number of cases I observed, young women stopped using contraception at a certain point in time without the partner's knowledge. Despite women's participation in public life and household decision-making it is still inappropriate for a girl to ask a boy out or propose marriage verbally. In discussions with young men, they thought it was an odd idea for a girl to propose to them but admitted that a pregnancy would force a boy as well as the couple's parents into commitments (Field notes

---

[22] This had also affected court trials on rape cases, as informants emphasised, as women found it hard to speak about the sex offence in front of mostly male judges (Field notes Kroeker MaKhotso: 10/2/2009). Although complaints have risen in recent years, it may well be that the number of cases has not increased and that women have started speaking out more (Motsoeli 2009).

[23] Available methods of family planning are as follows: male and female condoms, implants that last for five years, Depo-Provera injections, diaphragm and Intra-uterine device (IUD). Pills (oestrogen and combined type) are also available but not used as often, besides hormonal Emergency Contraception which features on some of the clients' expenses. Not all of those family planning methods apply to HIV-positive women due to possible drug interactions. Few women opt for a tubal ligation and even fewer men have a vasectomy. Abortions are illegal in Lesotho, which does not mean that they do not happen. Moreover, termination of pregnancy was recently legalised in South Africa (Nzioka 2003; Kaufman et al. 2000; Field notes Kroeker: 17/06/2008) and Basotho women may travel there if they cannot find a backstreet clinic in Lesotho.

Kroeker Theko: 15/04/2009; 21: 16/04/2009; 03/2010). Thus, the non-verbal option seems more common:

> MaMeli planned her pregnancy despite her unmarried situation. She moreover calls the father of the child her husband although no marriage ceremony took place and explains that the couple intended to speed up the process of negotiations due to their parents' reluctance. The couple had been engaged for quite some time, but MaMeli's parents disapproved of her liaison with a much older miner from their neighbourhood. Yet, a planned pregnancy hastened the process of marital negotiations due to the moral stigma of an unmarried girl with child (Field notes Kroeker 22: 25/11/2008).

In MaMeli's case the pregnancy resulted in a marriage, however, in many cases the strategy, and I particularly determine it as such, does not guarantee success (Field notes Kroeker 21: 16/04/2009). Counsellors in the antenatal care clinic, who also document the marital status of the client, criticise the increase in pregnant women who are yet to be married. However, many of them claim to be in a stable relationship and refer to their lover as a husband as soon as the relationship becomes public and they wait for his or his family elder's reaction (Field notes Kroeker 22: 25/11/2008, Field notes Kroeker 23: 28/01/2009). If the boyfriend is caught off-guard and does not intend to enter into a serious relationship (perhaps due to other commitments) he would then deny having caused the pregnancy and thus refuse her marriage request (Field notes Kroeker 9: 07/04/2009; Kaufman et al. 2000; Field notes Kroeker: 17/06/2008). To accept having fathered a child forces him to engage in family negotiations on marriage or incur a fine for seduction (Field notes Kroeker 21: 16/04/2009; Field notes Kroeker: 15/04/2009; 03/2010; Kaufman et al. 2000: 23):

> When a woman is pregnant for the first time, the options for her and her family are marriage or compensation for seduction. (…) Without marriage she has found herself in a situation where she has been dependent on her father, her brothers and the men in her life for support (Griffiths 1990: 11-12).

A client in antenatal care explains her situation accordingly:

> She fell pregnant and asked her parents to approach her boyfriend's seniors in order to arrange a marriage. The boyfriend, however, re-

> fused to be the father of her child and refused to marry her (Field notes Kroeker: 09/06/2008).

If the boy still denies his involvement with the girl negotiations will be delayed until after the baby is born and the outward appearance of the child may suggest affiliation and he will then be told to pay the fine (Field notes Kroeker: 03/2010). Notwithstanding this, many girls planned their wedding.

Kaufman et al. (2000), Griffiths (1990), and Boehm (2006) assume that the link between marriage and reproduction is slowly but steadily eroding. My interviewees argued quite the opposite. Basotho women are well aware that marriage and reproduction should ideally be considered as one (Field notes Kroeker 02/02/2009; 21/05/2009). The ideal family in their opinion consists of a married couple who live together with their children and entertain a close bond with extended family members for support and care, although men enabling this were described as hard to find and difficult to keep hold of (Field notes Kroeker: 02/02/2009; 01/03/2009; 19/07/2010). Young women nevertheless dreamt of eventually getting married to a husband who would care for their social and financial wellbeing, as well as father their children and, generally, Basotho women associated child-bearing with marriage and marriage with child-bearing. A child born within wedlock will belong to the paternal clan, while outside of wedlock the mother's family would be responsible for catering for the mother-child-pair in a social and financial sense. Child-bearing, thus, is not only associated with marriage but also with arrangements for support and care despite individualised marriage initiations. The difference between a relationship as boyfriend and girlfriend and as a married couple can be found in the support they can expect to receive, as LeRobong explains: "With a boyfriend you are only two, but with a husband you are with the in-laws, with the whole family" (Field notes Kroeker 19: 24/05/2009). Boehm's examples likewise indicate that an interest in marriage is high, only that relationships do not last (Boehm 2006).

> MaSepetlele, aged 28, came to town to work as a maid and became pregnant in 2005 by her employer. She quit her employment and took up a job in the textile factory not only to support herself in town, but also her aunt who minded the baby in the village, and her unemployed sisters. MaSepetlele's experience of being the breadwinner, as well as financial hardship, have both played a role in MaSepetlele's delaying or refusing marriage and having a second child. Now, aged 31, she found a man that she loved and expected to get married to him, may-

> be, she considers, she should impregnate herself without his knowledge with the sperm contained in the used condom (Field notes Kroeker: 11/06/2008-2012).

For MaSepetlele as well as for Leshome, who had supported her siblings' schooling (Chapter 4.5), their own desire for children or marriage came second to supporting family members. Both supported relatives in the rural area who were not generating income but had to look after children. Moreover, MaSepetlele and Leshome postponed their plans and intended to wait for a more financially and socially stable situation, including a supportive partner and eventually marriage. As women are now usually more educated and better equipped to support themselves financially, good 'husband material' is not so easily found. While women may take their chances in choosing a partner and 'trapping him' by pregnancy, gender relations still do not allow them to ask for his hand in marriage (cf. Haram 2004: 224). However, having a child can bond partners if a liaison looks promising to the woman.

Pregnancy: Navigating Between Conflicting Demands

Despite rapid social upheaval and an ensuing crisis in family life, children play an important social role for the individual and for the family network as a whole. Thus, in a woman's biography, childbearing is still a vital part of her social standing since it enables her to be fully recognised as a mature member of society (Ashton 1952: 30-31; Romero-Daza & Himmelgreen 2004). The advent of HIV/AIDS, which has a devastating impact on family life, falls into that time of crisis. Now, biomedical health practitioners and public health policy makers are also demanding rapid change. International and national health authorities aim at preventing new HIV transmissions and their behavioural recommendations try to initiate change in the most intimate sphere of human life: relations between partners and relations between mother and child.

HIV transmissions need to be prevented from one partner to the other. Therefore, HIV-positive or discordant[1] couples are expected to refrain from unprotected sex, which means intercourse without using a condom. Moreover, vertical HIV transmissions from mother to child shall also be prevented by means of medical intervention. Physicians argue that a pregnancy puts additional physiological stress on the HIV-positive woman which affects her fragile state of health (USAID 2006; Field notes Kroeker: 08/2008) besides potentially harming her baby. Consequently, policy makers argue that medical intervention and counselling are crucial for preventing horizontal (from partner to partner) as well as vertical (from mother to child) transmissions of the virus. Moreover, further pregnancies of HIV-positive women shall generally be avoided (I will discuss this aspect in length in Chapter 8).

From a demographer's perspective, Lesotho already represents a rather low fertility rate per woman in comparison with the rest of Africa, which corresponds with low life expectancy and high rates of both maternal and infant mortality. As a likely result of women's participation in the formal labour sector they are having fewer children on average and the overall fertility rate is decreasing. While the 1976 Census recorded 5.4 children born per woman on average, in 2009 the number had dropped to 3.3 children (MoHSW et al. 2010: 47). Nevertheless, the Government intends to reduce the total fertility rate even further. Lesotho's Government implemented a National Population Policy and defined targets aimed at the provision of adequate family planning services: contraceptive use of about 70% to 75% in

---

[1] One partner is HIV-positive, the other partner is HIV-negative.

married couples, and achieving the replacement fertility rate by 2011 (Tuoane et al. 2004). Its purpose was also to reduce the adverse effects of high fertility in Lesotho, such as high rates of male unemployment, limited availability of women for the labour market due to maternal responsibilities, and high demand of social welfare due to sickness and absenteeism.

In this chapter I shall draw attention to the communication between family elders and young expectant mothers as well as to the communication between medical staff and their clients. Both lines of communication hinge on power relations and therefore fall under the heading of authoritative knowledge. In the first part of this chapter I intend to outline how family elders approach their women regarding teaching and learning about sexuality and child-bearing. Many of their recommendations also need to be embedded into the historical context. Manifold local norms only make sense within a larger reproductive cycle starting with marriage, which shall therefore be explained, even though only particular aspects of it are performed today. However, they are not easily changed and their relevance needs to be explained in order to understand people's decision-making.

In the second part I will also present arguments expectant women receive in biomedical antenatal care and counselling. It is here that pregnant women are also screened for HIV and in addition to general information about pregnancy, delivery and infant feeding, women receive advice on how to prevent mother-to-child transmission of the virus. In biomedical facilities, the aforementioned facilities of social control, clients are trained to contribute to national and international public health policies. Demographic development and reproductive health are seen by health policy makers as key issues in a country which is tremendously constrained by the HIV pandemic (Adair 2007: 1; Singh et al. 2009: 30; GoL 2009 (b): 73). However, the communication between medical staff and their clients is somewhat limited due to communicative and organisational reasons as well as their professional interests.

Personal, familial and national interests are not necessarily in line with biomedical recommendations and I will therefore discuss conflicting demands in this chapter. Thus, I argue that women find themselves torn between medical practitioners and family elders, whose recommendations sometimes complement each other but are more often than not at odds. Hence, I will illustrate their arguments, instruments and how expectant mothers are directly or indirectly influenced by them.

5.1 Parental Authority and Ancestral Discontent

Family elders, men and women, are responsible for training the younger generation of the same sex to live a socially and morally good life and to perform rituals in a way that would please the ancestors. Elder next-of-kin are more closely connected by age to those who passed into that stage of mere spiritual life, which authorises them to control and supervise what needs to be done by the living lineage members to prevent the affliction of ancestral discontent:

> The ancestors, those relatives who have died, are considered to be guardians of their living relatives, and to afford protection, good health, and prosperity. However, if they are not honored in the appropriate way, or if they are neglected, they are likely to cause misfortune and illness (Romero-Daza & Himmelgreen 2004: 958).

Misfortune such as natural disasters, famine or livestock diseases, and the root cause of these, needs to be investigated by a traditional healer. If misfortune and disease can be attributed to ancestral discontent, as established by a healer, family elders will consult with the healer and negotiate with the ancestors on the rituals that will be performed for them. Young people will be advised accordingly on how to take part in the rituals and how to prevent ancestral discontent and thereby assure family well-being:

> The ancestors, collectively, represent and uphold social order and harmony, which is embodied in or preserved by various laws, customs and rituals, and personal qualities. These are to be obeyed, honoured or cultivated by the individual, family or larger society. Consequently, one enjoyed a good life – well-being for oneself, the wider family and community, as well as one's crops and animals. Conversely, to disobey or disregard the ways of the ancestors was to bring misfortune and illness upon oneself, as well as upon the family, community, animals and crops (Gill 1993: 51).

The fear of retribution was a major factor when instilling correct behaviour in young people and, hence, the role which the ancestors play in the daily lives of the Basotho people cannot be underestimated (Rosenberg et al. 2004: 348)

The *structure*, which Turner defines as the hierarchical order of a society, authorises how rites need to be performed properly (Turner 2005: 96). Elders memorise and authorise whatever is normative in their paternal clan culture (Kaufman et al. 2000:18) and the provision of ritual applications, which are handed down from one generation to the next, affirm an individual's integrity and respect. In short, interaction between the living and the dead relates to highly politicised interactions across generations (Comaroff 1985: 57-60; Ngubane 1976).

Rites of passage, the rites that accompany stages of life and mark life-changing transitions, entail the most crucial prescriptions in order to facilitate a successful life trajectory. As Turner described, prescriptions in rites of passage always involve the living and the dead. Rituals performed within these rites of passage follow clear structures and ought be followed accurately and with special care, including directives on foods to be consumed by neophytes, dress codes and religious-magical applications, servility, seclusion, physical pain, symbolic death and palingenesis (Turner 2005: 94-95). Some procedures among the Basotho, in wedding ceremonies for instance, already make reference to the rites of integration of mother and child following confinement, thus, a ritual process can vary in terms of time. Likewise, similar ritual symbols connect the dress code of neophytes in initiation, women becoming brides and women becoming mothers. Similarly, pumpkin seeds are used in rites of birth, coming of age and passing away. Particular dishes appear at the time of initiation and again in wedding ceremonies, and to welcome a child into the family. Smearing the face or body with ochre *[letsoku]* takes place in acts of marriage, childbirth and initiation (Rosenberg et al. 2004: 119), depending on clan affiliation. Only in this context can the behaviour of pregnant women and their family members be understood.

Among the Basotho, rites however differ depending on totemic clan affiliation. While Basotho people share the same language, political and legal system and strongly regard themselves as one nation, we still find evidence of ethnic differences when it comes to rites of passage. Basotho as a term solely described all people who inhabited the area known today as Lesotho and the Northern Free State in South Africa (Gill 1993: 27) whereas the tribes dwelling in this region did not necessarily share one culture. Thus, cultural differences in the rites of passage can be traced back to totemic clans, which were united by Moshoeshoe I in the times of *Lifaqane*. However, it is difficult to determine how many clans currently reside in Lesotho. I counted about ten to 15 different clans and totems, although there may be many more, especially since I only conducted my research in one district of Lesotho which had a high turnover due to labour migration. Cultural differences in the clans' rites and customs become particularly apparent in relation to rites of the beginning and the end of life, coming of age, and extending families through offspring or marriage involving practices which are passed down from one generation to the next[2]. All of these transitions involve the living as well as "those who sleep" *(Ba-robetseng)*, hence the neophyte is found in a situation determined as "in-between life and death"[3]. This "in-between" status is, across all clans, a precarious time. "In between life and death" (Sesotho: *Pakeng tsa lefu le bophelo*), a common proverb in Sesotho, describes the polluted[4] condition of a person in an uncertain ritual state.

Ceremonies of birth, initiation, marriage and death visibly entail variations depending on totemic clan custom as they vertically connect the lineage, whereby fulfilment of the rite indicates lineage affiliation and security. Hence, for issues concerning women, particularly matters of reproductive health, the mother-in-law, under normal circumstances the eldest female household member, holds the position of a lecturer, supervisor, and preserver of clan culture in the way she learned it when joining the husband's family. It is an integral part of her position to direct younger members, supervise appropriate behaviour and sanction failures. As with everything entering the work sphere from outside, a young person who arrives will also be "domesticated" and socialised by elder female family members on their particular lineage culture. Misbehaviour of subordinates may reflect badly on the elder's ability to teach younger members and affect the reputation and credibility of the house. Disquieting sicknesses in the family may therefore be a stigma, since sickness can be an indicator of ancestral discontent resulting from disrespecting moral values (Kücholl 1985: 15).

---

[2] Affiliation to a totem clan also plays a political part in local chieftaincy. Only direct descendants of Moshoeshoe I in a primogenitoral order qualify as chiefs *[morena]*. Royal *Koena*-families as the political elite used to marry their daughters endogamously into *morena*-families from other villages, while other clans practised cousin marriage (parallel as well as cross cousin) across clan membership (cf. Comaroff 1985: 49-50).

[3] "They (the relatives, L.K.) said, when I am pregnant, I am between life and death. It is better to deliver in a health centre or clinic where there are nurses and doctors" (ATCBM Sekameng 12/2091: 8/07/2008); "I need to be near the doctors because I am between life and death. (…) Maseru Private Hospital (…) is the cleanest hospital in Lesotho and many doctors and all things that can be needed during delivery (are available). All lives are safe." (ATCBM Matelile 11/2113: 15/07/2008)

[4] Pollution relates to a condition in which the living and the dead are involved, mainly in rites of passage. These conditions are surrounded by taboos and rites. For pollution see Douglas 1994, Ngubane 1976, Gausset 2002, Gausset & Mogensen 1996.

5.1.1 Between Life and Death

Female family elders supervise an expectant mother and make sure all rites are performed correctly. The eldest woman in the house, either mother or mother-in-law will be responsible for bringing the whole reproductive cycle, including the rites, to a successful end, before the cycle begins once more with a subsequent conception. Bledsoe clarifies:

> The most important fact about a pregnancy is its precariousness. Throughout, a woman should exercise care about what she eats, lest the child be deformed or be unable to function properly. (...) A woman who is pregnant must be careful not only about her own family's taboos but those of her husband's family, since the child is of his line (Bledsoe 2002: 78-79).

The rites Basotho sub-clans perform for mother and child actually start much earlier than with the first conception[5]. If the right order of marriage followed by pregnancy was obeyed, rites which are performed in wedding ceremonies relate to those performed in pregnancy and to those welcoming the wife back into normal family life after her delivery. In accordance with "The Ritual Process" (Turner 2005) the wedding could be translated as integration of a woman into her new family, whereas she is separated from her husband in the second half of her pregnancy starting at the liminal, most critical phase. Delivery marks the chore of the liminal, hazardous situation. Across many cultures "birth is universally treated as a marked life crisis event" (Jordan & Davis-Floyd 1993: 3) and during pregnancy or even before preparations are made for this life change. Unlike any other phase in human life, the first childbirth determines a transition from one social and physiological condition to another (Labouvie 1999: 66) as delivery marks a doorway into adulthood for the mother and a doorway into social being for the child.

> Socially the birth of the first child (…) is the most important and is hedged about with strict rites and taboos which are relaxed for the birth of subsequent children. (…) The birth of her first child also changes the mother's status. As childbearing is regarded as the main function of women, its fulfilment gives her greater standing in the

---

[5] "During copulation, semen (…) which is the vital substance, is thrown into the woman's womb (…). According to some, the vital essence comes from the Spirit of God. These two elements, the man's semen or "blood" and the woman's blood are not necessarily of equal potency and the child will take after the parent whose "blood" is the stronger." (Ashton 1952: 26)

> community. Moreover, she is considered to have completed her family's side of the marriage contract, and the cattle (*moato*) which had been held over from her *bohali* should now be paid (Ashton 1952: 30-31).

Becoming a mother is associated with a physical, social and spiritual time of transition; a crucial and dangerous time of becoming a new self. In this phase it remains uncertain if the outcome of the transition will be successful. It needs to be noted that not only the mother but also the newborn finds itself "in between life and death" as it shifts from its ancestral state into a social sphere of life. As with old people, newborns are closely connected to the supernatural world and Hazam points out that the movements made by the infant are gestures while in conversation with the ancestors (Hazam 1983: 33). The transition of mother and child, thus, confinement, marks the centre of a highly dangerous and uncertain time for both parties. Hopefully, this uncertain phase is succeeded by a successful arrival in the new phase of life. In this third phase, the mother-child-pair is integrated into society, which is also actively involved in bringing the transition to a successful end. Hence, the community welcome mother and child in their new situation[6]. Mother, child and community interact during the whole process of social change, thus, they act in and within an acting environment.

Rites and practices are of course in flux and not monolithic, but instead undergo innovation. Certain aspects of the ritual process have remained over time while others have vanished. Nevertheless, rites are performed despite globalisation, migration, urbanisation and other cross-cultural processes which bring along new ideas and concepts. In order to contextualise the rites I will now clarify the importance of some aspects that are performed today after conception, during the delivery and in early child-care.

5.1.2 Entering Adult Life

As in many cultures around the world an initiation ceremony marks the start of adolescence which ends upon entering conjugal adult life. Initiation

[6] Normative ways of interaction organise the ritual and involve the neophyte, his peers and the community. Turner distinguishes between *communitas*, which is the vertical peer group of neophytes, and *structure*, which comprises the horizontal, hierarchical order of society. Neophytes are about to move up within this hierarchy (Turner 2005: 96).
By social environment I do not specify whether I mean the horizontal or the vertical social strata, in fact, I am not even convinced that pregnant women in Lesotho are part of a horizontal group of neophytes, whereas structure definitely exists.

schools in Lesotho, which are nowadays, if at all, only attended by boys although in decreasing numbers, teach mainly about manhood and womanhood, marital rights and duties, sex education and the boys are also circumcised there (Ashton 1952: 46-50; Erny 1981: 154-155; Krings-Ney & Kotanyi 2009).Other topics include Basotho history, as memorised in songs and poems, warfare, and political and social responsibilities (Rosenberg et al. 2004: 118-11).

At least in theory, official premarital meetings between boys and girls have followed Ashton's notion of the early 1950s which are limited to festive dancing ceremonies of those who have returned from initiation school and are therefore available for marriage. Among girls, dance moves, which imitate sexual intercourse and behaviour in childbirth, were part of a girl's training in initiation schools. Thus, sex education would rarely include verbal teaching or, rather, verbally used terms would only be shared among same-age and same-sex members of the initiation group. Thereafter, a sister, cousin or aunt may teach younger family members informally. Today, few Mosotho girls attend initiation school at all and therewith this mode of education has disappeared. Besides sex education in primary school, teenagers learn from peers. In contrast to today, in olden times, traditional division of labour and familial supervision was meant to limit meetings between boys and girls. Work chores separated them geographically in their daily routine and even brothers and sisters did not sleep in the same compound.

In spite of sexual desires food taboos were placed upon adolescent girls. While there were no such restrictions for boys, girls between the onset of puberty and marriage (as well as pregnant women) must not eat animal intestines and eggs. It was believed that maidens will mature more quickly as the consumption will stimulate the growth of secondary sexual characteristics and raise sexual awareness (Sechefo n.d.: 19; Field notes Kroeker 21: 05/12/2008). Eggs particularly resemble the amniotic sac and consumption may, according to the narrative, result in a miscarriage or burn the girl from inside (Field notes Kroeker MaThloni: 10/01/2011). A limited intake of proteins was therewith associated with the prevention of teenage pregnancies (Romero-Daza & Himmelgreen 2004: 962)[7].

Livestock is slaughtered in all feasts of transition, birth, initiation, marriage, death, and the elder men, as keepers of the reserves, allocate these. In all generational rites certain parts of the slaughtered livestock are reserved

---

[7] I will come back to Basotho pedagogy in Chapter 5.4.

for particular people within the family (Comaroff 1985: 101; Gill 1993: 47) and only married women are allowed to eat the delicacy. Thus, a special meal of intestines from her sheep *[koae]* or beast *[mala]* is the special dish for a bride during her wedding ceremony (Ashton 1952: 68). It should be noted that she will only consume intestines with her in-law's family and not when staying with her maternal family since this meal signifies conjugal togetherness (Field notes Kroeker 21: 05/12/2008; 22: 11/12/2008; Maqutu 2005: 153). However, in urban households and also in boarding schools this taboo is neglected in this day and age, although many girls have heard about it.

The ritual cycle of pregnancy, delivery and infant care starts ideally with the wedding negotiations which mark an end to her adolescent life.

5.1.3 From Wedding to Weaning

One can never be sure that the ideal way of doing things was ever followed in the past or in the present. However, the norms of correct behaviour serve as a gauge against which the actual behaviour is measured.

According to custom, a boy would have indicated to his parents that he is now ready to get married instead of bringing a girl into the house which, as mentioned earlier, tends to be the custom nowadays (see 4.8). The initiated boy would have neglected his work chores and thereby announced his interest in marriage by disobeying his father's directives. Not milking the cows was particularly seen as non-verbal indication of maturity since he neglects his family's wealth and therewith announces his intention to start his own household and care for his dependents as opposed to being a dependent himself. The prospective groom entrusted his interest in a certain girl to his maternal uncle, *malome*, (cf. Erny 1981: 47-50) as he would not speak to his parents directly about his interest in marriage. I will revisit this idea of involving a mediator rather than confronting his parents directly, which would be considered disrespectful. His stubborn behaviour was sufficient proof of his intention.

Mediators apply in many situations which entail some tension within the family. *Malome*, however, has the role of inquiring on the boy's behalf and finding out if a certain relationship with a girl was likely to be approved by the family's decision-makers. Thus, it depends somewhat on his sensitive and trustful approach to mediate between members of different sex and generations. Only if the results of his inquiry are encouraging, the boy may dare to abduct the girl and elope with her. Even if *chobeliso*, the elopement, looks like a patriarchal way of bringing a young non-consenting girl under a man's control, it is in fact a done deal. Only the time is for both the girl and the boy's parents a matter of surprise.

The couple will spend the night at the patrimonial homestead and the family elders will meet to report this incident and debate on a fine for abduction. What sounds again like a punishment for rape is already a crucial part of the marriage negotiations. If both families agree on a marriage, overpaying the fine for defloration turns the payment into a first instalment of bride wealth. *Malome* thus discusses with the family elders, who then order him to approach the girl's family to inquire and arrange the marriage particulars. If the uncle returns from the meeting with the girl's elders with a shaved head and without the livestock he took with him, it signified that the offer was acceptable and further negotiations about the bride wealth *[bohali* or *lebola]* are to follow. Up to now, most of the communication took place non-verbally but gestures, behaviour and signs were equally understood.

The following negotiations on the bride wealth depend on the status, wealth, power of the girl's family of origin, employment and access to resources, and last but not least whether the girl had unlawfully produced a child already (Griffiths 1990: 16). Her reputation will be known in the village anyhow and the boy's uncle will additionally have made his enquiries.

Even before the actual wedding ceremony takes place a second instalment will be paid and the girl will elope again with her designated husband and from thereon in the couple lawfully consummates their relationship. Bride wealth payments will, however, continue over subsequent years and in many cases bride wealth is never paid in full. The debts guarantee a long-term relationship between the families and further instalments can be claimed in times of hardship.

During the wedding ceremony some clan elders give the bride a new name which is composed of the, yet unborn, first child's name and a prefix meaning "mother of..." (Sechefo n.d.: 22; Rosenberg et al. 2004: 399). This practice directly links a bride to the offspring she is going to produce and to the groom's family, who choose the child's name with reference to an ancestor or a current event. The bride will be integrated into her husband's family with a new identity and a new social status. The payment of bride wealth, as well as the new first and last name given by her in-laws, confirms their willingness to accept the bride into their bosom. The mother-in-law, for her part, accepts her duty to socialise the girl and all offspring the couple is going to produce at her compound (Mvududu 2002: 29). The groom will make efforts to build his own *rondavel* hut for both he and his wife on his father's premises.

Even today the *malome* still plays an important role as an entrusted mediator in all kind of conflicts between parents and their son. However, nowadays, his role in marriage initiation is somewhat marginal, given that young couples start their love affairs without a match-maker, but the maternal uncle is still involved in matters of generational relevance, such as *lebola* payments. Moreover, as part of the wedding ceremony, a sheep will be slaughtered which remains, to date, an integral part of every ceremony involving the ancestors' blessing. According to Maqutu, performing the rite has even gained importance as although marriage arrangements have become more individualised in recent years, familial approval is still well regarded (Maqutu 2005: 153-154).

5.1.4 Preparing for Motherhood

About a year into the marriage the ritual cycle demands that a couple takes their relationship to the next level. The integrative process of a bride that started with marriage only ends with the integration of her first child, which, in addition, confirms the marriage and proves it to be fully functional. Producing offspring as the woman's part of the marital contract is an integral component of family politics and elders will take care of pregnant and birthing women and help with early infant care to make the transition a success.

Pregnancy in the first year after marriage is part of a woman's "normal" biography and even today the first child is often born one year into the marriage. If there are no signs of pregnancy by the time of the first wedding anniversary family members will doubt the couple's well-being. What starts with good advice or mockery may result in the return of the bride wealth and an annulment of the wedding, if the wife cannot fulfil familial expectations (Rosenberg et al. 2004: 45). This puts pressure on young women who may have planned otherwise due to economic, educational or medical reasons. She will have a hard time in the family compound and present-day women may want to find employment in town to escape familial pressure. As usual in rites of passage, the authority of the experienced community members is paired with the inferiority of the novice, here the young wife, and she may not dare to speak up against female family elders.

If she gets pregnant, she will have to accept her subordination to her mother-in-law who will supervise her behaviour according to the rules she learned when she entered the husband's family. Taboos apply as for all rites of passage, such as the prohibition of restricted places, time, particular people or groups of people, as well as prescriptions on particular clothing, naming, sexual abstinence, food and social contact among many other aspects (Turner 2005: 95, 102-105; Gausset 2002). Otherwise, until about the seventh month of pregnancy, a woman will fulfil her domestic duties at her in-laws' house as usual (Field notes Kroeker 19: 01/04/2009). Then, in the last trimester of the pregnancy, she enters a transitional phase which lasts about six months. Around that time a pregnant mother returns from her marital home to stay in her maternal homestead (Sechefo n.d.: 27; Ashton 1952: 27-28; Romero-Daza & Himmelgreen 2004: 960; Field notes Kroeker 11: 01/12/2008), which is celebrated with a rite involving members of both families. A traditional healer belonging to the *Motloung* clan (Elephant totem) recalls her rite of seclusion during pregnancy:

> MaFumane was brought back to her maternal house in her 8th month of pregnancy accompanied by a young girl from her in-law's kin who is not yet engaged in sexual activity. She handed a red *selapa*-shirt to her and brought a sheep to the expectant mother's maternal home. Upon arrival the sheep was slaughtered and the young girl delivered the meat to her in-laws (Field notes Kroeker: 17/03/2009).

In some clans, the same shirt, which protected the mother from mishap, will serve as the child's first item of clothing (Field notes Kroeker 29: 10/05/2011; 13: 29/04/2009; Field notes 17/03/2009), which protects her/him from cold, as well as spiritual harm and signals a person's situation of in between life and death. Another informant from the *Mofokeng* clan (Rabbit clan) recalls:

> Her in-laws sent a young boy, who was not yet initiated and a sheep to her maternal family in her 7th month. She followed the next day with a young girl who was carrying a bag that contained a pink *selapa*-shirt and a *Seshoeshoe*-dress. In her clan, the s*elapa* belongs to the family-in-law and will be used by all daughters-in-law when first-time pregnant and her shirt also has a slightly different style: It merely covers the shoulders and crosses over the breasts. When the baby is born it will sit or lie in the crossed part close to the breast to facilitate drinking and keeping it warm. Moreover, as part of her prescribed dress code she was smeared with ochre for few days, given a necklace and she had to walk barefoot until she delivered.

> After she had bathed thoroughly and the sheep was slaughtered she put on the prescribed features every day and only washed and dried the *selapa* briefly at night (Field notes Kroeker 19: 27/06/2008; 15/03/2009).

Ngubane believes a marginal phase starts with conception and ends when post-partum bleeding stops (Ngubane 1976: 275), which is about the time when the mother returns to the marital home with the baby. Until then the *selapa* shirt is worn and highlights the mother's precarious situation. I assume that the red or pink colour of the *selapa* common to all clans enables the mother's liminal state to be identified from afar and warns passers-by, and the same connotation applies to a child, which is wrapped in the mother's *selapa* gown. In analogy, the house of a newly delivered woman is also decorated with red flags which notify and warn strangers of a hazardous areal (Hazam 1983: 33; Gay 1980: 52-53). In some clans an expectant mother also changed her outward appearance with the use of ochre. Covering the body in *letsoku* also applied in a rite which neophytes undergo in initiation ceremonies. The application of ochre indicates therewith ritual pollution and Ngubane argues that in doing so a pregnant woman not only protects parts of her body which are in contact with the ordinary world, but she also protects the world from her polluted state, as she is more likely to transfer dangers to others (Ngubane 1976: 275). In my interpretation, ochre also relates to a change of households, since it applies in the return from initiation school, upon arrival in marriage, when arriving with child but not after the delivery which is when she must stay in the house as she is highly polluted (Field notes Kroeker 24: 27/03/2009)[8].

LeTselela among others reported that the hair was also shaved off during pregnancy as is also the case in funerals for very close relatives of the deceased and for children until weaned, when they cut teeth respectively. Shaving the hair is also associated with a state in between life and death which the outward appearance indicates. Also, and maybe equally important, the shorn hair must be stored carefully in a safe place so that no witches can find it and use this dead body part for sorcery.

Along the same lines of argumentation, a prescribed outward appearance helps to prevent harmful practices. A few clans, for instance, recom-

[8] Tselela, who married a Ndebele clan affiliate, was even smeared with ochre again when she arrived at her in-laws' house as a rite of re-integration after confinement, which seems unusual among Basotho totemic clans.

mend for their *bakhachane*, a term referring to an expectant mother, to walk barefoot. Presumably this rite is meant to prevent women from doing any work far from the house, which would mean in the areal marked as "the wild" periphery, and spiritually dangerous environment (Comaroff 1985: 55). From the time she arrives at her maternal home until she leaves it after giving birth, the *bakhachane* shall rest (but not sleep during the day!) and not walk too far (Field notes Kroeker: 08/04/2009). However, expectant women may furthermore not be allowed to leave the house for medical check-ups in hospital or health centres. Therefore, traditional practices which mark the outward appearance are sometimes referred to as harmful traditional practices, since they prevent biomedical intervention. A nurse in Mafeteng Hospital recognised likewise, that the hot tarmac in summertime may crack and injure the bare soles of the feet and thus prevent expectant women from coming to the health facility. Moreover, she complains, walking barefoot may cause sickness or aggravate the mother's health and is especially inadvisable for HIV-positive women since their immune system is already compromised (Field notes Kroeker: 08/04/2009). Nevertheless, the *bakhachane* who stay in the hospital's compound until they give birth frequently go for walks bare foot to keep themselves busy, as I observed. Interestingly, and quite in contrast to walking barefoot, during the counselling sessions in hospital the nurse advises pregnant women to wear shoes with heels. A counsellor explains how the mothers should practice their balance and stand upright and straight in order to carry their increasing weight (Field notes Kroeker: 24/06/2008), although medical staff do not generally interfere with the ritual dress code. It is more common for medical staff to complain about the use of traditional medication in general and with pregnant women in particular.

Powerful objects such as talismans and bracelets containing medicine, regular baths with medicine, the burning of incense in the room where the mother and the child sleep, and also the use of nutritive techniques like special food and medicine protect mother and child from harm (Yovsi 2003: 70-75). The substances are used ritually in both a pharmaceutical and symbolical way (Turner 2005: 31) and often apply in various rites of passage. Some clans in Lesotho provide their expectant mothers with a necklace containing seeds, animal parts or powdered substances, which are all meant to safeguard against malevolent powers. Hazam assumes that Basotho healers tend to utilise animal parts in preventive health care as a means to balance metaphysical disorders, whereas minerals and plants apply in curative medicine

(Hazam 1983: 130, 139). This is due to the power of the pharmaceutical ingredient, as Ashton explains:

> The animal world is superior to the vegetable or mineral world, and man is superior to animals; therefore man is the greatest thing in the world. Consequently, medicines containing human flesh and blood will be superior to those which do not, and so it is essential that the strongest medicines should contain such ingredients (Ashton 1952: 307).

Human hair or other body parts, for instance, can therefore make strong medicine for the good but are used mostly for evil purposes. For expectant mothers, who generally need protective charms, plant or animal parts will suffice. However, since they are in a sensitive state in between life and death, they are also more likely to be affected by witchcraft which may harm them intentionally or accidentally. Therefore, pregnant women must be extremely careful about their finger nail clippings, hair trimmings, and excrement and take care to ensure that no one can get their hands on such items and gain power.

Expectant women do not know what the necklaces contain or what they indicate but refer to "our cultural issues" (Field notes Kroeker: 13/06/2008). The necklaces are provided by the paternal clan members according to their totemic clan rites, and Ashton explains:

> She may also wear a necklace of ostrich eggshell, threaded with her husband's clan beads, together with pumpkin seeds and a wildcat's claw or tail tip. This rite should bring luck and strength and marks the beginning of her seclusion. (…) The wildcat tail is associated by the Tlokoa with their totem. The pumpkin seeds are associated with birth and new life and are used in mortuary rites (Ashton 1952: 28).

Indeed pumpkin or other seeds used to be laid in a dead person's hand to allow new cultivation and prosperity (Sechefo n.d.: XX). According to clan custom, corpses will be buried holding seeds in the palms of their hands to start cultivation wherever the person rises again from the dead, another reference to a condition of "in-between life and death" (Ngubane 1976: 274; ATCBM Matelile 11/2113 15/07/2008). Meanwhile a necklace containing parts of ostrich eggs rather relates directly to the delivery, in particular to the amniotic sac referred to by Basotho mothers and counsellors alike as "egg". A vendor of traditional pharmaceuticals mentioned a traditional medication given to pregnant women which includes powdered ostrich eggshell and explained: "It is meant to help to have a smooth birth, it is given to pregnant women to allow the fruit to pass easily" (Field notes Kroeker: 19/06/2008).

Despite different approaches to assuring the well-being of the living, the dead and the unborn, applications are always handed down from the paternal grandmother for the mother and child to wear. Others use the same necklace time and again, which will be worn by all children of one mother. In either case, according to my interpretation, the necklace symbolises a bond between them (Field notes Kroeker 29: 18/11/2008; 16/01/2009). The child ends its transition either with weaning when the necklace will also be removed or, on the other hand, through signs of its maturity (Field notes Kroeker: 10/06/2008). Besides these material applications which are meant to prevent mother and child from harm, a healer may be involved to check for already present afflictions with evil powers, as this informant (I) explained to me (L):

> I: When I arrived at my mother's house, she asked, what I was doing to protect the child. I answered "Nothing". So my mother brought me to a *ngaka* to prepare *pitsa* for me.
>
> L: What did the doctor say to you when you have been there?
>
> I: He was throwing things on the floor and I was supposed to touch them. He didn't find anything evil against me. Then he put a mirror on my tummy and told me that I was in the eighth month of pregnancy. He said, although he didn't find anything bad, I should drink *pitsa*. He then gave me a drink he had cooked before and I drank it (Field notes Kroeker: 27/06/2008).

Ashton assumes that this *pitsa,* a herbal pharmaceutical drink, has the effect of turning the child into the right position "and ensure[s] an easy delivery" (Ashton 1952: 28). Conversely, I disagree with this explanation. From my observations, women receive a general *pitsa* starting with the last trimester which protects the child from any harm the mother may come upon accidentally, by negligence of preventive behaviours or by the force of others. Particularly doors, gates and windows are dangerous places. Powerful substances used either to prevent or cause witchcraft for example are usually applied at a door post or near a window and people in a sensitive condition should not expose themselves to that since the magical substances may have unintended side effects (Field notes 19: 12/07/2009). For example, LeRobong's child passed away suddenly at the age of six weeks without any signs of sickness. A counsellor attributed this to a Sesotho disease called *Matlala*, which is caused by a strong substance that affected the baby unintentionally. It can kill a person very quickly and with no visible symptoms. The substance can be applied at the front door to someone's house or to some person (Field notes Kroeker: 12/07/2009; MaThloni: 12/09/2009). For people who are extremely sensitive to health hazards, such as people in a liminal, polluted state (cf. Ngubane 1976), the substances may affect them instantly. If the pregnant mother lingers in the proximity of the door or window, so the narrative says, the baby may also hesitate at the "door" during delivery and not pass easily.

To assure a fast delivery a second *pitsa* containing different ingredients than the first one is applied as a routine intervention during labour, which, contrasting with Ashton's notion, strengthens labour pains. Ashton (1952: 28) and Peltzer et al. (2009 (a)) ignore the idea that traditional medication facilitates a short but strong, rather than an easy, less painful, phase of labour. According to my information, a bad delivery is characterised as a long phase of labour lasting several hours or even days. Prolongation may be a consequence of spiritual harm, and subsequently long or otherwise abnormal delivery refers to witchcraft afflictions.

5.1.5 Can the Ritual Cycle be Closed?

A ritual which takes place upon the mother's return to her marital homestead three to four months after confinement very much resembles her wedding ritual. The same dish of sheep intestines is served again in a ceremony which welcomes mother and child following seclusion for confinement. The ceremony confirms a lawful wedding, which was approved by the couple's ability to bear children, which thus confirms a successful amalgamation of two families and assures continuity of the patrilineage.

However, every ritual process entails uncertainty about whether it will succeed or fail. Despite precautions, misfortune may come upon the individual or the community. While men are afflicted with agnatic rivalry or sorcery if protective rites were not adequately fulfilled, women more often suffer from disruptions in their reproductive health (Ashton 1952: 26-27; Comaroff 1980). A fatal birth, for instance, captures what "in between life and death" implies: insecurity and potential harm of mother or child. Infant or maternal death while the mother stays in her paternal home therefore often relates to ancestral discontent and an incomplete fulfilment of rites. Secondly, witchcraft affliction, which may harm mother or child in that marginal phase of life, may also be related to inadequate or incomplete protection.

Moreover, in contrast to the "normal" biography of a woman becoming a mother, childlessness suggests some disorder in conjugal relations. The process which started with marriage cannot be concluded by integrating mother and child as proof of the successful amalgamation of spouses. Expectations and pressure will increase if a couple remains childless for a long time and a marriage may be considered unsuccessful unless conception proves fulfilment of marital obligations. Not having children would lead to a stigma surrounding the cause of this unfavourable situation. Eventually, a married but childless woman might be labelled as barren (*[nyopa]*) and infertility can be a cause for divorce (Ashton 1952: 26-27; Mvududu 2002: 14-16; Romero-Daza & Himmelgreen 2004: 960). My informant (M) explains:

> L.: Is it a stigma for women not to have children?
>
> M: Very, very much so. When they don't have children they are called *nyopa*, unmarried women are called *lefetoa*. Most women want to have children and also the social pressure forces them to have a child. When they are married you have to have some children (Field notes Kroeker: 19/06/2008).

In the absence of children a couple may be pitied for this unfortunate situation and the reason for it assumed to lie in some disorder of a physical, mental or spiritual nature. If the relationship remains childless next-of-kin may start to question the success of the match. No offspring would break the cyclic notion of life and death due to the close interlinkage of the beginning and end of life: "The cycle can only be broken by infertility of parents or the absence of children within the family" (Yovsi 2003: 70-75; cf. Turner 2005: 18-19, 59-60) which will involve negotiations of family elders. Robeli's family also interfered with her childless marriage, which had caused trouble.

> Robeli got married by the age of 20 in 2004. After the marriage remained childless for three years the husband started having an extramarital affair and his girlfriend fell pregnant. Robeli was presumed to be the cause of the childlessness while Robeli suspected him of being sterile. She assumed so since the husband was imprisoned when his girlfriend's conception must have happened. However, the husband accepted paternity and Robeli's father took Robeli home in 2007. Soon thereafter she entered a new marriage in April 2008 and presented herself being pregnant in antenatal care already in August (Field notes Kroeker 8: 14/11/2008).

While sexuality became a personal matter, offspring remained a crucial part of family and generational well-being. In order to avoid the pressure put upon women to bear children, an informant explains with tongue in cheek: "In-laws want to see children after marriage. If my brother wants to marry today, I would recommend that he marries a women that has a child already as proof that she is fertile and can get more children" (Field notes Kroeker Violet: 19/06/2008). Joking, she assumes that the expectations on the bride would be lower (cf. Maqutu 2005: 36). A counsellor adds: "the reason for a childless relationship would be considered on the man's part, which no one would dare to utter." (Field notes Kroeker Mathloni: 19/06/2008).

5.1.6 Are Ancestors Stronger than Pills?

Mafeteng District comprises 19 health facilities, including the district hospital and about 800 registered traditional healers which form the health care system. Besides the number of local healers (*ngaka, mathuela* or *sangoma*) and their representational body at the Ministry of Health and Social Welfare in Maseru, they receive minor recognition in the health hierarchy, which is dominated by the hegemony of western based biomedicine. In 1993 government employees stated:

> The lowest level of the health system is the widely spread number of Village Health Workers, Traditional birth attendants and Traditional Healers. They should be the backbone of the health system (Mafeteng Government Hospital 1993).

In a hierarchical order the sick person firstly approaches a lay person and is then referred to health institutions on a local, district and national level. Family, friends and neighbours provide advice on curative rituals and treatment for common diseases. Homespun remedies are known and many villagers grow some therapeutic herbs in their gardens and help out with their knowledge on preparation and dosage. The Basotho therewith treat "minor" complaints with self-medication (Hall & Malahlela 1989: 2).

The pyramid of the health care system, which also equivocates referral structures as foreseen by the health authorities, therewith included:

The sick person
↓
family / friends / neighbours
↓
800 traditional healers in Mafeteng District
↓
1 or 2 village health workers
↓
19 health centres in Mafeteng District
↓
10 district hospitals
↓
1 referral hospital

Pyramid of the health care system (Mafeteng Government Hospital 1993)

This pyramid has changed in so far as healers are no longer included. Notwithstanding this, health facilities of the biomedical or traditional school tend to be approached after first attempts at treating a disorder with these common means and local knowledge have failed. While biomedical facilities provide tools, a traditional practitioner's capital is trust, access to supernatural beings and personal relations with the family members of their community. In her ethnographic analysis of Lesotho's health care system, Kücholl states that ancestors "are ill-disposed beings who are mightier than the average human being and who are stronger than pills and infections" (Kücholl 1985: 39-40). This would suggest that traditional medicine should be higher in the health hierarchy than illustrated in the health pyramid diagram.

A family may approach one and the same healer over a long period of time, who then knows about family medical histories and social affairs among the client's next-of-kin. Moreover a healer combines a psychological and religious way of explaining misfortune in the family with technical and pharmaceutical interventions to re-install well-being (Kücholl 1985: 1, 39-40; Field notes Kroeker: 03/2007; 06/2008) and is therefore approached time and time again for many purposes. In fact, Basotho healers follow various traditional schools of healing depending on their training (Romero-Daza & Himmelgreen 2004: 959) and some specialise in the treatment of particular ailments. Those who have also undergone biomedical training even combine curative methods.

Traditional healers may in the case of a non-biological cause of disease, such as ancestral discontent or witchcraft afflictions, tackle the latter and provide religious explanations, rather than treating the symptoms. In contrast, biomedical practitioners mostly attempt to cure signs and symptoms of the affliction. Kleinman (2003) and Whyte (1997) thus call the biomedical approach symptomatic in contrast to the traditional healer's explanatory approach. Biomedical health facilities can consequently be considered defective because a patient is merely cured of a disease, which may reoccur since the non-biological, supernatural cause was not dealt with by nurses and doctors. Hence, the co-existence of both medical schools is validated and they are used alternatively or complementarily rather than in the order suggested in the health pyramid. Today, despite the continuous existence of around 800 registered healers, biomedical staff members have little or no respect for traditional healers and they are not considered as part of the health hierarchy. Counsellors affirm that clan-related rites remain in place and clients wish to follow them fully or partly whereas even local nurses state that "traditional things" no longer exist because "people are nowadays enlightened and modern". Counsellors rather assume that nurses deny that rites are in place and explain "maybe staff do not know about [customs] anymore or deny it" (Field notes Kroeker MaThloni: 19/06/2008; Violet: 19/06/2008; cf. Rompel 2006). Biomedical practitioners ignored spiritual, divine or witchcraft causes and condemned traditional healers and their medication (Field notes Kroeker: 21/01/2009). Instead they insinuated that biomedicine shall replace the body of traditional healing. Ngubane's assumption seems to hold true for the local context of Mafeteng just as elsewhere in Africa:

> All this contrasts sharply with the habitual disposition of the Western-type health agencies to look down on practically all indigenous methods of healing – not surprisingly, since the training provided in medical schools disregards the existence of African methods of cure. African patients, in contrast, see these as an alternative or as providing a complementary contribution to a sensible combination of methods for curing a given trouble (Ngubane 1992: 369).

In the 1970s Basotho healers were invited for training activities with the hospital staff. However, these activities apparently disappeared despite the healers' representation in the Ministry of Health as well as on a district and local level. To date, medical staff members are unaware that the healers have an association with a head office at the district administration. During the Ministry's annual meeting in Maseru in 2008 the National Association of Traditional Healers was represented in a fringe meeting. Regardless of the fact that traditional healers represent the only professional health facility in many villages, the representatives at that meeting were told to refer patients to rural health centres from which they may then be referred to the district hospitals in a hierarchical order. In the healers' eyes ignorance about their procedures and curative methods is blamed on biomedical practitioners and they view their profession as complementary to the biomedical school.

Last but not least, the health economy is also partly responsible for undermining traditional health professionals. The large and well-funded biomedical network achieves legitimacy through external donor organisations and international enmeshments. This also includes non-governmental organisations which are supporting heavily subsidised biomedical health institutions. Due to economic considerations, amongst others, traditional healers can therefore not compete with a governmental health infrastructure (Kücholl 1985: 32). However, healers would like to be seen as complementary health professionals, as Hazam stated in 1983:

> In some instances traditional Healers have stressed the dichotomy of Western and non-western spheres of healing. While these healers admit the adequacy, and sometimes the superiority, of cosmopolitan doctors in treating certain diseases such as measles, typhoid, or flu, they also maintain that there are areas of illness, which can be treated effectively only by traditional healers. Illnesses placed in this category generally include those attributed to witchcraft or ancestral intervention (Hazam 1983: 144).

In short, healers are responsible for a broad notion of health, which is also confirmed by the local terminology. The Sesotho term *bophelo* can be translated as both health and life and only from the context can the different meanings be determined, whereas in many cases there is simply no difference. Health is life and life is health and likewise disease and death has the same word stem *-lefu*. Therefore, a local notion of *bophelo* is generally inclusive and treated by *ngaka*, *sangoma* or *mathuela*, as outlined by Romero-Daza & Himmelgreen:

> The role of the traditional healers often extends beyond the treatment of physical and mental disorders, and covers the solution of interpersonal difficulties that may affect the harmony among family or village members. This role fits well with the overall Sotho conceptualization of "health" as a balance among physical, psychological, social, and spiritual aspects of life (Romero-Daza & Himmelgreen 2004: 959).

Therefore, healers in Lesotho, many of whom are trained in the Zulu school of healing, also do not necessarily restrict patients to one school of treatment or the other. Healers know that hospital staff members always insist on choosing one school of treatment, while healers focus on the different types of diseases and the fact that some of these cannot be treated by biomedicine. Therefore the patients should go to one facility for a certain disease and to the healer for another (cf. Ngubane 1992). Nne, being a client of both biomedical and traditional care, explained that the person whom a patient consults very much depends on the cause of an ailment:

> Nne is convinced that some diseases need to be attended by a traditional healer, while for others she may see a doctor in hospital. Her family elders will help her to investigate on the cause of the disease and advise her which doctor she will need to approach. If a treatment fails she reconsiders a second school of health and healing until she finds relief. Usually, she searches for the cause of her condition by herself and if she assumes malevolent powers to be involved a biomedical doctor may be able to treat only her condition but not the cause and the condition may be recurrent. Sometimes, if the traditional treatment does not help, Nne in addition visits her pastor who will treat her with blessed water, counsel her with proverbs from the Bible, and pray for the sick with the congregation. The pastor may also see "in the water" what someone is suffering from[9]. One time she also got a candle to light during the night and it helped her to get relief from the pains she had (Field notes Kroeker 4: 17/04/2009).

Patients in biomedical facilities usually deny having any history of traditional medicine. Various tools available to staff in biomedical "institutions of social control" allow them, however, to detect some traditional practices and thereby to exercise their social control. Therefore, patients have to weigh up their various interests. That being the case, it seems to depend on the person asked as to whether ancestors or pills are stronger. Biomedical staff argues against this idea and for the patients it is a matter of belief.

---

[9] Interestingly, traditional healers use the same method of divination, however, they arrive at different ways of treating pathological findings.

5.2 Teaching and Learning about Pregnancy

The traditional health system is indeed an essential part of the care for expectant women besides biomedical antenatal care. Pregnancy can be characterised as a special, but somewhat ordinary (in contrast to pathological) condition and clients considered counselling and medical check-ups as a crucial part of pregnancy. Antenatal care shall be defined, for the purposes of this study, as all procedures expectant women receive to monitor well-being in this crucial period in life.

In Lesotho, surprisingly high numbers of pregnant women attend antenatal care (ANC) in a biomedical health facility. 90% of expectant women attend an antenatal clinic at least once and 60% attend at least four times (MoHSW 2010: 105), which is the frequency that is recommended by government guidelines. Seeking information, first-time mothers are likely to come more often, while *multigravida* do not frequent pre-natal examinations or at least not as often. Younger women particularly seemed to appreciate education on biomedical issues and examinations to verify mother and child's well-being and it is not surprising that most women were between 20 and 30 years of age at the time they visited an antenatal care unit in Mafeteng's Hospital and clinics (Field notes Kroeker: 21/10/2008)[10]. A young pregnant woman in one of the rural health centres explained that she came in order "to be informed about how pregnant women should care for themselves". Therewith, mothers may view an antenatal clinic to be a school on pregnancy; an institution for learning about one's health condition which was the purpose of initiation schools in earlier times. Nonetheless, the antenatal care, which elder female family members or traditional birth attendants offered during pregnancy, was equally important.

Some women visited the clinic during their first trimester while the majority started during their 5th to 6th month of gestation. This late appearance in an antenatal clinic is due to the type of contraception many Basotho women prefer. Since the most commonly used hormonal injections suppress ovulation and therewith menstruation, a missed period cannot be taken as indication of pregnancy. Therewith many women consult the doctor for a pregnancy test due to morning sickness or when they felt the baby's first movements in the second trimester.

---

[10] The study, however, was not able to clarify whether older women are no longer attending ANC or whether they are no longer falling pregnant either by choice or because of their precarious health condition.

The standard protocol of antenatal care in governmental units offers the following examinations:

- General clinical and nutritional assessment,
- Pregnancy test,
- HIV rapid test and CD4 test for HIV-positive women,
- Hepatitis B and Hepatitis C serology,
- Urine is tested for urinary tract infection and protein,
- Weight is taken,
- Blood is taken for syphilis screening (VDRL) and anaemia test (Hb),
- Tetanus vaccination (TT),
- Physical examination for obstetric assessment (blood pressure, uterine growth and foetal well-being, pelvic exam including pap smear),
- Medical, obstetric, and family history is taken for the obstetric record, which includes symptoms of congenital infections,
- Drug history and the use of traditional medication, alcohol or cigarettes,
- Group counselling,
- One-to-one counselling for HIV-positive women (Field notes Kroeker: 27/01/2009; cf. GoL 2009: 24-25).

Ultrasound scans are not part of the protocol for government health centres but private doctors who are believed to provide higher quality services do offer them. Women who were able to pay for further examinations with a private doctor drove to Maseru for a check-up. Nevertheless, even those women also visited the government health centre in Mafeteng since the antenatal clinic usually served as a meeting point for young expectant women and a forum for discussing medical advice.

Depending on the time of year the number of clients in the antenatal clinic in Mafeteng Government Hospital varied between three and up to thirty women a day (Field notes Kroeker: 03/06/2008). Numbers of pregnant women were usually higher in the months between August and November. Many had conceived during the festive period when workers returned home to their families. From June to July, fewer women attended the clinic due to the harsh winter season which made it impossible to find transport to the health centres from some of the more remote areas. Others considered it too cold to spend the day waiting in a draughty hospital corridor. For those who arrived, however, the atmosphere was usually an enjoyable hustle and bustle and it was an arena of formal and informal, verbal and non-verbal interaction:

> Medical staff, counsellors as well as nurses of the antenatal unit, welcome the clients with a prayer followed by the "morning talk" in the corridor of the mother and child ward where the steps to be followed by the expectant women are explained. The mothers are waiting in the corridor until they are called into the nurse's examination room according to a waiting list and a physical examination takes place. Women are seated according to their time of arrival and the counsellors organise who needs to go next for check-up, counselling session and HIV-testing. In the counselling room the woman's weight is taken and each client receives a tub for urine, also blood pressure is taken and blood drawn for various tests. Women who have yet to receive a tetanus vaccine or who did not complete the advisable series of five shots will now receive injections. With a counsellor a blood smear reveals syphilis and anaemia results, thereafter, clients attend a health presentation and the HIV-negative mothers are released, while the HIV-positive mothers are referred to a one-to-one counselling session. Expectant mothers must carry a booklet called "Obstetric Record" as well as their health booklet "Bukana ea Bophelo" through all the stations and the results are signed in by the respective person. The communication mostly takes place via the obstetric record and the questionnaires it contains. Professional conversations between clients and nurses are rather limited, while there is more personal interaction between counsellors and pregnant women (Field notes Kroeker: 06/11/2008; 27/01/2009).

Young women did not usually mind long waiting times in the hospital corridors but spent their time exchanging with other women or listening to the general counselling. In fact, the hall provided a nutrient medium for a vivid exchange of experienced and first-time mothers on all aspects of pregnancy, delivery and mother-child-care and the crowd of waiting women took a dynamic part in discussions on the physical, psychological, spiritual and social well-being of mother and child and the various ways to achieve it. Consequently, biomedical antenatal care, community interaction and familial care must be considered complementary sources of information.

5.3 Female Clients in Biomedical Care

Women are typically those responsible for caring for sick and bedridden relatives at home; therefore, they are socially affected by disease to a larger extent than men (cf. Whyte 2005; Nyanguru 2005). As home-based caregivers women also frequently accompany sick relatives and are familiar with biomedical health facilities (Kücholl 1985: 32; Field notes Kroeker: 03/2007). In contrast, the notion of men being physically strong and valiant prevents them from approaching a facility where they may be considered sickly, weak and in need of care. Females, however, outnumbered men in the waiting rooms of all departments and receive health information through counselling sessions and personal exchanges with other patients and caretakers. Perhaps, due to their high engagement in health care women are also more aware of reproductive health constraints and accept HIV testing and counselling more easily than men.

From a cultural perspective, some topics of reproductive health must only be discussed with people of same sex or age, which may also prevent men from approaching a female doctor or nurse. In the antenatal clinic all the staff members were female which eased the communication between clients and staff on reproductive matters. Besides counselling on pregnancy, delivery and early infant-care other common health topics are likewise discussed since female clients are considered the gatekeepers to health, particularly reproductive health, at home (Booth 2004: 39, 41; Hall & Malahleha 1989: 10). The promotion of reproductive health by predominantly female medical staff speaking to women on their individual health needs is a mechanism which has been utilised by biomedical policies, despite the fact that women are carers in their families but not necessarily decision-makers in sexual matters. Nevertheless, women are in many cases if not infected themselves than at least affected by HIV-positive members of their household.

In 2007, the high HIV prevalence of 23% (CIA The World Factbook) affected the most (re-)productive segment of society, scourged reproductive health and presented a multitude of social challenges, high above other public health concerns.

After the first case of HIV was detected in Lesotho in 1986 a national commission was founded the following year to coordinate activities for preventing and controlling the epidemic. In the mid-nineties the Lesotho Government already recognised HIV and AIDS as not only a threat to public health but also as a general affliction of development in all sectors. The Ministry of Health and Social Welfare (MoHSW) of Lesotho had argued that the

HIV/AIDS pandemic had reached devastating proportions among the population, with one in four Basotho people already infected with the virus and by the year 2000 the Lesotho Government declared HIV/AIDS a national disaster (GoL 2007: 1) at a time when leading South African politicians were still in denial about the crisis in their own country (van Rijn 2006)[11]. In 2000 the MoHSW implemented an ambitious plan of prevention, treatment, testing and care and forthcoming national strategic plans to combat the spread of HIV thereafter which particularly focussed on the prevention of mother-to-child HIV transmissions. Overall, policy makers were eager to contain new HIV transmissions since it was expected that "there will be a rapid down turn in life expectancy as more people in the productive age group are infected by the HIV/AIDS virus and will eventually die. It will have a negative effect on the dependency ratio and the general life expectancy in the nation" (GoL 2000: 2). Moreover, the Ministry outlined that if the infected person is the main income generator a lack of revenue will affect the family as a whole. More generally, HIV/AIDS will have a negative impact on the quantity and quality of the labour force in the country causing negative economic growth (GoL 2000: 10-11). The way forward was consequently formulated following the preamble "The vision of the Lesotho National AIDS Programme (LNAP) is an HIV/AIDS free society" (GoL 2000: 14). At that time, many women were already family breadwinners and therefore additionally challenged in their role of caretakers for the sick. It was therefore imperative to prioritise women's health to enable them to support their family.

It was only from 2003 onwards that the World Health Organization (WHO) was able to offer a drug to prevent the transmission of the HI-Virus from mother to child in resource-constrained settings such as Lesotho. Medical trials had proven the effectiveness of a couple of drugs at preventing a transmission of the virus during labour and breastfeeding and the World Health Organization promoted one of them, the drug Nevirapine (NVR), based on safety, cost-effectiveness and its simple administration (WHO 2003). Women who agreed to have a HIV test during antenatal care were offered further counselling on HIV prevention. Those testing HIV-positive received medication from their 28th week of gestation onwards and were

[11] In contrast to South African politicians, senior politicians and representatives such as His Majesty King Letsie III, his wife, Queen Karabo, as well as the Prime Minister, Pakalita Mosisili, and his wife, First Lady Mathato, were the first ones to be tested in a nationwide testing campaign. Both Queen Karabo and the Prime Minister's wife were actively involved in initiating partnerships with bilateral donors and on a NGO level.

advised to deliver in a health facility where they would receive further treatment during labour and delivery. Furthermore, safe infant feeding practices were explained in the counselling sessions and women were advised to enrol in the family planning programme after giving birth to the baby.

This whole procedure including pharmaceutical intervention as well as examinations and counselling sessions was outlined in Lesotho's medical guidelines as of 2004. A policy was implemented and the 2004 guidelines on PMTCT were revised in 2009. In 2007 as well as 2011 smaller changes in the global policy were published in the form of an adapted national policy resulting from changes announced by the WHO.

The revisions to the 2004 guidelines signalled significant changes in women's rights to informed consent to HIV testing. While in the 2004 PMTCT guidelines HIV tests were advisable but needed written consent, the 2009 PMTCT guidelines no longer required the written consent of the expectant mother[12] (GoL 2009 (a): 8, 14). Therewith, screening for HIV became one of the standard procedures of antenatal care following an opt-out strategy (ARASA & HRW 2008: 39). Although this change in guidelines carried ethical concerns, it led to the envisaged result: almost everybody who underwent antenatal check-ups in a health facility was tested for HIV. In 2005, around 50% of the expectant mothers had agreed to be tested voluntarily for HIV in antenatal care and by 2009 96% were being tested (MoHSW & NAS 2009: 2, 17; GoL 2009 (b): 2). Medical personnel were encouraged to counsel clients to the point where they would agree to testing and referral (Field notes Kroeker: 06/2008) since women were seen as having a pivotal role in combating the spread of the disease due to their obligations in caring for the sick and in child-bearing.

Without medical intervention about one quarter of the babies born to HIV-infected mothers also carried the virus[13]. With the newly established PMTCT programme this figure was reduced to around 1-2% of babies contracting the disease (Cooper et al. 2002; Tonwe-Gold et al. 2007). Hence, on

---

[12] In Tanzania, many people living with the virus undergo testing while they are admitted to hospital, as Dilger states. The patient's consent was not obtained (Dilger 2010: 102-124). Whyte and colleagues also describe that in "Voluntary Counselling and Testing" – known as VCT – "voluntary" is being replaced with "HIV" ("HIV-testing and counselling") (Whyte et al. 2010: 80-101).

[13] MoHSW and GoL note "Without ARV intervention about 25-35% of HIV infected pregnant mothers can pass HIV infection to their babies" (HIV Testing and Counselling (HTC) training course, May 2004: 23)

an international level the WHO likewise argues in favour of early HIV testing in pregnant women. The target of PMTCT provision according to the Millennium Development Goals was 80% by 2011. This figure was already achieved in Mafeteng Government Hospital in 2008 where 84.4% coverage was reached when HIV testing was not yet a standard test (Field notes Kroeker: 23/06/2008)[14]. The following reasons were identified by the World Health Organization (WHO) for early HIV testing during pregnancy:

- Identifying HIV infection in pregnancy may enable women to access antiretroviral prophylaxis to reduce MTCT of HIV.
- Knowing a women's HIV status would allow counselling about feeding options.
- Knowledge of the HIV status enables women to make informed choices about future pregnancies and future fertility.
- In early pregnancy a termination may be offered to HIV-positive women where abortion is legal.
- A woman who knows about her HIV infection may seek early appropriate medical care for opportunistic infections and approach NGOs for ongoing HIV care and psychosocial support. HIV-positive women can be helped to adopt a positive lifestyle.
- Women who have had a positive test outcome may be able to share the test result with their partner and encourage counselling and testing.

Disadvantages of HIV testing in antenatal care as recognised by the WHO include:

- HIV testing may create disharmony in the family and an increased risk of violence against and abandonment of HIV-positive women.
- Stigma by community and health workers towards HIV-positive women.
- Frustration among health workers and clients if there are no resources to reduce the risk of transmission of the virus to the child.
- Additional workload and increased stress for health workers in the maternity service.

---

[14] The figures I quote stem from Mafeteng Government Hospital records from March to May 2008. 212 expectant mothers attended antenatal care for the first time in this three-month period. 179 accepted voluntary testing and counselling, which equals a rate of 84.4%.

- Increased need for privacy and space in a busy health facility (WHO 2001: 3-5).

The prevalence of women in Lesotho testing positive in antenatal care has plateaued in recent years, although at a high level of around 25%. Highest indications are found in the group of 30-34 years old with 40.2% (GoL 2009 (a): 1). Many HIV-positive women will be diagnosed for the first time while pregnant and thus antenatal care serves as an entry point for further counselling, treatment and care (WHO 2001: 2; Piwoz 2005). In Mafeteng Government Hospital the rate is at an even higher level of 28% (ICAP 2009) and all mothers who tested positive received counselling thereafter. Despite a lack of agency of pregnant mothers in the medical procedures in antenatal care the whole programme was very successful in reducing the so called vertical transmission.

Antenatal care in Mafeteng Government Hospital includes raising awareness on HIV and a HIV test on the first visit. HIV-positive mothers will receive individual counselling and blood is drawn for the CD4 count and clinical staging according to the WHO stages of HIV which indicate the mother's immunological status. Therewith they enter a state of uncertainty. Counsellors merely distinguish between those mothers with a CD4 count above 350 duplications and those below, since the CD4 indicates which treatment strategy to follow (GoL, 2009 (a): 22). A low immunological status, either due to a very recent infection or due to an advanced AIDS stadium, is assumed to increase the probability of a HIV transmission to a partner or an unborn child. Depending on this technological indication, the pregnant woman receives a package of medication to prevent the transmission to her baby. Counsellors will explain how and when to use tablets and syrup in order to allow for a pharmaceutical intervention even outside biomedical facilities. Given the fact that not everybody returns for subsequent antenatal visits or delivers at home HIV-positive mothers should be able to administer the drug by themselves.

The "minimal package" includes antiretroviral medications, namely Nevirapine (NVP), Zidovudin (AZT) and Lamivudin (3TC) as well as antibiotics (Co-trimoxazole). Antibiotics and the antiretroviral AZT shall be administered daily to the mother starting from the 28th week of gestation until seven days post-partum. NVP and an additional dose of AZT shall be taken by the mother at the onset of labour. The tablets need to be taken at least two hours before delivery but no more than twelve hours before delivery if they are to be effective. If labour is prolonged or stops the medication needs to be administered again. After parturition the mother proceeds with the daily AZT intake and additionally takes 3TC for seven days. The baby shall be given NVP syrup for seven days or one month. The length of administering treatment to the infant depends on when the mother started her tablets (GoL 2009 (a): 23-33).

One would need to keep in mind that these complex procedures take place while women are in labour, preparing or recovering from it. However, somehow it seemed that these prophylactic recommendations gave some of my informants guidance in a situation of anxiety and uncertainty. Medication helped to provide relief as it guaranteed some ritual intake and control in an uncertain situation. Notwithstanding this, not all women understood the instructions and were therefore not able to follow them correctly. Better educated women were more likely to understand some of the complex concepts of biomedical explanatory models, while less educated women had difficulty particularly when following the English terminology frequently used in the hospital setting. Compliance with treatment and counselling, however, was not necessarily higher among better educated women in urban Mafeteng, mainly because of the difficult interactions at the household level.

For others, the medication was a source of uncertainty and doubt. Besides the complex instructions the medication itself gave cause for confusion among the clients in antenatal care. Various pharmaceutical companies provide components of HIV therapy under different names, a fact that contributes to confusion among patients. Despite the same active component, tablets may vary in colour, shape, size and administration. MaRobong, one of my study participants, usually dissolved her AZT tablet in a sip of water for about 15 minutes since they were too big for her to swallow. After the pharmacy ran out of stock and she received the same tablet produced by another company, MaRobong was able to swallow it normally (Field notes Kroeker 29: 31/03/2009).

5.3.1 The Power of Medical Technology

While in traditional health and familial care trust in the person is an important factor, biomedicine bases its legitimacy on the use of technology. Personal relations between members of staff and the client do not seem to be a basis for a visit to the hospital or health centre. Both Kücholl and Jordan realise that the relationship between staff and patients in biomedical facilities is purposely based on professional distance and authority (Kücholl 1985: 66-67). Jordan adds:

> The physician's professionalism is expressed in his totally impersonal attitude toward the woman. He treats her as an object, a performance that is made possible by the fact that others isolate and shield him. He never has to deal with this woman as a person (Jordan 1997: 70).

Others concluded that in "technomedicine", which means biomedicine that is predominantly validated by the use of complex scientifically-based technology, a body is somewhat reduced to its functions. The power of medical technology derives from the use of technical devices that alienate patient and doctor. Social interaction and personal relations between patient and the machine operator are apparently less intense than the relationship between machine operator and machine. Medicalisation of health disenfranchises the patient and gives privilege over the patient's body to experts and their machines and thus biomedical staff gain strength and decisive power over clients with the help of scientific "evidence-based" operations. Technomedicine apparently "exalts practitioner over patient in a status hierarchy that attributes authoritative knowledge only to those who know how to manipulate the technology and decode the information it provides" (Davis-Floyd 1997: 8).

Examinations and tests allow one to reveal hidden, assumed or known information about the women's condition by means of tools and tests. Machines and techniques indicated seemingly "objective" information, while the mother's embodied knowledge was considered a rather "subjective" source of information. Access to information within the biomedical system is thus restricted to certain personnel that is authorised to operate the machines, receive the results and interpret them. Therewith a client is dependent on a transfer of information and it is the person-machine-group that knows more about one's body than the owner. Tests are taken, the procedures and results are rarely communicated except in a cryptographic way in the medical book, *Bukana ea Bophelo*, and although clients carry it through health facilities and medical staff note down personal information, information is not necessarily accessible to the client. Notwithstanding, in resource-constrained settings the machines may not be fully functional due to the inadequate supply of consumables while alternative ways of conducting tests are not part of health workers' training.

5.3.2 Knowing about Not-knowing

In the biomedical as well as in the traditional medical realm, authority is established by depriving someone of knowledge. In the biomedical field, however, according to a democratic, self-determined role of the client it is expected that he or she arrives at a decision individually. Patient confidentiality shall ensure that only patient and medical practitioner are informed about test results, medical counselling and medical intervention.

In the family and in the traditional health sector however, a patient is not expected to arrive at a conclusion individually but is usually treated within his or her social context and with a perspective on family or community well-being. Often caretakers are involved in decision-making while the sick person is not burdened with additional information. In the biomedical field a patient is not aware of his ignorance. Notwithstanding this, patients shall be convinced they made the right decision but can never be sure they received all relevant information.

In the medical field the training is based on a foreign western concept of medicine which does not necessarily coincide with the general knowledge and the local knowledge of the physical functions of a patient, or client, attending a health facility. Thus, clients and medical staff often speak from different perspectives and cultural backgrounds despite the fact that many nurses are locals and have been socialised in that context. However, their educational and professional background and their fluency in the English language, which is their language of tuition, separate them from ordinary people. In addition, the medical booklet contains merely encrypted information, which is therewith not accessible to the clients, as depicted in this short conversation between a client (I) and a nurse (A). I nevertheless need to add, that it was highly unusual and surprising for one of the women in the waiting hall to question medical staff about the procedures in antenatal care:

> I: Why did you take our urine?
> A.: I want to check your kidneys and liver.
> I: Why didn't you give us the results?
> A.: I wrote them down in the *Bukana*.
> I: Why didn't you give them to us?
> A.: They are for us, not for you. (Field notes Kroeker: 12/06/2008).

According to Ashton (1952: 300), in traditional medical understanding the liver is the seat of patience, the lungs of irascibility and the kidneys and spleen host the feeling of irritability. Whatever the clients thought about this brief conversation, it shows that the concepts of physical functions are not commensurate.

Secondly, the social background which challenged an exchange between client and staff, gender and work organisation, played a role in the provision of medical care. Being touched and examined by females, who are predominantly employed in the health and care sector, seemingly causes great unease in male patients. The rotating scheme moreover leaves patients uncertain as to who is going to examine them. Private as well as traditional health care facilities assure that the doctor or nurse is known to the patient personally. The health provider has established a reputation in the community and therefore gained respect and trust in his person. In government institutions these personal implications were subordinated to the technological means of examining, in contrast to the traditional health system which primarily places trust in the person and his/her abilities. By using medical technology biomedical staff is alienated from common norms of social hierarchy. Medical tools apparently provide a buffer between two people interacting. Moreover, most doctors were foreign or had studied overseas which provided them per se with a socially higher rank.

Lesotho does not have a Faculty of Medicine but nursing colleges. All doctors are therefore trained abroad and the government awards scholarships to Basotho citizens, although many do not return home afterwards due to the fact that their qualification allows them to work in all Commonwealth countries, including South Africa, where wages tend to be higher. By the time this study took place, Mafeteng Hospital was staffed with five doctors, two of which arrived from Zimbabwe, one from Pakistan, one was of local origin and another post was vacant after a second local doctor had left for further training. The rural health centres do not host doctors, but an American paediatric visited them one day a month to treat children.

Not only those health professionals from Lesotho, but those from other African countries, take South Africa as a stepping stone to migrate to higher paying countries. In order to mitigate a shortage of nurses who go abroad despite local training facilities, the Ministry of Health and Social Welfare advertises in Kenya where there is a surplus of trained medical staff but who then, after having completed a two year contract, either move back or follow the brain drain to further their personal career. Due to Lesotho's lack of resources, insufficient medical technology and limited career opportunities, difficulties experienced by staff to become familiar with the language, culture and harsh climatic conditions, it is not surprising that there is a high turnover of staff. Of course, this plays a part in comprehending patients' complaints and concepts.

Limiting knowledge to strengthen one's authority also applies for family elders and traditional practitioners. In either case the expert's exclusive knowledge allows him to acquire authority and to generate status over non-experts. Of course, the patient who approaches biomedical health facilities seeks the doctor's expertise and accepts a subordinate patient's role being a lay person. It is particularly this social dominance whereby medical staff holds exclusive knowledge which deprives patients from decision-making power despite the idea that in biomedical care a patient should be allowed to make individually informed decisions:

> A woman who enters the hospital is treated as a patient. From the time she is admitted, decision-making power and responsibility for her state rest primarily with hospital personnel and the physician in charge (Jordan & Davis-Floyd 1993: 46).

Browner and Press, who analysed prenatal care in the United States and its implications for the mother, consider technology a tool which confirmed women's bodily experience. Physical sensation needed to be endorsed by medical technology in order for the information to be used by medical staff. Women in antenatal care moreover accepted these tools as of higher informational value and "acquiesce to biomedical authority when it was backed by the power of technology" (1997: 113-131). For instance, according to physicians, the infection with the HI-virus cannot be diagnosed other than through biomedical testing kits and, hence, biomedical facilities remain the preliminary caretakers for those found to carry the virus. The exclusive access to information on a physically exhausting and highly stigmatised disease that affects the individual as well as gender and generational roles makes biomedical facilities powerful institutions and an essential part of the attempts to mitigate the severe consequences of such information on a condition that cannot be sensed. Suddenly, a person without symptoms becomes a patient in constant care. Between 2005 and 2008 the Ministry of Health ran a "Know Your Status Campaign" and therewith intended to provide testing and counselling to all Basotho citizens over twelve years of age. Furthermore, the campaign aimed at referring HIV-positive people to health facilities before their condition deteriorated and encouraged responsible sexual behaviour[15]. Many people who tested HIV-positive now approached medical units to receive antiretroviral treatment. The number of people in ARV treatment

[15] About 71% of all Basotho people were screened for HIV before the campaign came to a halt because of ethical and organisational challenges. Only two districts, namely Leribe and Mafeteng, achieved full screening and in Mafeteng District 13,300 people were tested (ARASA & HRW 2008: 47).

in the whole of Lesotho increased from 1,000 clients in 2003 to more than 21,000 clients by early 2008; numbers for which many health facilities were unprepared (ARASA & HRW 2008: 22). The campaign flooded biomedical facilities with large numbers of clients; many would not have otherwise known they were in need of medical care. Hence, clients and medical staff were overwhelmed by the consequences of the results provided by medical technology. In the aftermath of the campaign the number of facilities providing PMTCT was increased from 37 in 2006 to 179 in 2008 (GoL & NAC 2009: 42; GoL 2009 (a): 2).

Additionally, pregnant women in Lesotho had to undergo testing for HIV. Due to the standardised HIV test in the antenatal protocol, those women had to cope with a test result while pregnant, a time of insecurity and when in need of social and emotional support, yet also a time when they are considered highly receptive for health education (GoL 2009 (a): 14). They thereby accepted medical dominance when they were asked to give blood for an HIV test strip and as a consequence of the test result medical technology was a factor in decision-making and health behaviour. However, this factor alone may not increase the number of people who comply with the prescribed interventions.

In conclusion, medical technology may increase acceptance of biomedical care, however, it has no value without the social interaction with the patient thereafter. In fact the key issue is not accepting a test per se but in the stigma surrounding the test result. Due to the stigma attached to HIV/AIDS of having infected oneself as a result of an immoral sex-driven lifestyle and the disease being a just punishment, many individuals refrained from testing even if symptoms cannot be gainsaid (Ashforth 2010). Without comprehensive interaction it merely leaves patients in a confused and worried state.

5.3.3 Counselling to the Point of Accepting

The medical booklets carried by patients do not only serve as a medium of communication but also as one of the tools of supervision, which is part of biomedical authority. In fact, various performance mechanisms control the patient and therewith intend to produce compliance with medical prescriptions. In a medical field control can be in the guise of physical examinations, checking medical history, counselling, home visits, involving treatment supporters, administrative system to control compliance, follow-up appointment dates, physical marks such an inoculation scar, blood tests as well as interrogation and questioning. Administrative processes in the hospital, such as the birth register, calendars which schedule patients for a certain date, lists of repeat prescription dates, signatures and stamps serve as confirmation that the patient underwent the scheduled treatment. Meanwhile, compliance with the prescribed treatment rose when lay counsellors started bridging the gap between HIV clients in antenatal care and medical staff, and thus facilitated the communication.

Per definition, a counselling session in a medical environment involves a patient, respectively a client, and a professionally trained person who has some body of medical knowledge as well as interpersonal skills (Silverman 1997: 5-7). According to Silverman, counselling of people living with HIV/AIDS shall enable them to cope with life and with the treatment given in an institutional framework. Counselling, however, should be distinguished from advice-giving and from coercing someone. A counsellor shall present different options, which are discussed with the client, who may in the course of counselling decide with the counsellor on what is the best option in his or her situation. In contrast to advice-giving, counselling is, according to Silverman, not biased *per se* but rather an interactional information exchange (Silverman 1997: 5-7).

Notwithstanding, counsellors fulfil an ambiguous role. On the one hand, they inform clients about potential risks, here the risk of producing an unhealthy child; while on the other hand, counsellors shall not impose their opinion and allow the client to choose freely (Wahlberg 2009: 90). Weighing up the odds during decision-making can easily be biased by the information given to someone and by the personal interests of the person giving such information. Yet, Williams et al. describe that "the boundary between choice and coercion is not a clearcut one for health practitioners" and that "slippage (...) between these concepts" may occur (Williams 2006: 3). In conclusion, Williams doubts that there is such a thing as unbiased information in the counselling sessions proceeding antenatal screenings:

> Partly in order to dissociate itself from eugenics, antenatal screening values the principle of non-directiveness as a key feature. It is believed that client autonomy can best be encouraged within this approach, with only the client's values being discussed within the counselling process (...). Doubts, however, have been expressed about how achievable non-directive counselling is in clinical practice (Williams 2006: 3).

Lesotho's guidelines stipulate non-directive counselling for HIV-positive women who are expectant or recently delivered. During monthly work evaluations of the counsellors in Mafeteng Government Hospital, the numbers of women who came for HIV counselling and those who attended family planning on referral were compared. Cases of women who arrived for their second PMTCT treatment due to a new pregnancy were also discussed in full and with regret by medical staff during these monthly evaluations. Observing these meetings, I learned that counsellors were pushed to discourage HIV-positive women from getting pregnant in their counselling session (Field notes Kroeker: 12/07/2008). Consequently, there was no means for the clients to decide against pharmaceuticals, biomedical attention or contraceptives (see also Chapter 8). In accordance with my observations on this practice one of the counsellors in that particular facility explained to me that clients receive "counselling to the point of accepting" biomedical care and if a client does not agree "we will try again another time" (Field notes Kroeker: 06/2008).

This position of authority a counsellor exercises over a client results in various implications. On the one hand, the counsellor has access to personal, health- related information which the client cannot access by herself, i.e. a HIV test strip. Moreover, a counsellor guides the client through the health facility and refers her to other units. Hence, the client is somewhat dependent on the counsellor and, thus, expected to follow orders the counsellor gives. Notwithstanding this, HIV/AIDS is a life-long condition which implies that clients and counsellors will also be in on-going interaction. Indeed, this situation is not free from hierarchy. It can be doubted to what extent a client can enjoy a right to full information and free consent. Apart from the relationship, the procedure also controls clients.

One would assume that educational attainment influences compliance with biomedical treatment. However, in our quantitative survey (ATCBM study) this was not confirmed. Interestingly, formal employment rather correlated with adhering to biomedical advice. Women in formal employment were more likely to reside in a smaller household community comprising only one generation or only their own young children. Hence there was seldom an elder female companion as a source of information and caretaker. Small household communities thus correspond with a lack of complementary information in pregnancy whereas a visit to antenatal care was an important source of information. Moreover, not only examinations as such, but the interaction in the facility, influenced the decisions a mother eventually made on pregnancy, delivery, infant feeding as well as on self-care.

Physicians' and demographers' interest in reducing the number of off-spring born to HIV-positive women was, however, rather based on certain aims of an economic, public health and demographic nature. Yet, some of these hidden interests showed in the counselling sessions where some aspects of coercion were applied. Coercion can be subtle and unintentional or, as in Lesotho, paired with authoritative knowledge and as part of professional health care. Written documents steered clear of a rhetoric which would violate reproductive rights, however, certain aims were to be met and thus the outcome of the counselling session was already set: medical staff would in the course of counselling presumably consider individual rights as secondary to their work targets and governmental demographic aims. However, an evaluation of patients' reasons for defaulting with treatment conducted by the Mafeteng Government Hospital staff revealed that about 60% of the cases were actually due to mistakes of an administrative nature (Mafeteng Government Hospital 2008). Clients had been transferred to other clinics or had already passed away without anyone in the hospital noting it down[16]. In 2008, supervision of staff, particularly in terms of paperwork, became more restrictive and work performance, opportunities and challenges were discussed in monthly meetings. An external organisation, the International Center for AIDS Care and Treatment Programs (ICAP), supervised the work of all those involved in the prevention of mother-to-child transmission of HIV. Now, there are hardly any opportunities for clients as well as staff to avoid supervision from within the hospital, which, of course, cannot solve structural problems.

5.4 Authoritative Knowledge and the Control of Misfortune

In general, child-bearing mothers were barely able to explain the rationality behind particular traditional or biomedical practices and struggled to come to terms with either of them. Preventive measures play an important role in traditional care with respect to witchcraft prevention, talisman and charms. I asked a client in antenatal care about her necklace:

[16] Due to this major finding, staff refrained from publishing the results (Field notes Kroeker: 3/2007). However, people living with HIV who miss medical appointments ("treatment defaulters") are few in percentage compared to western countries (Field notes Kroeker: Lennemann 2007).

Client: I don't know what it is for, but my mother-in-law gave it to me.
LK: What is this?
Client: It's the tail of a nakeli [wild cat], but I don't know why she gave it to me.
LK: And that one? (pointing to the rope, which looks like a twisted band made of plant fibre).
Client: I don't know.
LK: Was it a special situation when she gave it to you? Like the wedding or were you sick?
Client: She gave it to me before I was going home to my parent's house.
LK: Why did you go home to your parent's house?
Client: Because I was pregnant (Field notes Kroeker: 27/06/2008).

Enlightenment about certain topics of traditional health care, as we will see, does not take place in a prospective way, but as the need occurs, exactly as Jordan and Davis-Floyd (1993) described in Yucatan: "Whenever possible, her teaching is demonstrative rather than verbal. (...) She does give practical advice about nursing, especially to a first-time mother" (Jordan & Davis-Floyd 1993: 33, 42). As the authors (1993: 178) recognise for traditional birth attendants in Yucatan, this also applies in the Basotho context: knowledge is transferred by showing, watching, imitating and experimental learning at the point of time when this knowledge comes into use.

In hospital, however, counselling was preventive and explanatory. For instance, medical staff caution expectant mothers against the use of traditional medication and warn against side effects (Field notes Kroeker: 10/06/2008):

> Usually we tell the people, they should leave these things aside and only take the hospital's treatment. (...) You know, [the client] said the Basotho-doctor cooked the *pitsa* and had it ready for her to drink. You don't know what they mixed. (...) We don't know their recipe, they might mix the eggshell with other herbs and sometimes they don't have a limit of giving something. Additionally, you don't know whether the drinking water is safe, maybe it's not the herbs, but the water that makes people sick. It can be harmful to the person. And I think the clients might lie. They sometimes don't know about it but sometimes they also lie. [The client] might not have told all the things

> they were doing to her. So they won't tell you what they got from the healer. Therefore we advise them not to take anything from them (Field notes Kroeker: MaThloni 27/06/2008).

Counsellors and nurses warn expectant women that traditional infusions may induce pharmacological interactions or on the other hand "flush out" the active substances of biomedical medication. In either case the probability of a HIV transmission from mother to child presumably rises (Field notes Kroeker: 19/11/2008). From a biomedical perspective, traditional medicine appears to be more part of the problem than part of the solution in caring for the sick.

"Teaching" in the hospital implies a theoretical and prospective focus. In the household, elders (thought they) knew about the general situation of their next-of-kin and presumably took aspects they found relevant into consideration. Accepting an elder's authority, experience and knowledge, young people considered it disrespectful and offensive to question an elder's advice. Despite ignorance, youngsters were widely scared of non-compliance with crucial preventive practices since they could not predict the consequences.

As the example shows, it is a hard task for young pregnant women to "teach" elders about their pregnancy and to pass on information that shall be taken into consideration in decision-making. Moreover, it is not clear who needs to be informed about a piece of information such as a positive HIV test result. Does it affect elders who make decisions or is it, as considered in the hospital, a secret between doctor and patient?

> Robong, a 19-year old girl, who, according to a home-based model of communication, does not speak openly to family elders, insists that her positive HIV-test shall be taken into consideration when caring for her and the child. She expects her elders to give her good care and advice once they know about her infection with the virus, however, Robong struggles to talk openly and she actually hoped that sister, mother or boyfriend would check her medical booklet, which she leaves lying around openly in the hope that they will find out about her status by themselves (cf. Mogensen 2010). Four weeks after the baby was born still no-one had checked her *Bukana*. Moreover, she did not dare to lecture her mother on her infant care when they jointly took care for the baby on the weekends. She did not want to appear as a troublemaker particularly since her family was more concerned with the fail-

> ing marriage negotiations. Sensing an urgent need to get the message about her HIV-status across Robong needed to find someone to speak openly to her elders and eventually invited a counsellor from hospital to her place. She therewith complied with norms of communication and hoped that her maternal elders adjusted their behaviour and advice to biomedical recommendations (Field notes Kroeker 19: 07/11/2008-16/04/2009).

Even with traditional healers, patients hardly speak about themselves, but the healer being the expert asks the patient questions or the oracle provides further information (cf. Whyte 1997), which also plays a part in the client's timidity to ask questions to a biomedical doctor. Quite in contrast to Basotho care, clients in the hospital are expected to be frank and open about everything of relevance, in particular their reproductive activities. In biomedical care, however, a body seems to be divided into various fractions and different doctors are responsible for their part. For instance, antenatal caretakers only take care of pregnancy-related issues while in the Tuberculosis unit the affected organ is monitored by a different specialist. Health information is usually given for a particular body part but not for the whole body or the body in its social relations. Hence, whatever is of relevance to the medical caretaker may be rather limited. Familial advice mostly concerned social, spiritual and physical harm to the individual or the community as a whole whereas biomedical advice concerns physical, biological disorders. In short, biomedical care aims at securing *bophelo* (health), whereas the family considers *bophelo* in its broader translation of "life". With regard to their understanding of *bophelo* elders take a different approach to health care. For instance, the pink *selapa* gown provided by the patrilineage will warn passers-by of the mother's transitional state "between life and death". It shall indicate to others that a woman is expectant and therefore prone to witchcraft which may come upon the child. Elders from the matrilineage, for their part, provide the expectant mother with *pitsa* when in labour, which safeguards her from harm and facilitates her delivery. Responsibility for both mother and child is therewith shared between the two clans; the one of the mother and the one of the child. Fulfilling certain protective rites therewith corresponds with a certain time and place. In this context it is not only a right but also a duty of experienced females to assist verbally and practically in preventing misfortune. Making sure that the mother fulfils her duties, obedience and reproduction, hinges on the welfare of two clans. Therefore, active involvement of family members during pregnancy, delivery and child-care appears as a social obligation to the other clan and sign of love and care for a young woman. Most young women merely mentioned that neglecting rites or health advice would leave the baby sick or disabled (Field notes Kroeker: 08/04/2009; Gill 1993: 51; Romero-Daza & Himmelgreen 2004: 959; Bledsoe 2002: 78-79; cf. Sargent 1989: 115) and the blame may lie with her caretakers.

While in hospital counselling sessions patients shall be made aware of certain risks and how to be "a compliant client", explanations at home are merely meant to force adherence without understanding the connection between rule and reason. A major task of a community of female household members who surround an expectant next-of-kin is to keep her busy and interrupt behaviour which is associated with harm. Basotho pedagogy intends to encourage certain behaviour, whatever means it takes. Therewith narrations and causations may not have any rational correlation and it is more important that a youngster complies than understands. Being ignorant of the actual underlying cause of something forces young people to follow. This can be more easily illustrated with a second example: the prohibited nutrients, for instance, were associated with sexual intercourse and teenage pregnancy, yet, the narrative about these foods was merely meant to scare girls from tasting them:

> For example, youth were not supposed to eat eggs and intestines because they would be too mature and become interested in sexual activity and it was thought to be a means of contraception, because there was no other means despite abstinence. (…) If young girls were told the explanation why they are not supposed to eat proteins they might like the idea of being sexually active and mature and hence become interested to eat those nutriments largely (Field notes Kroeker Theko: 28/07/2009).

A child out of wedlock would have affected the family and options to negotiate the bride wealth.

Expectant mothers are usually surrounded by experienced women who supervise, comfort and assure them, meanwhile women who lived in small households rarely knew about elder women's advice and made decisions for themselves unaware of the risks they may be exposed to. Even if the pregnant women knew about certain norms or practices they neglected some due to a lack of supervision.

Pedagogy in a biomedical facility is somewhat different. During the sessions where questions from clients are expected and appreciated, clients particularly took the opportunity to raise issues of traditional advice for expectant women in order to question their validity but hardly ever questioned medical practices:

> While we were sitting in a group counselling session MaRobong turned to me and inquired whether we have those kinds of traditions in Europe. I deny. She resumed that our children were still not disabled, which was proof to her that this advice does not correlate with the child's health. She asked herself then, what would happen, if she does not wear charms or only refuses to comply with the dress code for pregnant women. However, she did not dare to take it off. She wore the *selapa*, a necklace and walked barefoot as she was told by her mother-in-law (Field notes Kroeker 29: 07/04/2009).

In antenatal care, however, the nurse refutes any rationale albeit she cannot explain the reason behind traditional advice (Field notes Kroeker: 24/06/2008). Clients were made aware that traditional rites do not have any reason, although only the explanations given, not the hidden intention, were discussed. Therewith, biomedical staff somewhat undermined familial care and control and diminished the elders' authority.

Jordan argues that certain aspects in a discourse on the "right" behaviour in pregnancy, delivery and child-care gain value, which qualifies the statement as decisive and authoritative despite alternative opinions or feeling. Conflicting opinions, however, need to be balanced against each other by the recipient and due to the relationship to the speaker:

> The central observation is that for any particular domain several knowledge systems exist, some of which, by consensus, come to carry more weight than others, either because they explain the state of the world better for the purposes at hand (efficacy) or because they are associated with a stronger power base (structural superiority), and usually both. (...) *The power of authoritative knowledge is not that it is correct, but that it counts* (Jordan 1997: 56, emphasis in original).

For the clients, however, two systems of expert knowledge are in competition. In conclusion, traditional and biomedical harm and the prevention thereof are inseparably intertwined in a patient's behaviour. While some recommendations of a biomedical and traditional kind conflict, others remain untouched, however, it is rather dependent on supervision than on arguments. Hence, all the aforementioned women complied with elders' advice for pregnant women (mostly due to fear of sanctions) but used biomedical advice complementarily, such as Peli:

> In the counselling session in antenatal care Peli cries and refuses to start antiretroviral treatment since her husband prefers traditional medication. She argues that he is the head of the household and she respects his authority, moreover, her husband pays for her traditional antenatal care with the healer, Peli argues.
> Peli's mum received counselling in hospital when Peli was there for her delivery. The mother agrees to biomedical treatment and suggests that the daughter shall stay with her as long as she wants after the childbirth so she can supervise compliance. The grandmother promises the counsellor that she will take care of administering the 7-day course of Nevirapine-syrup to the baby and supervise Peli's feeding practice for up to six months.
> Caught between these options represented by two people in authority, Peli is convinced that "the Sesotho treatment and the hospital treatment fight each other". She finally decides to take traditional treatment for herself and biomedical prophylaxis for the baby. Aged three months the child develops a common Sesotho-disease called "pulsing fontanelles" (*puoana*). The disease relates to witchcraft affliction and the child receives traditional treatment as a cure since biomedicine does not provide treatment against the cause of it. Peli then decides to leave the mother's home and abandon her supervision to treat the child traditionally (Field notes Kroeker 2: 18/10/2008-19/05/2008; cf. Sargent 1989: 5).

MaNne in contrast decided to avoid parental supervision altogether and rely on biomedical care:

> MaNne complied with traditional practices according to her mother-in-law's custom when pregnant with her first child. Though, after four months the baby passed away and her husband believed that she must have missed some of the traditional measures and she did not perform them properly. MaNne, in contrast to her husband and his family, concluded, though, that the first child had already died of AIDS and not as a consequence of her neglecting customs. In order to prevent the same thing from happening twice, he now wanted her to go for the hospital

> treatment as an alternative. Consequently, with her current pregnancy she did not even go to visit her family but stayed in town close to the hospital at all times (Field notes Kroeker 24: 27/11/2008).

Biomedicine and traditional medicine do not address the same harms to which expectant women are exposed and it would be safest for the mothers to use traditional and biomedical care complementarily for the sake of physical, spiritual and social prosperity (Sargent 1989: 19). It would not be wise and even ethically disputable to neglect important means of controlling uncertainty. However, certain norms consequently need to be broken as the mothers cannot adhere to all of these and the guiding principles given by elders or staff and this caused uncertainty rather than control.

In fact, many expectant women, particularly *multigravida,* doubted certain aspects within both explanatory models. Non-compliance with an elder's orders may be understood as disrespect and failure of subordination and young women were anxious about losing face if talking openly or were scared about losing support and love. Even if a pregnant woman has contrasting information at hand she will perhaps comply with the recommended behaviour of authorities, in spite of better knowledge, argues Sich (1983). Sich assumes that a young person therewith lets another person in a dominant position keep honour and face. Thus, in generational debates young people comply with directives for the sake of showing respect and honour. Notwithstanding, supervising subsequent fulfilment of taboos, rites and rituals on the one hand and biomedical compliance on the other is far from perfect. Thus, study participants' agency concentrated on taking steps to avoid the supervisory powers as well as the resulting sanctions (Field notes Kroeker 14: 04/12/2008).

In summary, it is due to the notion of *bophelo* as life or as health from which caretakers, family members as well as medical staff, assess the situation. Biomedical health carers follow a rather scientific-technological approach to pregnancy and HIV, while the client and her family mostly see a spiritual and socio-emotional side of the reproductive life. The perspective governing which condition receives preferential treatment also seems to differ depending on this approach. While biomedical staff apparently focuses on HIV as a priority, I hypothesise that within the family women are considered pregnant in the first place and, provided next-of-kin are informed, the mother carries the attribute of HIV as a secondary piece of information. In the hospital, my informants were HIV-positive in the long-term, while being temporarily pregnant in addition to the infection. Consequently, while in a biomedical setting PMTCT as a technology is rather considered an emergency option to prevent the infection of the child of a HIV-positive mother, mothers may view PMTCT in a rather more positive way. PMTCT provides an opportunity to have a HIV-negative child irrespective of the mother's condition.

Delivery: "In between life and death"

The perception of danger in labour and birthing, which appears as an intercultural constant, is accompanied with tools and aids for dealing with these perceived risks. A "good" and thus "safe" birthing process for mother, child and community likewise deserves manifold considerations and preparations, including decision-making on the best place to deliver, who will assist during the passage, what mode should apply and what material and immaterial tools must be used. Thus the standard birth practice, both in a traditional or biomedical notion, entails material as well as immaterial artefacts in order to disarm potential harms. Notwithstanding, since biomedicine and traditional obstetric care tackle different causes of misfortune, different technologies apply depending on the place of birth. The labouring mother and her supporters prepare in advance in order to make the birth a success and, here again, notions differ as to what this entails. Thus, despite different perceptions on complications during delivery and success in birthing, Floyd and Sargent (1997) note that birth requires assistance from experienced (or professional) experts, who guide and supervise the progress, evaluate it and thus advise on how to proceed. Birth attendants' authoritative knowledge is a crucial part of the standard protocol for deliveries in the biomedical sphere as well as in familial care. The place of birth is synonymous with what a good delivery needs to be and equally needs to prevent, consequently that which is undesirable in birthing.

In the locality of Mafeteng women basically have four different birth facilities to choose from: two biomedical facilities and two places where traditional deliveries take place. Besides the urban district hospital, families may opt for a delivery at one of the rural health centres[1]. Traditional deliveries are performed in a traditional clinic where a healer practices as well as in private houses, where Traditional Birth Attendants (TBA) or elder females come to assist at the labouring mother's homestead. Generally, in Lesotho, just over half of the labouring women receive help from biomedically trained

---

[1] None of the women in my ethnographic study contemplated a delivery in a local health centre. To complete the picture I nevertheless mention the health centres in the list of birth facilities and present the arguments of the ATCBM study participants who attended antenatal care at one of these. Unfortunately, quantitative data from the Ministry of Health and Social Welfare does not distinguish between the hospital and the rural health centres, which makes it difficult to support or negate my impression that health centres are unpopular as places to give birth.

nurses or midwives in one of the health facilities during confinement. 59 % deliver in public or private biomedical facilities, while 40% of the mothers delivered their baby at home (MoHSW 2010: 109)[2]. In the district of Mafeteng about 55% of the babies are delivered under biomedical supervision and the higher the number of antenatal visits the more likely it is that women will return to the hospital or health centre for their delivery.

For women who learned about their HIV-positive status their worries about harming the child (as well as about birth attendants) may have added to their considerations. Consequently, the test may have unravelled a crucial aspect which influences the decision-making of the mother, although maybe not of those who are making decisions on the mother's behalf on where to give birth.

In order to allow a deeper analysis on why a particular place is favoured, I intend to describe the four above mentioned facilities in more detail. I argue that in most cases the families make a decision, although some expectant women also used hidden strategies to influence decision-makers. This chapter intends to present factors that are decisive for the preferred place of delivery. I will conclude with a case whereby, despite many considerations, for births affected by misfortune, different places of birth had to be tried.

6.1 Shifting Places

Despite the high number of biomedical antenatal care attendees according to the counselling records, the number of clients registered in the maternity ward is not commensurate. More women enrol in antenatal care (92 %) than deliver in the hospital (59 %) in spite of the fact that biomedical staff usually advise against home deliveries and characterise them as unsafe due to unsterile conditions and a lack of expertise of lay midwives (MoHSW 2010: 103, 109; Field notes Kroeker 4: 14/11/2008). Decision-makers who are in charge of an expectant mother may argue, in contrast, that biomedical facilities are unsuitable for a delivery because of unknown birth assistance and shifting from one place to another while in a sensitive condition. Secondly, the register shows that the majority of women who attended the antenatal clinic at one facility actually delivered at another. For instance, women who attended

---

[2] The number of deliveries outside biomedical facilities may be higher since women may conceal the fact they delivered their child at home.

antenatal care in a rural health centre decided to travel to the hospital for confinement.

Delivery, the most crucial and hazardous part of procreation, entails manifold preparations and considerations to allow for its best possible result. Prohibitions and prescriptions in gestation, delivery and the early post-partum period already foreshadow the uncertainties one may experience. Thus, elderly and experienced decision-makers are involved in highly politicised and crucial decisions on life and death, and conclude on what mode and place of delivery suggest safety and success. Elder female family members, who already mastered the transition themselves and hence fulfilled the requirements of a mature member of society, approached the mother and taught her about what was involved in reaching this status (Yovsi 2003: 19). Those who had delivered children and thus learned about the dangers will therefore fully cater for the expectant next-of-kin and many expectant mothers were seldom considered to have a say in this debate but rather waited for an elder's decision on this crucial question of delivery care (ATCBM Kroeker: 16/07/2008). Grandmother, expectant mother and child are therewith merely part of a three-generation matrifocal group of support and care (Gay 1980: 53), in which the maternal grandmother's attitude towards the birthplace of her grandchild as well as other safety preparations drove the decision. Trevathan states:

> The larger historically rooted social group may have already made decisions about where birth is to take place, what position the woman will be in when she delivers, what "artefacts" will be used during delivery, who receives her newborn infant, and how she may or may not behave during labour and delivery (Trevathan 1997: 80).

In accordance with elder ethnographic descriptions on Basotho culture, my study revealed that particularly first-time mothers move to their maternal homestead when delivery approached (Ashton 1952: 30; Gay 1980: 52; Kuecholl 1985: 58). The majority of women, even in the urban proximity, did indeed change residence in their last trimester of pregnancy (cf. Romero-Daza 2004: 961), however, they rarely knew why they were advised to do so.

In the event that the expectant mother usually lived at a distance from the health facility, which elders preferred as place of delivery for their offspring, the mother may change residence a second time towards the end of her pregnancy in order to stay with a mentor who lived closer to the facility. Meanwhile these mentors were also advised by elders to do so and therewith facilitate what the elders had decided: Nnoe, for instance, when pregnant for the first time, was sent to her elder sister who lived in Mafeteng town within walking distance of the hospital, whereas Robong was no longer supposed to stay on her own. Following her mother's instructions, Robong moved to her elder sister's house, which was not only closer to hospital, but more spacious than her house. However, Robong moved back and forth to her house since she did not feel comfortable there. Nne also felt uncomfortable and shifted time and time again from one grandmother's house to another's. The one whose house she usually stayed at kept on sending her back to the other one who was a traditional healer and birth attendant and Nne made up excuses, pretending that this one had sent her back home again. LeTharo had intended to stay at her house but had to move to her brother-in-law's home after discovering some witchcraft affliction that drove her out, and meanwhile, LeNne preferred to move from her rural mountainous homestead to stay at her sister's urban rented accommodation. She had delivered her first and second child in a home delivery with the assistance of local elders, but after testing HIV-positive during her third pregnancy, she decided on a hospital delivery. Later she changed her mind and travelled to the traditional clinic after having enjoyed her sister's care and biomedical antenatal examinations (Field notes Kroeker 14: 04/12/2008). Others coming from remote areas decided to move to the hospital's expectant mother shelters where they would not be surrounded by family members and, while Ashton recognised differences between the first and subsequent deliveries, my study could not confirm this. Subsequent children were, as the study revealed, also more frequently born at the mother's marital home or a nearby health facility, while Ashton concluded, in contrast, that after a first child had already confirmed the social status a mother receives in child-bearing, subsequent children tended to be delivered at the patrilocal residence or at the couple's neolocal homestead (Ashton 1952: 29; cf. Ansell & van Blerk 2004; Field notes 3/2007).

Nevertheless, the expectant mother who attended antenatal care in a biomedical facility will have been questioned on where she intended to deliver. Due to biomedical practitioners' frequent disapproval of home deliveries, clients in antenatal care who anticipated a home delivery usually hid this information from medical staff or referred to easily acceptable arguments related to financial means, transport and the sudden onset of a previous delivery to justify giving birth within traditional care. This is either because the women are ignorant of "traditional" arguments in favour of home deliveries or as a strategy to avoid a discussion with the counsellors as to why they must not deliver there. However, these three arguments, finance, transport, and labour advancing quickly, must be analysed in more detail.

In a society that largely depends on familial networks and single people who generate income for many relatives, access to finance depends on negotiations. Larger expenses need to be discussed and money will eventually be allocated for one enterprise or the other. The delivery of a child must be considered as an enterprise, which calls on those who have access to money and its allocation, although different delivery options also demand different amounts of money. Since the eldest female supervises the household expenses and allocates the money, her opinion also plays a part in where an expectant mother delivers. Unless the expectant mother generates her own income, she will be dependent on her family's (or in-laws') financial resources, and it is consequently her in-laws' decision whether to provide money for the delivery. And in many cases it does not necessarily seem to be a question of available funds, but rather the preference of the household heads.

A delivery in a government hospital or health centre was usually assumed to be more expensive than a home delivery with a traditional birth attendant. However, this is not necessarily a valid argument since the price for a hospital delivery is fixed and only transport fees need to be added. Whereas a delivery with a traditional birth attendant is about 80 ZAR for a female baby, which is cheaper than a baby boy (around 90 ZAR) (ATCBM Kroeker: 10/07/2008; Field notes Kroeker: 20/01/2009), the hospital charges 70 ZAR for the delivery service plus a daily fee of 15 ZAR depending on the number of days a mother stays in hospital (as of Nov. 2008)[3]. A Caesarean Section in a government hospital will cost about 130 ZAR plus a daily fee, with a stay normally lasting seven days post-partum. In contrast, however, birth attendants in the villages in many cases allowed the family to owe the fee, negotiate the sum and pay in instalments, whereas a mother would not be able to leave hospital before settling her fees. If she or her family is una-

[3] According to my observations the fees in the hospital altered a little as well, since nurses, respectively accountants, made a little money from charging ignorant mothers of baby boys more than mothers of baby girls. While a mother of a boy paid 79.90 ZAR for one night in the hospital and the delivery, a mother of a baby girl was charged 70 ZAR for the same time and service (Caesarean sections are about 130 ZAR). LeTselela paid 50 ZAR for a delivery in the traditional facility where she delivered a boy, but she did not stay there for longer than one day (Field notes Kroeker 16: 04/03/2009; Fieldnotes Kroeker: 08/04/2009).

ble to pay, she will have to stay longer which further adds to the sum owed. Giving birth in a private hospital may cost exceedingly more than an average monthly income and very few families consider it an option. In a private hospital a C-Section costs about 3000-3500 ZAR (Field notes Kroeker: 18/11/2008). By comparison, a local laywoman may not ask for any financial compensation for a home delivery but consider it neighbourly solidarity to help.

Therefore, the decision between traditional birth attendant and biomedical delivery may not necessarily be based on financial arguments. Either decision-makers were ignorant about the actual costs or mentioned the higher costs to strengthen their preference on the place of birth (Field notes Kroeker: 10/06/2008; ATCBM Kroeker: 14/07/2008; 08/07/2008). Out of respect and politeness, expectant mothers waited and accepted suggestions from their seniors as being in their best interest, just as a mother concisely explains: "the parents are those taking the decisions and holding the money" (ATCBM Kroeker: 10/07/2008). Yet, even if expectant women disagreed they respected decisions made by their elders (ATCBM Kroeker: 14/07/2008). The case of a mother from the rural Sekameng catchment area, where transport to hospital is not only onerous but also expensive, illustrates the decision-making process:

> It was not my intention to give birth at home. There were financial problems, not enough preparations were done by the family for me to give birth at hospital (ATCBM Kroeker: 15/07/2008).

However, behind the scenes, financial constraints were not necessarily the main reason for a home delivery in the parent's argumentation either, merely money allocation was a means to justify it publicly. Another woman from the same area tried to influence her elder's decision due to her disagreement and also ended up delivering at home:

> The expectant mother expected to deliver in hospital, while her mother-in-law did not see any need to schedule money for a hospital delivery. When the expectant mother took up a job to generate money for a hospital delivery herself, elders insisted. Her parents were convinced that working during her pregnancy was a bad idea, moreover, they considered a home delivery to be just fine (ATCBM Kroeker: 09/07/2008).

Women in formal employment with smaller household units in urban areas do not usually pass their earnings to the head of household but decide upon its use more independently. Elder women recommended rather than decided on where these women should deliver, moreover, financially independent women chose to stay away from elders if they expected disagreement on certain matters such as the place of delivery.

While women were not necessarily aware of the reasons elders had for their decision, mothers often gave excuses to biomedical staff that a home delivery occurred due to the fast onset of labour which made travelling impossible. Pregnant women were not sure about their due date and were caught by surprise when labour started. Secondly, strong and fast labour pains as well as burdensome and unreliable transport had made it impossible for them to get anywhere else, such as to a health facility, in due time. Some health centres are not within easy reach of the villages and the hospital is inaccessible, and yet biomedical staff stressed the need to go there for confinement. Transport with private cars has to be arranged in advance and is very expensive indeed.

In Lesotho, as in many biomedical facilities around the world, calculating the expected date of delivery depends on the first day of the last menstruation. The method of calculation presumes a regular cycle, however, due to the most common current method of contraception in Lesotho, Depo-Provera injections, ovulation is suppressed or irregular as the cycle recovers. Women may therefore conceive during the first fertile days after missing the date of a subsequent injection, in spite of not having had a menstrual flow or a regular period. The calculated date of conception and subsequent delivery might therefore be calculated inaccurately. Ultrasound scans can confirm or disprove the expected due date in line with the visible development of the foetus, but in Lesotho ultrasound scans are not part of the standardised check-up in antenatal care. Consequently, the expected due date remains more or less a matter of guesswork[4]. For the families this means that miscalculations in the expected date of delivery may inhibit a timely allocation of money for the delivery as well as travelling to the preferred place of delivery in due time[5]. Spontaneous deliveries indeed happen more often than not after

[4] If a mother is two weeks over the due date labour will be induced by injections. Due to frequent miscalculations in the expected date of delivery an ultrasound scan has to confirm the baby's maturity first (Field notes Kroeker: 25/11/2008).

[5] Employed women also go on maternity leave starting from the day the child is born and not before since they do not expect the calculated due date to be accurate. Since maternity leave

the administration of labour pain-inducing *pitsa.* As a result, delivery approaches fast while the women are unable to get to the health facilities. Staff in rural health centres thus complained that women who intended to deliver there sometimes gave birth on the way when labour progressed quickly due to the medication administered.

Regardless of wherever a delivery eventually takes place, those with access to funding had a major influence on the decision. However, men in Lesotho were excluded from these debates in contrast to Sargent's observation of men in Northern Benin. While Sargent argues that the husband's education and social status played a part in the decision on where his wife was to deliver (Sargent 1989: 73, 206), Basotho men were not expected to interfere in women's issues. A nurse explains:

> In most cases in our culture, men do not decide whether the woman delivers at home, the decision can be made by the mother-in-law, or the in-laws whoever. Those are the decisions for the women, not for the men, they must not be involved in [decisions on] delivering and pregnant women (Field notes Kroeker Mampho: 22/03/2007).

In any case, many partners were not living with their wife at that time, but may perhaps have had an indirect influence on deciding on the place of birth in urban areas when living as a nuclear family, yet, the mother in most cases would have own income and make her own decision.

6.2 Option 1: The Safe Sanctuary

Especially in some of the mountainous regions of Lesotho, biomedically trained staff would rarely be accessible and transport is frequently onerous. The more mountainous the geography, the more likely it is that an expectant mother will deliver at home[6]. Yet, even in urban areas, home deliveries are current but in small and decreasing number. The decision to deliver at home, however, does not solely depend on a lack of access to a health facility but

---

terminates after 2 months, regardless of the day of delivery, some women prefer to work until the delivery day in order to spend two whole months recovering rather than waiting for the birth (Field notes Kroeker 24: 30/4/2009, 24/11/2008).

For the calculation of the expected date of delivery, see also, Jordan and Davis-Floyd 1993: 54.

[6] In the district of Mokhotlong only 48% of women deliver in biomedical facilities. In the Thaba Tseka district the numbers are even lower (42%) (MoHSW 2010: 109).

on a myriad of factors surrounding the mere act of giving birth and perceptions of potential mishap.

To understand why home deliveries were part of the safety precautions for mother and child as well as for the maternal lineage, one needs to recall the traditional arrangements of the settlements and the core of the female sphere. Despite the fact that architecture had changed, arguments for home deliveries relate closely to the women's safe sanctuary inside the house and its vestibule. Individuals in an insecure transitional stage, such as towards the beginning and end of life, as well as during confinement and marriage, remain in the house until their situation stabilises and greater distance is gradually allowed over time. Comaroff reminds us that

> Birth was a subsocial process, occurring in domestic seclusion and ending with the ritualized reincorporation of mother and child into wider community. Like death, it was associated with the floor of the house, with planes below the normal level of social interaction. Birth established a personally individuating link between mother and child, itself the matrilateral relations (Comaroff 1985: 97-98).

Consequently, during deliveries, the chore of liminality, women were supervised by elder female relatives, well known villagers or a traditional birth attendant, hence, people from the inner circle that are trustworthy and familiar. On the other hand, men, prepubescent girls, or unfamiliar people were explicitly excluded from the birthplace. Besides excluding certain individuals, certain places were also not recommended for labouring and new mothers. The delivering woman was advised, for safety reasons, to stay in or close to the house while in the polluted condition between life and death, in fact, some even remained in bed for anything from a few days up to a week (Hall & Malahleha 1989: 50) and should not be exposed to spiritual harm outside the centre of the compound. She will initially go no further than into the vestibule[7] before she has recovered from her polluted condition and exposes herself to other people's views and interaction.

> The backyard (segotlo) was (...) the privileged sphere of the woman of the house and of her children and matrilateral kin (Comaroff and Roberts 1981: 50); an enclosed sanctuary where these kin consorted and ate together without risk of contamination by rivals, and where they were protected by the female "living dead" (badimo) buried beneath

[7] *Segotlo* in Tswana-language = *Seotlo* in Sesotho; *Badimo* (Tswana) = *Balimo* (Sesotho).

> the floor (…) in the segotlo, too, raw food from field and bush was prepared, cooked, stored, and apportioned, and the young nurtured and raised (Campbell 1815: 184). It was in other words, the site of the transformation of presocial elements into more decidedly social form (Comaroff 1985: 57)[8].

The place was fenced with reed which shielded the areal of solely female activity, and to warn those approaching the house from afar flags were raised in the colours of the totemic clan to indicate the pollution. Particularly strangers and men must avoid the house where a newly delivered woman stays because of the sensitive condition of its resident. Strangers cause harm due to "their bad conduct" and trampling everywhere, and they are apt to cause evil to the infant (Sechefo n.d.: 27; Romero-Daza 2004: 961). Ashton notes: "If a man deliberately ignored the warning signs outside her hut and approached a fresh mother and her new-born babe, he would be regarded as a sorcerer, trying to kill the babe by his action" (1952: 289). Ngubane adds that a woman who is affected by a high intensity of pollution is not only prone to affliction but also affects others accidentally (Ngubane 1976: 275). Even agnatic males must not enter until the umbilical cord has fallen off, while the seclusion from affinal relatives, in particular the husband, will even last for some months after confinement and until the mother returns to his house. In the meantime, the infant remains inside and the mother must cover herself up well when leaving the house (Ngubane 1976: 275). Eventually she will leave the safe premises and move again to the marital homestead after some months, crossing the bush as a wild, hazardous and "unmarked sociomoral universe" (Comaroff 1985: 51) which surrounds the known realm in concentric arrangement.

Quite in contrast to this notion on safety, women who delivered in hospital arrive there when already in labour and under normal circumstances leave one day after the birth. Journeys to and from the hospital take place at a highly hazardous spiritual time. Notwithstanding this, a geographical shift entails a shift of social supporters and therewith affects those who supervise the "correct" process.

---

[8] Male living dead populate the *kraal* where old men were laid to rest, or as an act of euthanasia, were laid to be killed by their beloved cattle (Field notes Theko 7/2009).

6.2.1 The Birthing Process

As part of their care and while being less prone to spiritual hazards from strangers, elders will run errands until they authorise when a new mother is ready to leave the close proximity of the house again (Hall & Malahleha 1989: 50). Still at that time, which belongs to the actual birthing, taboos as means of prevention apply to recently delivered women, who are called *mot-soetse* (plural: *bomotsoetse*):

> *Motsoetse* (...) means a woman who has recently given birth, is still nursing her child, is sexually continent and therefore ritually pure. It ceases to be applied after about six months (...) During this period, the *motsoetse* is under the complete control of her parents who feed her, nurse her and provide for her medical attention (Ashton 1952: 29).

The delivery, as the most crucial and dangerous part of the whole transitory experience has to take place in the safe house which only trustworthy wom-en, who will not harm the mother, are allowed to enter. Trust in the person from within the community and whose reputation is known seems to be one of the major features of a home delivery before trust in technical support (ATCBM Kroeker: 08/07/2008). Therefore, a trustworthy and well-known birth attendant is an integral part of the obstetric team among Basotho wom-en. Sargent (1989) emphasises that in Northern Benin, a labouring woman receives the highest merit for having undergone a solitary delivery without the help of a birth attendant. About half of the women in Sargent's sample delivered without birth attendants, which allows the mother to destroy the child if she finds signs of a witch-child (Sargent 1982: 209-210; cf. Einars-dottir 2005). However, a birth attendant was close to the labouring mother and could be called on when help was needed (Sargent 1982: 345).

In Lesotho a birth attendant will be present at all times. Family elders will call a birth attendant at the onset of labour and she will stay until the uncertain situation is over (Field notes Kroeker 4: 04/12/2008). LeNne re-members that the home was made comfortable for the event of upcoming birth. While she was uncertain about the procedures, she was familiar with the place, water was warmed and the fire kindled. Her mother had called in some elder women, among them the traditional birth attendant from their village who LeNne knew and whom she trusted.

Birth attendants in both Northern Benin and Lesotho were elder multip-arous women who assisted deliveries without any specific formal training.

Their expertise derives from experience and practical learning by doing. On the other hand, we also find professional midwives in the communities, who trained as traditional healers (cf. Sargent 1982: 60-63). In Lesotho, village chiefs appoint one or more of them, who receive training within the government health system[9] besides their traditional vocation and formal training with the healers' association. Laywomen as well as trained traditional midwives attend deliveries at the labouring women's maternal home and their main task, thus, was not only to help during the actual delivery as in a biomedical facility, but also to provide trust and confidence, hence, to secure the situation as such. Hermon, an old woman who delivered her ten children in home deliveries, explained that she preferred psychological support as offered by traditional birth attendants while in pain over the medical technology offered in biomedical facilities. She recalls that her mother kept her busy with household activities like cleaning and washing during the gaps in her contractions, before the pauses became too short and she squatted down to deliver (Field notes Kroeker: 15/03/2009).Other mothers in home deliveries mentioned a dorsal position, since they found it more comfortable or the birth attendant asked them to do so[10]. Then the birth attendant instructed the mother not to start pushing too early and determined when pains and position were just right to start, and a healer explained that she therefore observes the mother and therewith recognises from the woman's eyes whether the pains have just started and when they are getting severe (Field notes Kroeker 4: 04/12/2009). According to her observations she will also decide when to interfere if the water does not break in due time and to manually turn the child from a breech into a head-down position (Field notes Kroeker 4: 04/12/2008; cf. Jordan & Davis-Floyd 1993: 27). However, it is usually

---

[9] The public health nurse of Mafeteng Government Hospital disputed that any training sessions had taken place in the last year since there was no curriculum authorised by the Ministry of Health and Social Welfare. She mentioned, however, that in some other districts training sessions were offered without standardised curriculum.

[10] Jordan suggests that the traditional midwife Dona Juana does not advise on the position of the mother in labour and delivery: "Dona Juana says that every woman must buscar la forma (find her own style). For her, the midwife's function is to assist with whatever method the woman comes to find best" (Jordan & Davis-Floyd 1993: 42). The authors also list manifold arguments against the use of the lithotomy position in birth (1993: 85). Schiefenhövel (1983, 2005) and Kuntner (1983, 1985, 1995) also mention that the birthing mothers in non-western societies preferred vertical positions such as standing, kneeling, sitting and squatting. The mothers changed freely between those positions depending on their choice and comfort.

the birth attendant's task to take care that the labouring mother is kept busy and to administer pharmaceuticals to open the uterus.

The uterus had closed after conception and encapsulated the menstrual blood, which fused with the men's *mali* and therewith produced the child (Ashton 1952: 26). In Sesotho, the term *mali* conceptualises ejaculate as well as blood. Yet, in labour, the herbal infusion, *pitsa*, opens the uterus again and therewith facilitates delivery (see Chapter 5.1.4). This second *pitsa*, different from the one women received in traditional antenatal care, induces strong labour pains and abdominal cramps (Field notes Kroeker MaThloni: 09/02/2011), and one informant, MaNne, was convinced she had received a *pitsa* containing mercury which counsellors confirm (Field notes Kroeker: 14/12/2008)[11]. Whether the traditional medication indeed contained mercury or herbal pharmaceuticals or not cannot be confirmed here. However, the infusion is meant to induce severe labour pains in a short time. LeNne recalls, for instance, she had unbearable pains as a consequence of the *pitsa* she had received. At the same time, her birth attendant started massaging her during contractions to comfort her as well as to examine the child's position (cf. Jordan & Davis-Floyd 1993: 27; Sargent 1989: 195). The attendant rubbed her abdomen with balms and ointment prepared in advance, although other healers or midwives, according to reports, also applied warm compresses, which LeNne did not receive. Finally, and thanks to the infusion, contractions only lasted for a few hours before the child was delivered. *Pitsa* thus helps to open and close the uterus quickly and therewith protect women from spiritual misfortune which may enter during that time window.[12] In analogy, Sargent and Bascope describe:

> Local women and midwives share the notion that a rapid delivery is much to be desired as birth is a dangerous time. The sooner it is over,

---

[11] I am not sure though, whether the reference to mercury indeed means the chemical element or, once again, is a recipient design word construction. Considering the chemical element mercury, the German Public Health Office, *Bundesamt für Gesundheit*, warns that mercury resolved in water may dilute and affect the central nervous system and when consumed over some time small amounts cause cramps, shaking, agitation and the like. In unborn children mercury may cause mental impairment (Bundesamt für Gesundheit 2009).

[12] Witchcraft can also affect a newborn while the fontanelles are not yet fully closed. These openings seem to be pathways which allow witchcraft to enter the body. Maternal or infant death always relates to witchcraft affliction unless the mother was found to have neglected rites and taboos during pregnancy (Sargent 1989: 29, 115; Field notes Kroeker MaThloni: 09/02/2011).

> the less time the mother and child are exposed to risk (Sargent & Bascope 1997: 191).

Along the same lines, Jordan mentions a time window of maternal sensitivity surrounding birth in Yucatan:

> Immediately after the birth, mother and infant are considered extremely vulnerable to the influence of spirits from the bush. During the birth, doors are kept shut and all cracks are stuffed with rags in order to keep these spirits out (Jordan & Davis-Floyd 1993: 42).

In Lesotho, as soon as the baby was born birth attendants shared the tasks of caring for mother and child. One attendant instantly sucked "the wax" (*Vernix caseosa)* with her mouth to clear the baby's mouth and nose (Field notes Kroeker: 09/07/2008)[13]. If the nose was blocked birth attendants caused the baby to sneeze in order to ease the air supply. Thereafter the birth attendant cut the umbilical cord as long as the baby's thigh and fixed the cord tightly with a thread (Field notes Kroeker 4: 04/12/2008; Field notes Kroeker Maluela: 20/1/2009). LeNne then received the baby to kiss and cuddle for bonding between mother and child. Following her observations, though, not all mothers are expected to kiss the baby first, often the baby is brought when washed and dressed and after the afterbirth was delivered. For the delivery of the afterbirth LeNne was offered a big pot of *pitsa* again to clean her from inside (Field notes Kroeker 14: 05/12/2008; cf. Griffiths 1990: 25)[14]. LeNne appreciated the *pitsa* which she received post-partum since it relieved her from the abdominal pains she felt after the delivery. At the same time, the traditional birth attendant massaged her womb again. A healer suggested this procedure in case the placenta did not come easily. The massage

---

[13] If the baby makes rattling sounds when breathing it is believed that the vernix was not removed properly. The wax that is still left in the throat will cause that sound. Removing the wax with finger or spatula, an old midwife complains, does not completely remove it, while old healers had techniques to remove it completely and therewith prevent the noise. A nurse agrees that according to her understanding the wax that is left in the baby's windpipe can cause those kinds of coughs and noises (Field notes Kroeker: 26/01/2009). Sucking the wax, however, seems to have died out even among birth attendants, and all informants referred to "the olden days" when it was carried out. Nurses also knew about it but reported this practice to be old-fashioned.

[14] This kind of medication may also have the connotation of cleansing from evil spirits and dangers surrounding the mother, however, this assumption was not explicitly mentioned in interviews and conversations. One mother mentioned that she received peppermint tea as a cleanser directly after giving birth (Field notes Kroeker 1: 27/10/2008).

follows the same moves as during delivery (Field notes Kroeker 4: 04/12/2008). Post-partum, the mother's abdomen will be wrapped tightly with a cotton or wool scarf to facilitate postnatal recovery, hence, to close the womb (Field notes Kroeker 19: 06/04/2009; cf. Jordan & Davis-Floyd 1993: 44).

To be on the safe side, all potential harms shall be taken into account and traditional healers and midwives suggested that expectant mothers should attend antenatal care in the biomedical clinic, where problems may be found which a traditional healer can neither foresee nor treat. With a normal delivery, however, labouring women shall stay at home where traditional birth attendants will offer help for "traditional problems" such as spiritual harms, whereas in the health centre physical dangers will be treated by means of medical technology (ATCBM Kroeker: 10/07/2008).

6.2.2 Safe Disposal of Human Body Parts

In the context of a home delivery good care for mother and child also implies concern about the safe disposal of the afterbirth and umbilical cord. In Basotho culture human body parts and waste may be utilised by jealous people to cause harm to the owner and hence the Basotho take good care of dead body parts such as hair, fingernails and the like, which thus go into the backyard, *seotlo,* the sanctuary of the female ancestors. Comaroff suggests that the floor relates to the ancestors buried in its soil, and certain places in the compound are associated with their security. The *Totobolo* refuse area contains ashes from the house as well as children's faeces as they must not move too far from the inner circle of the homestead when going to the toilet. The afterbirth and umbilical cord will also be buried thoroughly in this place protected by female ancestors.

Kuntner mentions that in the state between life and death one part (that is the child) will live, while a second part, the afterbirth, dies. In various cultures this latter part is also animated and shall be buried, and thus be treated as an entity along with the living body (Kuntner 2004). The dead part would include the placenta, umbilical cord as well as the product of an abortion, miscarriage or a newborn which passed away while the mother was still in seclusion. If the child dies before the umbilical cord falls off, it will be considered as nothing other than water and not fruit. The rituals that apply therefore somewhat relate to those taboos of menstrual blood; miscarriage, early infant death or menstruation are considered as missed opportunities to conceive (Gausset 2002: 634; cf. Ngubane 2002: 274-284). The woman additionally finds herself in a polluted condition which does not allow sexual intercourse and she must firstly be cleansed, which may involve treatment by a healer if witchcraft was detected as the cause of the disorder (Field notes Kroeker 28: 05/12/2008; cf. Kaufman et al. 2000: 16). If a man disrespects the taboo and sleeps with a woman who has not been cleansed after an unfruitful birth, he will die from her pollution since her blood will be hot and dangerous for the man just like menstrual blood (Gausset 2002: 628-650; cf. Ngubane 2002)[15]. If the woman undergoes cleansing it will also end the ritual reproductive cycle and she will thereafter move back to her marital home. The husband will understand from her early return without child that something went wrong[16].

Practices changed due to living and housing conditions in town. The architecture, especially in the urban area, had changed significantly and does not necessarily allow for rites of good care for the mother, child and dead body parts. Urban rentals host known and unknown people and inhabitants may move in and out, hence, *malaene* do not provide any safety but are a melting pot of the familiar and unfamiliar. This fact may contribute to the low number of home deliveries in urban areas. Moreover, room limits, lack of possibilities for spiritual safety and familial care as well as insufficient space to hold everybody involved in obstetric practices make home deliveries unfavourable.

Burials of human body parts must not take place in rented accommodation and urban residents decide instead to take the umbilical cord to their "real home", which is synonymous with their maternal home, where residents will handle it with care. Stillborn children are also often taken to a family's home, although interestingly enough, after a hospital delivery freshly delivered mothers or their relatives did not ask to take the placenta home to bury it, but it was simply thrown away and burned in the hospital's incinerator (Field notes Kroeker: 13/06/2008). Hospital midwives did not recall any case when families had asked to take the afterbirth home to bury it

[15] I was not able to investigate menstrual blood and taboos since none of my close female friends had their period due to the method of contraception. Men, however, they recalled, would fear females at their time of the month and ask "Do you want to kill me?" in the event they found out (Field notes Kroeker: Theko 5/2009).

[16] A father is likewise not informed about the successful birth of a child but will receive this message through a rite, which is rigorously performed today: in the event of the birth of a baby boy the father will be beaten up by brothers and friends and if his offspring is of the female sex, the father shall be doused with water (Ashton 1952: 29; Sechefo n.d.: 26; Field notes Kroeker 24: 5/2009, Makhotso 5/2009).

properly. It might be that in a hospital setting the abundance of human body parts cannot be traced back to the individual persons and hence no harm can be directed towards the owner. Therewith hospitals are somewhat spiritually safe, whereas rural health centres are dangerous. Due to the fact that fewer women deliver in health centres, families may be more concerned about the safe disposal of body parts within the village. People who are jealous and intend to utilise bodily material for evil purposes, may have better access in the health centres.

While practices of burying the placenta have vanished in urban areas, it remains a great concern of urban women to bury the stump of the umbilical cord safely. Mothers were eager to keep it safe until they found a good place for safe disposal as it may otherwise be used for witchcraft. LeMeli's mother-in-law recalls:

> In the old days the cord was put in a mouse- or rat hole to make sure it is eaten up and not misused by anybody else. Since the son's house does not have a mouse hole, they threw [the umbilical cord] in the pit latrine to make sure no one gets hold of it (Field notes Kroeker: 13/01/2009).

Urban women, like my study participants, were more influenced by hospital counselling and less by elder family members. Moreover, some families with residences in urban areas are already in their second generation of hospital deliveries. Nevertheless, being a target of witchcraft remained a constant fear (Sargent 1989: 213).

6.3 Option 2: Rural Health Centres

Apart from a large network of traditional healers and birth attendants, rural clinics also offer biomedical care. The district of Mafeteng provides 18 such local clinics, which serve as satellite clinics in relation to the district hospital. These clinics, respectively health centres (H/C), cover more remote places with biomedical health care and may refer patients for treatment to the district hospital in Mafeteng. While ten of the clinics work in close collaboration with the hospital under government management, a further eight clinics served as missionary health stations under the Christian Health Association of Lesotho (CHAL) until 2007.

Despite higher charges in missionary clinics and limited services they were quite popular in contrast to some government health centres as they combined religious and physical considerations of health and healing similar to traditional healers and had a similar understanding of *bophelo* as life (Field notes Kroeker: Mampho: 11/07/2008). On the other hand, CHAL clinics lacked other technological infrastructure. Depending on space, equipment and staffing some centres were not prepared for deliveries; Catholic missionaries moreover do not provide family planning. Other centres were not equipped for HIV/AIDS medication until they came under the supervision of the Ministry of Health and Social Welfare for finance and quality assurance, which improved infrastructure and service significantly. Some of the Christian as well as some government clinics, moreover, received additional staff from Médecines Sans Frontières (MSF), who started providing HIV treatment and counselling through lay counsellors in 2008. Mothers2Mothers, a South African based NGO, also started in Lesotho's hospitals and health centres in 2008. Both NGOs provide counselling to HIV-positive people with a peer educator-approach, although the latter, Mothers2Mothers, counsels predominantly pregnant and infant feeding women with HIV. This programme started in Mafeteng Government Hospital in June 2007 and in five rural clinics shortly thereafter, and was extended to further rural clinics in 2009. Litsoeneng Health Centre, as one of the clinics which provides counselling for HIV-positive mothers as well as delivery services, should serve as a showcase.

Litsoeneng Health Centre is situated in the outer rural part of Mafeteng District on a windy and desolate plateau close to the South African border. The geographical coverage of the clinic includes 31 villages with a total population of over 7,000 people and the longest distance to the clinic is approximately two hours' walk in an area with poor infrastructure (Mafeteng Government Hospital 1993)[17]. Due to the remote setting the health centre does not have a tarmac road or telephone coverage. The only connection consists of an uneven path on which a private car owner offers transport to and from Mafeteng town once a day, unless the road becomes impassable after heavy rain. For patients and pregnant women this mode of transport was impractical or unfeasible, especially since the fare was high at around 20 ZAR (2008).

Litsoeneng Health Centre was erected as part of a government initiative in 1986 and started operating in March 1987. Most health centres built within this initiative comprise two examination rooms, a storeroom for instruments with a locker for PMTCT and HIV prophylaxis and a storeroom with

---

[17] Since no new health centre has been erected in the area, I assume these numbers to still be more or less valid.

a fridge and other medication, and offers preventive and curative services including family planning. Unlike many health centres, Litsoeneng provides a separate delivery room, which is well-equipped with two beds, a bathtub, toilet and shower (which is used for storing boxes), a cot and all kinds of emergency tools for delivery, that are awaiting sterilisation. Although Litsoeneng offers delivery services, other health centres may not do so in the absence of electricity, space, running water or staff to attend women at night and after hours. Besides these limitations, informants generally had mixed feelings about giving birth in rural health centres and preferred either a home delivery or the district hospital, which is able to host women in waiting mother shelters even in the run up to their delivery. Despite the fact that some pregnant women attended antenatal care in Litsoeneng and other rural health centres, they were not popular for deliveries and clients frequently criticised the limited opening hours. A expectant woman in antenatal care complained: "We discover a problem, that at 6 pm you will find the clinic closed, while you are in labour pains after some time. It's a problem to find help" (ATCBM Kroeker: 08/07/2008). Also health centres are not open during weekends while the hospital still operates, as this woman outlined: "I might have labour pains on Saturday and they are not working on weekends" (ATCBM Kroeker: 12/07/2008). Indeed, some missionary health centres did not have night security and consequently a nurse refused to open the gate at night due to fear of crime (Field notes Kroeker: 10/07/2008). At the same time, medical staff members were bound by the Ministry not to practise outside the health facility, such as helping in home deliveries.

In addition to arguments concerning inadequate staff, an unfamiliar atmosphere and safety, I encountered a major problem in confidence and trust in biomedical health centres on a personal relations level. This was mainly due to the Ministry's work schedule, which allocates nurses on two-year contracts at a particular health centre on an alternating placement. Of course, rural areas were less popular as workplaces amongst nurses, while health centres close to town or the hospital appeared more appealing, leaving unfamiliar and foreign staff to work there. This rotating system, however, prevents a social engagement with the community, which patients often mention as crucial for good medical care and trust. Yet, patients considered good terms and trust in caregivers as an important precondition for quality service and for delivery in particular. Thus, missionary clinics were more popular since the faith-based health centres keep their staff for longer and the church affiliation created a bond with community members. Moreover, sharing ideas on health and healing in a religious as well as a physical sense seems to facilitate a trusting relationship despite the poor conditions and lack of equipment in some missions. The bad reputation of biomedical staff in government health centres, which were rather new in the area, also played a part, while missions had been there since the 19th century and were well accepted.

Mistrust and disapproval of government health workers may also have been part of the local policy as documented in older reports by Mafeteng Hospital on the erection of rural clinics. In some instances the community protested against land allocation for erecting a health centre. This attitude may have been fuelled by missionaries as well as traditional healers who feared competition and mobilised the community to protest. In spite of this disapproval of health centres as birth facilities, the other services they provided were well attended.

6.4 Option 3: Mafeteng Hospital Maternity Ward

The Maternity Ward at Mafeteng Government Hospital was constructed in 1986. The ward has a long corridor with wide doors at both ends, one opening towards the hospital compound and a back-door towards the garden. The facility provides beds for three women in advanced stages of labour, about ten beds for post-partum women and ten for prenatal mothers. At the time the study took place the rooms were spacious and all equipment was fully functional. Mafeteng Hospital's Maternity Ward also comprises a separate examination room for sick mothers with two beds and a small room used for counselling, a premature baby unit with baby warmer, an incubator and photo therapy techniques and a room used for ultrasound scans. Approximately five to eight deliveries are performed a day, most of them as normal vaginal deliveries. Although most women do not consider a caesarean section on demand, they can be performed in a nearby theatre and three study participants opted for it due to their HIV-positive status[18].

---

[18] However, according to a hospital policy, a woman who has delivered by "scissor" (Caesarean Section) before, will have two subsequent deliveries of this type and shall not get pregnant thereafter (Field notes Kroeker: 19/01/2009). Especially very short women and women with complications in pregnancy may be told beforehand that they will deliver under narcosis. Unfortunately I did not get hold of the policy guidelines and this information is based on what I was told by counsellors and midwives. The guidelines may have also given some hints on mother and child care after delivery. According to a student midwife and a nurse, some babies are also under narcosis when delivered by caesarean section depending on the anaesthetic,

Recently, "waiting mother shelters", which provide accommodation for up to an additional 15 expectant women, were erected within the hospital compound. The shelters guarantee direct access to the maternity ward via a back-door. Mainly expectant women from rural areas which lack transport or women at risk of complications chose to stay in the shelters in close proximity to the delivery room since they preferred the hospital to the local clinics (Field notes Kroeker: 08/04/2009).

6.4.1 A Quest for Physical Safety

Patients' arguments in favour of a delivery at a biomedical facility were mostly related to the availability of equipment and trained staff in case complications occurred. Clients who intended to deliver in the hospital mostly considered:

> The hospital is a safe place because if any problem occurs, doctors will be near compared to home (ATCBM Kroeker: 11/07/2008; 15/07/2008; cf. Sargent 1989: 38).

In contrast to home deliveries, personal relations did not play a big part, while technological equipment did. The possible allocation of treatment for the mother and vaccinations for the child qualify the hospital over home births, hence technological ways of intervening were highly appreciated by the expectant mothers and their relatives, who usually made the decision. This stands in stark contrast to those women who preferred to deliver with birth attendants they knew and trusted such as the decision-makers of LeNne and Hermon. However, as in western countries, delivery preferences changed over time and depending on cultural preferences.

While some birthing cultures facilitated a natural birth experience with little or no technological intervention, others preferred technology to reduce pain and labour such as in hospital deliveries in the United States (Lazarus 1997: 128-158). Davis-Floyd & Sargent describe the extent to which the "modern" way of birthing affected procedures in biomedical maternity rooms:

> By the 1940s (…) the progressive, "modern" way of giving birth was to divorce oneself from outdated servitude to biology by giving birth in the hospital under total anaesthesia. Likewise, the progressive par-

---

though I wonder what the guidelines foresee and how this relates to the practice (Field notes Kroeker: 11/07/2008; Mpho: 08/04/2009).

> enting of infants became defined by the bottle and the scheduled feeding instead of the breast. (...) By the late 1960s, the progressive, "modern" way of giving birth was the "natural childbirth" (...) that initially presented a radical and heretical challenge to the dominant orthodoxy of total medical control. Throughout the 1970s and early 1980s, the rhetoric of "natural" or "prepared" childbirth defined the "modern" birth.
>
> In this postmodern era, we have gone beyond (...) the systematic elimination of lay midwifery, the demise of breastfeeding, and even "natural childbirth" to an enormous range of options and historical shifts. These include the presence and active involvement of fathers during pregnancy and at birth; the renaissance of midwifery and of breastfeeding; the spread of freestanding birth centres such as the one in which Trevathan worked; the rising popularity of home birth and water birth; and even "unassisted birth" (Davis-Floyd & Sargent 1997: 9).

Jordan and Davis-Floyd (1993) compared the degree of medicalisation of child birth in Yucatan, the United States, the Netherlands, and Sweden and recognised different levels of technological intervention of labour and pain relief in the standardised practice. Personnel in the US considered birthing as a rather pathological situation, which also justified the standardised use of medical technology in the course of labour and delivery. Sweden also proffers a high level of technology with standardised pain relief medication and minimum distress for mother and child. Yucatan and the Netherlands show higher rates of home deliveries attended by trained midwives, instead of doctors as in the US and Sweden. The Netherlands, with scant technological intervention and the basic idea of a "natural birth experience", suggested increased comfort for the mother paired with the lowest infant and maternal mortality rates. In Yucatan, manual instead of technical interventions were applied to assure a successful birth result. Besides a traditionally trained midwife, lay assistants, who were close community members, were actively involved in the birthing process. The mother for her part was also considered an active part of the obstetric team whereas, in contrast, in highly technological settings medical staff rather authorised birthing procedures (Jordan & Davis-Floyd 1993). Thus, mothers who favoured a biomedical delivery focused on technological options in the event of complications during birth, which is regarded as more important than being close to home or amongst family members. Medical staff for their part emphasised their authority due to the complex birth procedures, which would disqualify lay persons as birth attendants. They criticised conditions as unsafe due to unsterile conditions and the substandard expertise of lay midwives[19] (Field notes Kroeker 4: 14/11/2008; Jordan & Davis-Floyd 1993: 149).

In both the biomedical staff and their client's perception, physical harm that was detected in antenatal care, irrespective of the cause, was related to biomedical trained attendance. Particularly an infection with HIV was seen as a risk that must not be managed by traditional birth attendants but biomedically trained staff. Moreover, pregnant women with complicated deliveries, to which women carrying the HI-virus belonged, should refrain from a delivery in a health centre which was also not well-equipped when it came to complications (Field notes Kroeker Makoa: 11/07/2008). Counsellors and nurses hence appealed and encouraged women who attended antenatal care in a rural health centre to deliver in hospital and staff particularly promoted the new waiting mother shelters in the hospital to mothers from rural areas.

As outlined before, antenatal care serves as a source of knowledge on pregnancy and delivery as well as confirmation of the well-being of mother and child. Hence antenatal care indicates risks other than the spiritual risks a healer will be able to detect in a complementary way. If a risk is detected by either, healer or nurse, an expectant mother will approach them again for further consultation, check-up and treatment. The information expectant women received about their condition in antenatal care influenced their preference on where to deliver. In some cases, expectant mothers remained in hospital after complications were discovered in antenatal care, and in the event they moved back home many returned for a biomedical delivery. MaThloni confirms this to be a general rule:

> If the nurse tells the expectant mothers that everything is alright with her and the baby, they would go to the traditional birth attendant, that is, the traditional healer for deliveries. If they expect any complications they would consider coming to the clinic for delivery (Field notes Kroeker: 12/07/2008).

---

[19] Although I did not get to talk to birth attendants in the villages but only in the traditional clinic, I assume that their skills were underestimated rather than non-existent, as Jordan also realised: "It became apparent that the midwives, who in the environment of hospital-based training courses often appeared stupid, illiterate, and inarticulate, showed a completely different face when engaged in doing their work in their own communities, where their skills were acknowledged and respected" (Jordan & Davis-Floyd 1993: 149).

Even though clients do not necessarily have to stay in hospital after being diagnosed with minor abnormalities, some clients did so and favoured a hospital delivery as a result. Along the same lines, women who experienced complications during a previous home delivery (either in their own history or with family members) preferred a hospital delivery thereafter. Physical difficulties were positively correlated with a biomedically attended confinement, as also confirmed by Sargent in her study in Northern Benin (Sargent 1982: 295). In Lesotho, a switch from traditional to biomedical birth attendance often had some history in a loss of trust in the respective birth attendant. Trust in medical technology replaced this in the hospital setting in the event of complications during birth. One pregnant mother tells me:

> She is currently pregnant with her eighth child which she is going to deliver at the hospital. Six of her children were delivered at home but the last child was delivered in the clinic after encountering complications that led to the infant's death. She comments: "It is necessary to deliver at the clinic these days, because there are so many diseases that are not cured. I reckon that for pregnant women it is necessary to deliver in the hospital, because the village health workers don't take HIV/AIDS serious at all" (ATCBM: Matelile 16/07/2008).

Another girl aged 21 lost her first baby after having a home delivery. Yet, she blames her relatives for not having taken good care of her during delivery and refers to her bad experience as a strong argument for having a hospital delivery. Moreover, she tested HIV-positive in her antenatal examinations and therefore decided she required some medical attention. Her family supports this decision due to the unsuccessful home delivery last time which resulted in the baby's death (ATCBM Kroeker: 10/07/2008).

HIV was the most common disorder that was detected in pregnancy after the test became a standardised practice and posed a strong argument for a biomedical delivery. Almost 28% of the women in antenatal care in Mafeteng Hospital were found to carry the virus (ICAP 2009) and many mothers assumed HIV to be a disorder that needed biomedical attendance, which may have resulted from the introduction of special counselling for HIV-positive mothers in 2007. In short, mothers who tested positive in antenatal care recognised this to be a risk and were hence more likely to decide in favour of a biomedical delivery, and at least some facilities recognised an increase in the number of hospital deliveries thereafter as well as a significant decrease in the number of HIV-positive infants born in Mafeteng Government Hospital

(Field notes Kroeker: 01/2010)[20]. However, as in the abovementioned case, elders may not have considered HIV as an argument. While many expectant mothers were concerned about a HIV transmission, the difficult decision-making process at home due to their interaction with elders challenged young mothers. In particular, young women were anxious to disclose the test result, however, without disclosure it was difficult for them to present arguments in favour of a biomedically supervised delivery. As a matter of fact, disclosure of the seropositive status to elders and decision-makers may also result in a loss of reputation and some family elders were informed about antenatal care findings by checking the medical booklet, just as Robong had attempted (Chapter 5.4). Others hence used hidden strategies to convince their relatives of their exigent wish to give birth in a biomedical unit and other complications served as a means to the end when convincing elders.

6.4.2 Decision-making Agency: MaRobeli

HIV-positive women, who preferred to deliver at one place but were afraid of raising their point with elders, sometimes found creative ways of dealing with the situation. However, some found themselves in a vulnerable situation that scarcely allowed for an open dispute with their relatives. For one, they often depend on their family financially, but secondly, being with child as well as being sick entails a strong reliance on support from a large social network. Losing reputation and face may weaken the support granted by members within that network. Therefore, MaRobeli, who had tested positive and with pregnancy related high blood pressure (pre-eclampsia) in antenatal care, convinced her in-laws to let her have a hospital delivery and further medical check-ups without discussing her status with them:

> When I meet MaRobeli, aged 25, for the first time, she did not give the impression that she was unhappy about staying in the hospital. In the contrary, she seemed to enjoy the community, visited other wards and ran errands for less fit patients. Later I learned that she had tricked her mother-in-law to letting her stay in hospital since MaRobeli feared her mother-in-law would prefer a home delivery for her. Hence, MaRoboeli wanted to take over control over the decision without having to discuss her health condition.

---

[20] It, however, needs to be added that the above mentioned study on maternal and infant mortality included the whole of Lesotho, while both my studies only addressed women in the urban lowlands of the Mafeteng District.

> In antenatal care she had learned about her HIV-positive status and high blood pressure. MaRobeli did not expect her in-laws, particularly the mother-in-law, to understand about HIV and PMTCT, while she wanted to adhere to the counsellor's advice due to an earlier miscarriage, which she related to an undetected infection. She therefore preferred the waiting mother shelters as her residence even though she could have been treated in her local health centre while staying at home. During the festive season, when her husband was home, she moved back there temporarily. Shortly after Christmas and after he went back to the mines MaRobeli was back in the hospital. She had told her in-laws that minor pregnancy pains had commenced and that she felt dizzy again. Whenever she needed to go for a check-up in the hospital and requested the bus fare she pointed at high-blood pressure check-ups, though she was well aware that she underwent an examination of her immune system due to HIV. Again she stayed in the hospital for observation without any onset of labour. On the 19th of January she gave birth to twin boys, one of which passed away. After the delivery she moved to her maternal home where she expected to stay as long as possible in order to comply with the PMTCT advice on infant feeding without her mother-in-law's interference.

Perhaps due to intensive counselling during several visits to the health facility and the counsellors emphasising that a mother who does not comply with biomedical recommendations harms her baby[21], many expectant mothers made efforts to give birth in the hospital even if their relatives were not supportive. Moreover, women who attended counselling several times were more familiar with the facility and staff, which increased their confidence in them. In conclusion, most of my HIV-positive study participants opted for a biomedically supervised setting as shown in the following table:

---

[21] Du Plessis, a Senior Scientist of the South African Medical Research Council quotes Wilton to support her argument for preventing offspring in HIV-positive women: "Someone who understands the disease and is logical will not want to be pregnant and will consider the test results when making family planning decisions". Wilton (1997) emphasises that blame is often attached to any women who falls pregnant in her HIV-positive state: "But concern for the baby always outweighs concern for the mother, and a mother who, along with giving life, gives her baby a fatal illness becomes the opposite of a mother" (Wilton 1997 in: Du Plessis 2003: 84).

Education	Hospital	Home	Health centre	Trad. clinic	Number
Primary (Std. 1-7)	7	2 +1 ?	-	1	11
Secondary (A-E)	14	-	-	1	15
Tertiary	3	1 ?	-	-	4
Total	24	3+2 ?	-	2	30

Place of Birth (Fieldnotes Kroeker 2008-2009)

Some apparently concealed where they delivered their baby. Especially those who gave birth at home may have lied and from interviews and observations I conclude that five women may have delivered at home even though only three told me so.

6.4.3 Delivering on the Maternity Ward

The delivery room at Mafeteng Government Hospital provides three beds for labouring women whose progress can be easily monitored by one staff member. Yet, Mafeteng Hospital provides its maternity ward with two members of staff: a registered nurse and an assistant nurse but they were often understaffed for the five to eight deliveries per day (Field notes Kroeker: 26/02/2009). In order to better manage the work load for birth attendants a few organisational and architectural amendments were indispensable.

In the middle of the corridor of the maternity ward a niche provides a space where staff gather, the mothers' obstetric books are collected, and from where all rooms can be easily monitored. Through glass windows it was possible to look into the rooms, yet, most of the times the curtain of the delivery room was closed. For other rooms it was possible at any given time to monitor mothers and their children. For the same reason, there are also no room dividers which would give some privacy to the labouring women or those recovering from their delivery. For women in severe labour pains who had already moved to the labour room it was therefore possible to interact with two further women in the same condition. One nurse attended up to three deliveries at the same time.

Furthermore, one nurse will check the opening of the uterus of all labouring mothers from time to time and perhaps allow little walks in the corridor until the contractions come closer together. When the time arrives the mothers will generally shout and the staff will check once more. Notwithstanding, depending on the work rota the nurse may also be male, although I did not hear any complaints from mothers about the gender of the midwife. Yet, there was a general staff shortage and particularly in the case of an emergency nurses from all wards will be called at once leaving other patients by themselves. In one instance I observed, the nurse had to handle the delivery of the woman on her own, despite the fact that several women usually populate the delivery room in the advanced stages of labour, leaving the nurse to run outside and find an assistant.

Usually, the nurse only arrives for the actual delivery, prepares her tools and arranges the mother in a position which allows good monitoring. The mother will lie on a plastic lining, which provides a flap at one end to collect water, blood and afterbirth and hence needs to be positioned in a functional way close to the end of a normal bed since beds with foot rests were not available. Due to the infrastructure and the need for nurses to monitor the birth process closely only one birthing position applies: a dorsal position (lithotomy position). In biomedical health facilities in Europe a lithotomy position applies as the most common position and missionaries favoured this position within their health facilities overseas, while in home deliveries other positions were preferred (Sargent 1989: 176; Cosminsky 1986; Kuntner 1985). Bio-mechanically, a dorsal position puts more pressure on the perineum and therewith enhances the likelihood of an episiotomy, while in home deliveries, in an international comparison, vertical positions apply such as standing, squatting, kneeling, and sitting as well as (lateral) lying down (Schiefenhövel 1983: 41-56; Field notes Kroeker: 09/06/2008; 15/03/2009). Binder-Fritz summarises debates surrounding birthing positions favouring shifts during labour and delivery:

> In general, an upright position of the body effects a shorter duration of labour due to better efficiency of labour, while a combination of particular vertical positions of the woman in labour is mostly considered more comfortable and shortened the duration of the delivery (Binder-Fritz 1995: 98)[22].

Jordan, who attended several deliveries when accompanying a traditional midwife in Yucatan, described two usual positions for delivering women:

---

[22] The German original reads: "Eine aufrechte Körperhaltung bewirkt im allgemeinen durch bessere Weheneffizienz eine kürzere Wehendauer, wobei eine Kombination zwischen den einzelnen vertikalen Körperpositionen von der Gebärenden meist als angenehmer empfunden wird und auch zur Verkürzung der Geburtsdauer beiträgt" (Binder-Fritz 1995: 98, translation mine).

lying in a hammock or squatting in an upright position. Tearing and other complications were rare in the home deliveries Jordan attended although many mothers were delivering for the first time (Jordan & Davis-Floyd 1993: 35). She also relates this to the fact that women were actively involved in decision-making on the most comfortable position. A traditional birth attendant would suggest a position, however, it was up to the mother to change to a more comfortable one, unlike in the hospital where a dorsal position is enacted to enable birth attendants to access and supervise the mother's abdomen and private parts at all times (Jordan 1997: 55-79)[23].

In Lesotho, biomedical staff explained that they use a dorsal position despite known disadvantages. A nurse explains:

> We have heard that they are squatting at home, (…) and here in the hospital they are lying on their back. That's not the most comfortable position, but we are using it in the hospital (Field notes Kroeker Mampho: 22/03/2007).

While the dorsal position remained the most widely used in Euro-American teaching hospitals, the sources of authoritative knowledge in developing countries, the standardised utilisation of technology changed the birthing experience for women significantly.

The mother will receive a sign from the nurse on when to start pushing. She must not push too early despite the impulse to bear down since it would cause, in the nurse's opinion, great pressure on the child. Early pushing would also exhaust women and they are hence encouraged to withstand the pain. The nurse in the meantime will stand ready at the end of the bed to receive the child's head as soon as she pronounced the mother ready to push (see also Jordan & Davis-Floyd 1993: 157). Davis-Floyd and Sargent 1997 compare this way of delivery with home deliveries and conclude that in less technologically supervised birth settings women *deliver*, whereas in highly technological facilities, such as hospitals, women *are delivered.*

When the child is delivered its sex is announced and the *vernix* covering nose and mouth will be removed using the finger or a spatula. The umbilical cord is clipped and the child is handed to the mother for bonding. The nurse will wrap the child with a towel and dress it with clothes provided by

---

[23] I will not enter the debate on birthing positions here, since for this study authority in decision-making is what matters rather than the consequences, unless related to PMTCT. Nevertheless, I am aware of the link to Foucault's panopticon (1991), an institution of supervision and control which signifies means of impersonalised power.

the mother until the afterbirth is delivered and an episiotomy is sewn. The mother receives cotton wool, which she also had to provide, to dab further bleeding. She will then climb from the table, dress herself with her blanket, and walk to the post-natal room where the baby is also taken. The order of tasks may vary depending on staff, birthing procedure, and the number of women delivering at any one time.

While all deliveries I attended were supervised by a nurse, some other women reported that they were left alone, unaware of what to do and when to push. The possibility of having to deliver on one's own scares mothers who therefore prefer home deliveries, which, as a matter of course, allow individualised attention (cf. Sargent 1989: 63, 210).

Jordan stresses that this attitude relates to the technology used during birth. In a biomedical facility with technological procedures such as foetal monitor, episiotomy, forceps, epidural anaesthesia and the like, authoritative knowledge is rather hierarchically distributed (Jordan 1997: 55-79). The hierarchy consists of doctor, nurse, assistant nurse, intern and last, but not least, the mother, as depicted in the flow of communication. While in Lesotho no particular tools or machines are involved in the standardised birth, the staff's authority, without a doubt, resembles the one in Jordan's example. She contrasts this notion with observations in Mexican home deliveries attended by a traditional assistant. As suggested in narrations of home deliveries in Yucatan and Lesotho, a rather different distribution of decision-making authority applies. The birthing mothers took active part in decisions, while her knowledgeable assistants merely gave recommendations on the birthing position. Jordan described this as a rather horizontal flow of authority in contrast to hospital deliveries (Jordan 1997: 60, 72). The personal relationship between assistant and woman in labour seems to be a factor in these contrasting notions. While familiar women supervise their family's offspring in a home delivery, in a hospital the nurse's care is out of detached professional interest, not personal concern.

Trevathan points out that the emotional support of a caring delivery team, as a home delivery team assures, contributes to improve the biomedical success in birthing. Of course, a close relative or familiar birth assistant will treat a woman in labour in a different way than an unfamiliar nurse in a sterile biomedical facility. By all accounts, trust and individual care seem a crucial argument in home delivery.

> As many have pointed out, the most important service provided by birth attendants in most world cultures is emotional support for the

> birthing woman. (...) For millions of years the birthing female was the most important member of the "obstetrical team," but today her knowledge about her body is often suppressed and "managed." In many contemporary birthing settings it is assumed that the woman has nothing to tell about her body or the birth and that only the machines and medical gatekeepers have the knowledge necessary to produce a healthy baby. (...) Recent work by John Kennell, Marshall Klaus, and their colleagues suggests that not only does emotional and social support contribute to more positive feelings about birth, it also serves to improve the biomedical outcome of birth (Trevathan 1997: 83-84)[24].

Jordan and Davis-Floyd (1993: 67) make the same criticism: "In short, it appears that the importance of human companionship during labour and birth has been vastly underestimated by the Western biomedical community". Indeed, relatives caring for the mother individually will only be seen in the post-natal room, while the labour room is the exclusive meeting place of labouring mothers and staff.

Despite the availability of technical instruments which help in emergencies, expectant women and their families feared that an understaffed maternity ward and overworked nurses may leave the mother in labour to deliver on her own, a great fear in a most crucial phase "in between life and death". Besides the frightening atmosphere of an unfamiliar place, such as the maternity ward of a hospital, mothers and their next-of-kin feared that nurses would not arrive in time for the delivery or only at the last minute. Although narrators easily over-exaggerated their stories and blamed biomedical staff for having caused unsatisfactory situations, rumours about insulting, careless treatment by nurses and negligence during labour, whether true or false, were many and significantly influenced fellow women. Indeed, frequently avowed concerns amongst peers discussing the place of delivery had a major opinion-building influence on decision-making. Especially the idea that women in labour would be slapped, insulted and scolded by moreover unfamiliar people, in an anonymous and sterile environment without privacy and without the support of relatives, put expectant women off (ATCBM Kroeker: 08/07/2008; cf. Sargent 1982: 336; Sargent 1989: 53, 210).

Medical staff, for their part, admitted that particularly first-time mothers do not behave in the required way in labour. Disappointment, if biomedical

---

[24] Reference is moreover made to Frédérick Leboyer's works on birth without violence.

advice was not taken, was sometimes evident and led to frustration amongst staff, especially in times of high workload and when working with uncooperative colleagues or facing staff shortages. In this dilemma, two sisters, who both have one child which was delivered in hospital, summarise:

> We discovered what all mothers discover there. The nurses leave you alone, you don't know what to do with your first pregnancy they insult you and sometimes even slap you. (...It) is now that I know what to expect in my second delivery, but I am even more afraid about having complications while delivering at home. I definitely want to go to hospital, even if the baby is coming fast. I don't want to deliver with untrained people (Field notes Kroeker 14: 23/11/2008).

Therewith, the debate on the place of delivery basically boils down to a debate on trust in good care due to personal relations with the birth attendant, versus good care due to available technology in a biomedical setting, which would not be available at home. Home delivery is preferred due to social and spiritual safety as well as trust in good familial care in a frightening situation. Being surrounded by family members at this anxious time would comfort the mother, while loneliness would increase tension. Since during a delivery, which entails supernatural forces and dangers, harm can happen to mother, child or relatives, this may be considered a reason for a home delivery. In contrast, a preference for the hospital as a place of delivery primarily entailed trust in medical technology and professional expertise, and good personal relations was a secondary factor as a mother of three said:

> I always chose the hospital, where I knew many people, so they will treat me very well and look after me" (Field notes Kroeker Sylvia: 09/07/2008).

A 43-year-old mother of four delivered all her children in the hospital but attends antenatal care in her local health centre. She believes that the antenatal service is good there "but she wouldn't deliver here because she does not have a good relationship with the nurse". Her husband also does not trust the nurses at the clinic. The same reason led to the decision of a husband from a village out in the rural part of Mafeteng District: "There are some we are not on good terms with, so I don't want my wife to be helped by someone I dislike". In both cases the women travelled far to give birth in hospital.

LeNne does not share traditional notions on pregnancy and delivery and gathered most of her information through the hospital counselling sessions, nevertheless delivering there seems unfavourable to her and she found a birth facility that combines both schools of care (Field notes Kroeker 14: 25/02/2009).

6.5 Option 4: Giving Birth at the Traditional Clinic

Since 2000, a traditional healer, who is specialised in midwifery, runs a birth clinic about 15 km outside of Mafeteng town. The compound is decorated with colourful flags, while analogous houses of recently delivered women are marked with reed to warn passers-by[25]. Her compound is well connected to a tarmac road, visible and widely known throughout Lesotho according to her own statement. Apparently, she receives clients from all districts of Lesotho as well as from beyond. Most of Maluela's clients attended antenatal care in a biomedical facility beforehand and move to the traditional clinic in their last trimester, instead of moving to their parent's house. Some mothers thus stay for several weeks while others only arrive in time for the delivery.

> LeNne derived from a remote village in the South Eastern district of Qacha's Nek and came now to Mafeteng while pregnant with her third child. She had known about her infection with HIV for some years and had also trained as a peer educator for people living with HIV. While still in Qacha's Nek LeNne attended antenatal care twice at the district hospital but then decided to move to her sister living in the urban area of Mafeteng in her 7th month of pregnancy.
> Due to her training LeNne was eager to prevent a transmission of the virus to the child but also feared a delivery in the hospital since she had delivered twice at home and had appreciated the atmosphere there. LeNne stresses that hospital staff may be rude and shout if she does not behave according to their expectations and she is afraid that the way she is used to is not appropriate in the hospital. At home she was treated individually, while in the hospital she doesn't have a personal treatment but is one amongst others. On the medical side she neither wants to have an episiotomy. At home no one would bother about sewing after a natural tearing[26]. When she had received a high

---

[25] The colour of the flags, white and red, refers to the ancestors and the colours of her totemic clan (Field notes Kroeker: 10/06/2008).

[26] Tearing is also rare in non-biomedical deliveries in Europe in contrast to biomedical settings where about two thirds of the women experience an episiotomy. I am not sure whether there are biological or traditional conditions in Lesotho that are able to prevent tearing in

> CD4-count above 500 duplications and PMTCT medication to administer by herself in labour and after delivery she decided to be safe in the traditional clinic of Maluela (Field notes Kroeker 14: 25/02/2009).

In accordance with Browner and Press' observations, women in prenatal care "rely on their own embodied knowledge more heavily than a clinician's opinions; in contrast, they acquiesce to biomedical authority when it is backed by the power of technology" (Browner & Press, 1997: 127). LeNne accepted biomedical care and technology to confirm her well-being and decided then for a more comfortable treatment at Maluela's traditional clinic. It turns out that most of Maluela's clients attend a biomedical antenatal clinic before they deliver in the traditional facility, while they fear ill-treatment from hospital staff. Ironically, the nearby health centre (about 2 km) is not equipped to perform deliveries (Field notes Kroeker Maluela: 21/01/2009; Mathato 21/01/2009). In contrast, the traditional clinic is spacious and well equipped. Maluela's compound contains two *rondavels* with the usual reed fence that creates a shaded vestibule and various rectangular buildings. One of the houses serves as waiting mother shelter for about 15 expectant women at that time, an examination *rondavel*, a delivery *rondavel*, and a self-catered kitchen in a clean and well maintained condition. Just as the nurses in the rural clinics, the healer stays at the compound and she or her daughter are available day and night to assist in the delivery. Maluela delivered her six children in a biomedical hospital before she became a healer and therefore combines biomedical experience and traditional knowledge in her facility. The examination in the traditional clinic includes the same tests as in biomedical care (Field notes Kroeker 14: 25/02/2009; Maluela: 21/01/2009). The healer likewise performs a vaginal examination with her finger[27], uses gloves, and examines breasts and abdomen with her hands. However, an exchange of patients and information between the traditional and the biomedical facility only exists gradually and only if complications occur or are expected. Some clients at the facility told about a recent case in which Maluela organised transport for a client to be taken to hospital when the healer recognised difficulties (Field notes Kroeker 14: 25/02/2009). Yet, she

---

Basotho women. However, a relaxed atmosphere, longer time for the tissue to stretch slowly and massages with special oil or balm can prevent episiotomies. All conditions which are provided in home deliveries and with traditional antenatal care.

[27] Jordan (1993: 28) observed that Dona Juana, a traditional midwife never performs vaginal examinations and believes that the midwife's hands should stay out of the birth canal. In Lesotho, medical staff and traditional birth attendants perform vaginal examinations.

must have observed these difficulties through her examinations, since clients denied that their medical booklet was checked.

The healer will inform the mother how far along the child is and approximately how long it is going to take, listens to the child's heartbeat, and examines the baby's position. Just as in a biomedical facility, Maluela provides the same instruments, disposable knifes and gloves and recommends a dorsal position. Surprisingly, however, she disapproves of using *pitsa* unless a mother is unwell and labour needs to be induced (Field notes Kroeker Maluela: 21/01/2009; Mathato: 21/01/2009). In that case Maluela receives this information through her ancestors. Whatever complications a client experiences, she also has to go through and "experience" it for herself at the request of her ancestors. Through her body she will know how to help the parturient mother (Field notes Kroeker Maluela: 21/01/2009; Mathato: 21/01/2009). For the actual delivery Maluela has two helpers: two doves live in the *rondavel* which is used for maternity and Maluela explains that they will start cooing whenever a mother is almost due to deliver. Maluela will then visit her waiting room and accompany the respective woman to her delivery room:

> LeNne explains that the doves cried when she was in labour and Maluela brought her to the delivery hut. The labour pains then stopped again and the baby was easily delivered onto the floor. She observed that the healer used rubber gloves and a disposable knife for cutting the umbilical cord.
>
> After the delivery first the *vernix caseosa* was taken from the baby's nose and mouth. Maluela did not suck it like other healers told, but used her finger for removal. The umbilical cord was tied with a thread and Maluela washed the baby's face. She then put it aside to massage LeNne's womb. This time, in contrast to her home deliveries before, she did not receive traditional medication to deliver the placenta. After the mother was cared for the baby's *vernix* was peeled off and collected into a little container, before the baby was washed. LeNne was told to bath the baby with it, since it brings good fortune to the baby's life.
>
> After Maluela had bathed the baby boy he was brought to suckle. They then had to shift to another room, so that the delivery room could be cleaned. Afterbirth and cotton wool that was left in the delivery room was then disposed into a special toilet that only Maluela uses, while waiting and delivering mothers use two separate ones on the compound (Field notes Kroeker 14: 25/02/2009).

According to Mathato, the district healers' representative, traditional midwives should check the medical book and direct HIV-positive mothers to the hospital. However, as a matter of fact, the *Bukana* is not regularly checked, since Maluela receives the information about the women's conditions through her ancestors and the HIV status is of no interest to her.

> Being a peer educator and spending much time in the expectant mother house with 13 other women LeNne brought up the subject of HIV, though, the healer did not want to discuss it with her. LeNne, who intended to comply with her PMTCT-treatment nonetheless decided to be secretive about the tablets. By the time her labour pains started around 10 p.m. she administered her tablets from the hospital package. LeNne administered the second dose of ARV for the baby boy again secretly the morning after (Field notes Kroeker 14: 25/02/2009).

I tell LeNne in a later conversation that Maluela emphasised that she does not deliver HIV-positive women but instead refers them to hospital. She apparently knows the mother's status through the ancestors. LeNne laughs: "she is lying if she knows through the ancestors. She didn't ask me about it, but delivered me in her clinic".

Despite LeNne's disrespect for Maluela's mindset she was satisfied with the delivery. LeNne kept the umbilical cord to take it home to Quacha's Nek district and bury it at her house. Despite that fact she was staying in Mafeteng at the time of her delivery she disapproves of leaving a body part at her sister's rented accommodation.

6.5.1 LeTharo's Bad Delivery

Interestingly, the absence of traditional hazards encouraged a hospital delivery, as a sterile hospital setting may also be free from invisible, traditional harms. Thus, the hospital would be a safer place for a delivery, whereas at home witchcraft may harm mother and child if the traditional preventive procedures are neglected. The disregard for spiritual harm in a biomedical facility was mentioned by some interviewees as an advantage, such as by a 22-year-old. She was staying with 6-8 people in the household and had already had a baby, which had passed away a year after. Now, in her third month of pregnancy, she states: "I want to deliver in hospital, although I do not know how to get there, because at home there are people who will bewitch me" (ATCBM Kroeker: 18/07/2008). To prevent this mishap a second time, she should go for the hospital delivery to be on the safe side this time.

However, she got into a conflict with other expectant mothers in the waiting mother shelters over stolen belongings. She assumed that, following a quarrel, their relatives tried to apply witchcraft to her while staying in the shelters. Some power loaded item was attached to her door, however, this time it did not harm her or the child.

Witchcraft affliction in pregnancy was a constant fear and Sargent also mentions that families, irrespective of what their educational background and life style indicated, feared malevolent powers sent by jealous fellows. The means to control this was nevertheless a problem, too. The accurate fulfilment of prohibitions and prescriptions shall assure well-being of mother and child, however, on the other hand one must also not over-do it (cf. Whyte 1997: 29). MaMong, for example, believed that traditional protections can sometimes bring about evil instead of preventing it. That is also why she does not want to use anything like traditional medication or charms but relies solely on prayers for herself and the baby (Field notes Kroeker 21: 16/04/2009). LeTharo, nevertheless, experienced witchcraft in her house despite her prayers:

> LeTharo, who is an evangelical pastor by profession, and especially confronted with malevolent powers, also prayed a lot for herself and her child: While she was pregnant her husband fell victim to criminal violence and passed away weeks after due to the head injuries he had suffered. Just before this incident LeTharo was tested HIV-positive in antenatal care, a very surprising and confusing situation, which she denied to be true. She therefore assumed witchcraft to be involved in these recent bitter changes in her life. Due to her strong Christian belief she disapproves of traditional re-instalments of health and well-being. LeTharo suggests praying as the only means to fight witchcraft and prevent harm which is caused by jealousy and greed.

MaKhotso, a pastor's sister, explains accordingly that "true" Christians believe in the existence of witchcraft, but use a different approach to fight its harms. True Christians believe that prayers will help protect them from harm and believers therefore refuse traditional schools of health and healing (Field notes Kroeker: 08/12/2008).

> LeTharo did not take any traditional medication during her pregnancy but realised malevolent powers of witches around her premises. LeTharo felt the heat in the house, which usually surrounds witches

> and also saw them with their cats in her dreams. Wicked people also must have placed faeces in front of her house.
> Eventually, the pastor left her parish to stay with her brother-in-law. Despite this attempt to avoid the afflicted premises, she found herself in labour for five days.[28] After she could not get rid of this witchcraft affliction by moving place, she had to shift again to the hospital where LeTharo eventually had to deliver by caesarean section after labour-inducing injections did not work either. A private doctor[29] diagnosed that she had been bewitched and advised her to refrain from breast-feeding since her milk will also be affected and hence poisonous for the child. LeTharo eventually accepted treatment to cleanse her from wicked powers and feed the child with milk formula only. Retrospectively, she also relates the darkness of her amniotic fluid, dark debouchement, a long labour, and her bad birthing experience to witchcraft (Fieldnotes Kroeker 13: 29/04/2009).

Similar to LeTharo, MaMong is also convinced that too much protection can have the opposite effect and consequently attract evil, although incorrectly applied medication can also provide opportunities for witches. For LeTharo, staying at home did not work and the hospital delivery was not good either.

Notions differed on the appearance of witchcraft in hospital settings and Binder-Fritz (1995) cautions, however, that a hospital is a place full of spiritual hazards. Firstly, it is an unfamiliar place, secondly, a place of sick people and thirdly, one where people die. Therefore, a hospital is a highly loaded place where behavioural taboos must protect the living, especially sensitive people in between life and death such as newly delivered mothers and newborns. Neither mothers in Lesotho nor in Benin (Sargent 1989: 38) shared this notion. While some tried to neutralise witchcraft affliction, others avoided places where harmful substances are placed. Perceptions on where this may be and how witchcraft may be prevented remained somewhat blurry to them but their family elders may have made a decision on the safest place taking various dangers into account.

In any case, several mothers did not like living with other women in a transitional and therewith polluted condition in the waiting refuges provided

---

[28] "Five days" seemed to be a rhetorical figure LeTharo mentioned in the interview after her return to Mafeteng. As she was not around during the time of labour and delivery, I was not able to visit and talk to her.

[29] She avoids the term "*ngaka*" or "*sangoma*" and prefers "private doctor" although there is no doubt that her practitioner follows a traditional school of health and healing.

by the hospital. Reasons for that were, however, not necessarily associated with witchcraft but other causes. Some expectant women disliked staying in the huts due to discomfort, shared rooms and the use of traditional medication that can have harmful effects on room-mates and passers-by. Others argued that their personal belongings would be stolen by fellow mothers or their visitors since the shelters cannot be locked (Field notes Kroeker: 10/07/2008; 08/04/2009). Moreover, some women missed their relatives' care and assistance in household activities, while in the shelters cleaning and the like would be shared amongst all pregnant women providing comfort and a sense of community. In conclusion, the decision on where to deliver was never an easy one, something which some mothers enjoyed handing over to those who knew from experience.

Options for Safe Infant Feeding

In many African societies, long-term mixed feeding is the cultural norm for various reasons. Breastfeeding is an essential part of infant care and about 95% of children in Lesotho are nursed for a length of time along with an early introduction of additional food stuff (MoHSW et al. 2010: 138). Aside from the nutritional aspects, breastfeeding undoubtedly entails a social inter-linkage and with respect to the bond between mother and child, breastfeeding gives the baby a social home. Desclaux and Alfieri even identified breastfeeding to be a most essential feature of "good mothering" in Sub-Saharan Africa (Desclaux & Alfieri 2011). Nutritional, as well as social and emotional reasons for mother and child, support breastfeeding of an infant, whereas non-breastfeeding is associated with stigma and may even reveal a mother's HIV status (Desclaux & Alfieri 2009; Moland 2004: 94). Notwithstanding this, breastfeeding, as with pregnancy and delivery, underwent a medicalisation. Along these lines, Davis-Floyd and Sargent (1997), Kneuper (2003) and Binder-Fritz (2003) criticised the notion of contraception, child-birth and infant feeding as medical events which are consequently controlled and supervised by health professionals.

For HIV-positive mothers manifold aspects need to be taken into consideration. Besides social and nutritional aspects, there is the additional risk of transmitting the virus to the child via breast milk. Undoubtedly, learning about one's HIV-positive status nevertheless affects the mother's behaviour. Kisanga assumes that people who know about their status are more likely to be motivated to look after their own health and that of their partner, to seek more information about HIV/AIDS, and to make informed decisions about their lifestyle, including sexual behaviour, child-bearing, and specifically how they feed their infants (Kisanga 2000: 9). Additional biomedical counselling for women living with HIV impacts upon the mother's attitude towards the feeding practice. Studies have showed that even the mere knowledge of infection with HIV and that the virus can be transmitted through breast milk alters the preferred feeding method (Gottlieb et al. 2004) and mothers ignored the medical and non-medical benefits of breast feeding. A significant number of women, however, who tested HIV-positive, considered replacement feeding with commercial formula during pregnancy as a good alternative to breast milk. Even if the World Health Organization's recommendation stipulated otherwise, they fear infecting the baby when breastfeeding exclusively (Moland 2004; Desclaux & Alfieri 2011). Moreover, the stigma of having HIV as well as the culturally normative mixed nutrition for a baby (Desclaux & Alfieri 2011) significantly challenged HIV-positive women. The next example illustrates the dilemma of a young HIV-positive mother with respect to the complex power relations in her impoverished multigenerational household and when interacting with medical staff:

> A twenty-year-old girl with a tiny baby enters the counseling room of a rural health center in the southern Lowlands district of Mafeteng, Lesotho. Her thin, pale baby is six months old, but seems much younger and does not move much, as she sucks on a piece of orange the mother holds. The infant tested HIV-positive at the age of six weeks and has now been brought for a confirmation test. The mother tested positive in antenatal care and received a short course treatment while in labor and under delivery.
>
> The counselor asks the mother about her feeding practice and she explains with hesitation that she has only given replacement food to the baby. The counselor insists that she does not believe her. The client starts crying and admits, that both her grandmother and mother told her to breastfeed and gave the baby other foods to supplement the little amount of breast milk the girl provided. A health counselor advised her repeatedly not to mix the baby's food, so she stopped breastfeeding for a short period. However, her grandmother and her mother were adamant that the child needed breast milk and they beseeched her to start again. She relented and resumed breastfeeding. The counselor now tells her again to cease breastfeeding, although it is obvious that the baby girl is malnourished.
>
> A nurse and two counselors discuss the case vividly following this interaction. The nurse complains about the client's non-adherence to exclusive breastfeeding, which is advised to prevent the transmission of the virus to the baby. She argues that patients simply lack comprehension. One counselor suggests summoning the grandmother in to counsel her on exclusive feeding options. The second counselor insists that if the child is already HIV-positive anyway, the mother could carry on mixed feeding in order to prevent further malnutrition, as the family does not have the means to afford formula milk. In order to secure the life of this malnourished, HIV positive infant, her HIV infection was in the end viewed as the more manageable risk in the face of more imminent hunger (Field notes Kroeker: 12/06/2008).

Breastfeeding is not self-explanatory but an interaction which mother and child have to learn and get used to. Therefore, the assistance of people who are experienced, such as midwives or female relatives, is essential, particularly if faced with additional insecurities. Mother and grandmother do their best to care for the young mother and her baby and it is common that the household community as a whole supervises the child's development holistically, considering the care needed to "make a child "heavy," healthy, and strong" (Dettwyler 1988). At the same time new parents in the role acquisition phase can seem frequently overwhelmed and frustrated by child care alternatives as role models may offer conflicting information in formal and informal learning about early child care (Riordan & Auerbach 1998: 693). We also need to bear in mind that information, either transferred between generations within a family or by health care professionals, owes to a particular school of thought. Here, mother and grandmother give advice that owes to traditional knowledge on resilience in an area that had experienced precarious food security situations ever since (cf. Kroeker & Beckwith 2011).

In this chapter on infant feeding I will explore biomedical recommendations and cultural norms, including advantages and disadvantages, prescriptive and comprehensive arguments, as well as uncertainties and possibilities influencing young urban mothers in their choices. The first part includes biomedical and traditional arguments on breastfeeding in general. The second section of this chapter talks about HIV-positive women and their options for infant feeding. The third section discusses how HIV-positive women put these options into practice.

7.1 Global and Local Arguments in Infant Feeding

From an anthropological as well as from a biomedical perspective, breast milk is considered highly beneficial for the child's development and well-being as well as mother's recuperation, bonding and birth spacing (Maher 1992; Stuart-Macadam & Dettwyler 1995: 8, 10; Desclaux & Taverne 2000: 37). For the infant, breast milk offers a myriad of health benefits, and the Government of Lesotho states accordingly:

> Breastfeeding is sufficient and beneficial for infant nutrition in the first six months of life. Early initiation of breastfeeding (breastfeeding within one hour) (...) helps to stimulate breast milk production and provides all of the nutritional requirements of a young infant. The high concentration of antibodies in colostrum, the first yellowish, highly

> nutritious milk that is present right after delivery, protects the child from infection before the child's immune system has matured. Early initiation also encourages the bond between mother and baby and helps to maintain the baby's body temperature. Breastfeeding also helps the uterus to retract, hence reducing postpartum blood loss of the mother. Prelacteral feeding (giving something other than breast milk in the first three days of life) is generally discouraged because it may inhibit breastfeeding and expose the newborn infant to illness (MoHSW et al. 2010: 135; cf. Yovsi 2003).

Beyond biomedical research, benefits of breastfeeding are, of course, also known worldwide. Whereas biomedicine solely considers the physical aspects of breastfeeding, local notions do not distinguish between arguments for the physical, emotional and spiritual well-being of mother, child and the family, as Moland previously criticised in 2004 in the case of Tanzania by stating:

> The current national and international policy guidelines on infant feeding in HIV positive women do not fully recognise that breastfeeding is a practice that involves much more than a physical and psychological relationship between two individuals. Neither do the guidelines sufficiently reflect the fact that infant feeding choices are never made in a social and cultural vacuum. The social relationships surrounding and conditioning breastfeeding involve much more than the relationship between mother and child. Breastfeeding is embedded in a social system involving relationships of control, power and authority. It is integrated into a universe of symbols about the female body, about sexuality and reproduction, about motherhood, and about belonging (Moland 2004: 87).

Differences in the biomedical and local notions revolve around preparing the mother for lactation, length, frequency and timing, breastfeeding method, who will breastfeed the child, introduction of complementary food, and complete weaning (Desclaux & Alfieri 2009; Leshabari et al. 2007; Leshabari et al. 2007 (a)). In the biomedical context, breastfeeding should be initiated within thirty minutes after birth, as suggested by the Baby Friendly

Hospital Initiative[1], in order to stimulate milk production (UNICEF n.d.). In contrast, in some parts of Africa the preparations for lactation start earlier than just after delivery. In order to reduce the time needed to wait until mothers had milk, a healer's wife in Lesotho advised preparing a balm to rub on the mother's breasts in order to initiate timely lactation and desensitise nipples in preparation of a suckling child (Field notes Kroeker: 07/2008). Also, Binder-Fritz (1995) explains that the nipples of Maori women in New Zealand were massaged and therewith desensitised before the child was born:

> It was usual from about the 7th month of gestation that a female relative massaged the areolae of the expectant mother with various herbal oils in order to make them more resistant against external stress during breastfeeding. Not only in rare cases this led to lactation in these women already during pregnancy (Binder-Fritz 1995: 96).[2]

Some mothers or mothers-in-law in Lesotho likewise suggested massaging the nipples starting from the seventh month of gestation, when the expectant mother left the matrimonial house and entered the transitional phase. Apparently, during that time a traditional birth attendant offers to massage the womb and breasts as part of traditional antenatal care and preparation for delivery. Although this might still be done with traditional birth attendants, the practice seems to be disappearing in urban Mafeteng. None of my study participants indicated that their breasts were massaged in preparation or that colostrum should not be given to the child, as stated by Ashton (1952: 29). In contrary, all the children I saw were breastfed without milk being expressed in advance and without complaint from elder family members who would expect it to be so. In contrast, Ashton assumes that the early initiation of lactation is part of the preparation for the baby and implies the idea that the first yellowish milk, the colostrum in biomedical terms or *lebese la litlobo* in Sesotho, must not be given to the child. *Lebese la litlobo* was not suitable for a newborn (Ashton 1952: 28-29; cf. Liamputtong 2011: 2). Some mothers interviewed by Fjeld

---

[1] The Baby Friendly Hospital Initiative was launched in 1991 by the WHO and UNICEF (UNICEF n.d.). 15,000 hospitals worldwide are listed as baby friendly, among them Mafeteng Government Hospital.

[2] "Etwa ab dem 7. Monat war es üblich, dass eine weibliche Verwandte auch die Mammillen der Schwangeren mit verschiedenen Pflanzenölen massierte, um sie widerstandsfähiger gegen die äußere Beanspruchung beim Stillen zu machen. Nicht selten solle es bei den Frauen dadurch bereits in der Schwangerschaft zur Laktation gekommen sein". (Binder-Fritz 1995: 96; translation mine).

and colleagues in Zambia likewise considered colostrum as "only water" which made the child sick, while others stressed only benefits for the baby (Stuart-Macadam & Dettwyler 1995: 9; Fjeld et al. 2008). Almroth and colleagues found that newborns in Lesotho were fed with water when the mother was not yet ready to lactate:

> Water as a supplement or replacement for breast milk was recommended and given first at birth "before the milk came in". A nurse explained that "when breast milk was not well established, we encouraged mothers to give sugar water." A mother remembered when her baby was born: "She got glucose, because I did not have any milk" (Almroth et al. 2000; cf. Fjeld et al. 2000).

Some family elders introduced water or sugared water during the first hours or days after birth. Different reasons were mentioned in literature and in the course of the field work: firstly, the child was thirsty, but milk was not yet available and water would bridge the gap, secondly, water or glucose water would release the meconium and allow important gastro-intestinal functions (Field notes Kroeker 4: 4/12/2008)[3]. Therewith a mixed infant diet was introduced right from the beginning (cf. Desclaux & Alfieri 2011).

---

[3] Various reports by biomedical facilities cite traditional practices as an obstacle to PMTCT adherence in Eastern Cape, South Africa: 'Sometimes babies do not receive nevirapine 72 hours after delivery because of the belief that the new born baby should be given isicakati (a traditional drink) as their first feed for a couple of days; some mothers are not allowed to go to hospital 14 days following delivery as they are to receive home-based postnatal care (efukwini) provided by their families and some people believe that the new born baby should be taken to ilawini, which means to a "coloured" traditional healer to make sure they get a relief of evil spirits' (Phaswana-Mafuya 2008).
As with many articles, biomedical staff members unfortunately do not discuss the value of these practices, but accuse these home remedies of being harmful practices which hamper biomedical success.

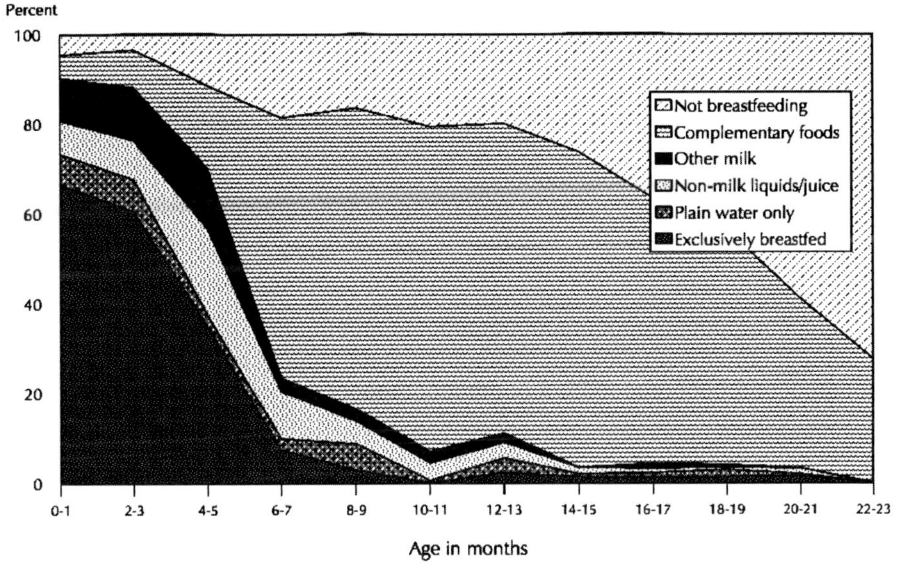

MoHSW et al. 2010: 139

As a home remedy and biomedical rehydration solution, sugared water or sugar and salt solutions administered to the child relieves constipation and diarrhoea. The children's medical books indicate glucose as well as glucose and salt water as a home remedy to treat these complaints. Healers may also use this *pitsa* to treat children who had failed to pass motion after two to three days postpartum or treat other common childhood diseases. However, procedures are not standardised, despite training through the healers' district office (Green 1985). In both the biomedical and the local discourse, thus, sugar water has the connotation of being healthy as it secures good digestion, prevents dehydration and the baby happily drinks it because of the sweet taste. Due to these generally beneficial implications many infants predominantly drink sugared water throughout the day. Mothers in Lesotho use water anyhow as a supplementary drink to satisfy the baby and sugar to "give the water some taste" (Field notes Kroeker 25: 31/03/2009). For HIV-positive women, however, this cheap and easy home remedy is not advised by medical counsellors since it interferes with biomedical recommendations for preventing HIV transmission.

7.1.1 The Bottle-Breast-Dilemma

Long-term mixed feeding is common practice in Lesotho. The mixed diet enables a mother to supplement her breast milk shortages with other nutriments. According to Ashton (1952: 33-34), in addition to breast milk, infants are often given other food, such as cow's milk, liquid unfermented porridge or a dish made of maize. Nowadays, the same type of infant feeding is reported (cf. Thairu et al. 2005). For instance, Lesotho's Demographic and Health Survey of 2010 suggests that 61% of the children are exclusively breastfed, while another 36% receive water, milk or other liquids additionally even during the first and second month. The number of children who are exclusively breastfed falls significantly after two to three months, while the number of children who receive mother's milk and complementary foods other than water and milk escalates. More than one third of children receive breast milk and complementary foods even above the age of two (MoHSW et al. 2010: 138).

International organisations recommend, mainly for nutritional reasons, that all infants should be fed exclusively on breast milk from birth until 4-6 months of age. Thereafter, children should continue to be breastfed, while receiving appropriate and adequate complementary foods, until they are two years of age or above (WHO & UNICEF: 1990).

The implementation of artificial baby food changed common notions on breastfeeding. Especially in more well-to-do families, complementary feeding with commercial formula implied a high social status, similar to Jordan's observation of a Yucatan mother's notion:

> Bottles constitute a status symbol, an expression of the parent's progressive attitude. Generally speaking, however, bottles are still seen as supplemental to breastfeeding, providing additional nourishment to the child, rather than as a replacement for the breast (Jordan & Davis-Floyd 1993: 43).

In her introduction (2011: 1-23), Liamputtong presents authors who correlate class and gender with breastfeeding practice. Some analysed breastfeeding rates were lower among low-income mothers and they may feel relegated to low social class. Middle-class women, in their opinion, were able to afford the time and take long maternity leave which would not be an option for low-class women since they would depend on a quick return to work for financial reasons. Others, with whom I will side, argued that low-income mothers breastfed due to its inexpensive provision when compared with artificial products. High-income groups, on the other hand, argued in favour of the benefits of prolonged breastfeeding since they agreed to it from a more scientifically-fuelled point of view, whereas middle-income mothers weaned quickly, enabling the mother to generate income (Field notes Kroeker: 10/2009). Bottle feeding in Lesotho also partly signalled financial security and good infant care, and some family members even considered western commercial products more beneficial than breastfeeding (Field notes Kroeker Laura: 06/06/2008). Advertisements by companies discovering the African market must have contributed to this notion, however, public health organisations opposed the milk formula industry.

Since the 1970s good infant feeding practice in resource-constrained settings was revised by international organisations in order to reduce the worrisome trend of commercial formula as a replacement for breast milk. Nestlé had invented artificial infant food around 1890 and promoted it widely throughout the post World War II baby boom (Dettwyler 1995: 39-74). International organisations such as The World Health Organization (WHO) or UNICEF as well as non-governmental organisations such as La Leche League International (LLLI founded in 1956), The Infant Formula Action Coalition (INFACT), The International Baby Food Action Network (IBFAN), amongst others, set up campaigns to promote breastfeeding worldwide as the most socially and medically beneficial choice for a mother and her child. The debate became known as the "bottle-breast controversy" (Desclaux & Taverne 2000). While INFACT initiated a boycott of Nestlé products from 1977-1984, IBFAN worked on an International Code of Marketing of Breastmilk Substitutes with the WHO and UNICEF which was ratified in May 1981. One hundred and eighteen WHO member countries (excluding the US) agreed to the non-binding instrument of consumer protection, and IBFAN declared itself a non-governmental surveillance organisation to monitor the implementation of the code. It stipulates that the marketing of replacement food must be reduced and women not dissuaded from the idea of breastfeeding. The Innocenti Declaration stipulates:

- No advertising of any of these products to the public.
- No free samples to mothers.
- No promotion of products in health care facilities, including the distribution of free or low-cost supplies. (…)
- No words or pictures idealizing artificial feeding, or pictures of infants on labels on infant milk containers.
- Information to health workers should be scientific and factual.

- All information on artificial infant feeding, including that on labels, should explain the benefits of breastfeeding, and the costs and hazards associated with artificial feeding. (…) (WHO & UNICEF: 1990).

The worldwide trend of breastfeeding promotion also reached Lesotho. In the 1980s, a government awareness campaign of the newly established "Breastfeeding Committee" was launched encouraging women to breastfeed for as long as possible with the slogan "Breast is Best."[4] A minimum of two years was considered necessary to secure the child's nutritional status and elderly mothers were advised to "encourage [their daughters-in-law] to identify minor breastfeeding problems so that they should not wean their babies, but should treat the problem while continuing to breastfeed" (Mafeteng Government Hospital 1993: 15).

The campaign sought to champion the normative practice of long-term breast feeding while discouraging women from introducing commercial infant formula. The "baby milk scandal" revealed that baby food companies apparently undermined breastfeeding by commercial exploitation of the market. Campaigns blamed companies for making mothers and children irreversibly dependent on expensive commercial products once lactation stops, while especially in developing countries, with limited access to safe drinking water and refrigerators, this feeding practice led to the death of large numbers of babies (Maher 1992: 3). The WHO is concerned that an estimated 9.5 million children worldwide pass away before their fifth birthday and two thirds of those deaths occur during the first year of life, many of them associated with diarrhoea and malnutrition. Due to the poor quality drinking water in many resource-constrained countries, which mothers nevertheless use to prepare formula milk for their babies, they are at risk of contracting intestinal infectious diseases. Moreover, drinking vessels, bottles and the like must be handled carefully and hygienically, which in many countries proves impossible. Lesotho, however, is blessed with plenty of safe drinking water from the mountains. 80% of the population have access to

---

[4] The internal document did not give any reference to the initiators of the campaign, although I can only assume that the unmentioned initiators of the Breastfeeding Committee had some affiliation with the WHO and the implementation of the International Code of Marketing of Breastmilk Substitutes. Writing in 1985, Green mentions a "Breast is Best" campaign to have already been in place in Swaziland for a number of years (Green 1985). Avishai (2011: 24-25) also mentions it with reference to Kukla (2006) who again refers to campaigns of the mid1970s.

clean wells or taps and the water does not need any further treatment such as boiling or chemical purification (MoHSW et al. 2010: 19). However, in accordance with the guidelines for resource-constrained settings, counsellors and nurses in Lesotho cautioned against using baby bottles, teats and dummies, as a nurse explains:

> [Mothers] should not use teats or dummies to feed the child, it is even written on the breastfeeding policy sheets that are pinned up on the wall. (…) Basotho women are careless. [They] don't clean the teat regularly and also they don't exchange it often enough. Then the baby gets diarrhoea and they come to the hospital. We therefore advise them not to use the teat at all. We want to see the babies drinking from the mug from day one onwards (Field notes Kroeker Makabello: 07/05/2009).

Particularly women who have insufficient fuel or who cook using firewood cannot be expected to heat the bottles until they are sterilised despite safe drinking water, a counsellor adds (Field notes Kroeker MaThloni: 16/04/2009). The WHO therefore suggests that infant mortality could be significantly reduced with a good breastfeeding practice. Leading organisations in public health and breastfeeding promotion recommend exclusive breastfeeding followed by twelve months or more of complementary breastfeeding and other nutriments (WHO et al. 2010: 6). In Lesotho's health centres mothers are accordingly advised to breastfeed exclusively for six months, for both HIV-positive and HIV-negative mothers. For HIV-negative ones, no further advice is usually given.

As of the present day, in Mafeteng Hospital, the Innocenti Declaration is displayed in the mother and child ward, the labour ward and adolescent corner, where the HIV-positive (expectant) mothers' support group meets. Manifold posters from UNICEF, and the Ministry of Health amongst others, use both pictures and words to inform on infant feeding practices and some are also available as leaflets for clients to take home. Counsellors refer in their morning talks to the posters where applicable and simultaneously use these as teaching materials and decorative elements. As a matter of fact though, in the international as well as the national arena, the whole controversial debate has been dumbed down since it solely concerns nutritional aspects of infant feeding (Maher 1992: 4).

7.1.2 Further Concerns of Breastfeeding

In practice, the permanent introduction of additional food in Lesotho can usually be dated to around months four to seven after birth (cf. Desclaux & Alfieri 2011). Women who work in the formal sector, of course, start much earlier since maternity leave consists of only six weeks off. In order to support these mothers nevertheless, 22 factories in the clothing sector in Lesotho provide a workplace programme which allocates money for a hospital delivery and milk powder supplies for employees irrespective of their HIV status[5]. HIV-positive mothers who have an opportunity to receive milk powder free of charge often comply closely with HIV testing and counselling advice. For them, not only generating income but also milk supply ties them to the employer (Field notes Kroeker: 11/02/2009). Those mothers who are not employed in the textile sector can barely afford the cost of breast milk substitute and mostly rely on the normative practice of mixed feeding.

As indicated in the example at the beginning and the graph, Basotho children receive mixed nutrition from an early age onwards. Family elders, usually the child's paternal or maternal grandmother, take care to introduce other products when the child is mature enough to take them. The first complementary nutrition after water or watery solutions usually consists of goat or cow's milk, maize porridge (Sesotho: *Lesheleshele*), or pre-chewed adult food (Field notes Kroeker: 10/06/2008; cf.: Ashton 1952: 34). Apart from the practical reasons, grandmothers and other experienced women insisted on mixed feeding since additional nutrients familiarise the infant with this diet. From a certain age onwards milk would leave the baby hungry and it should also be able to digest adult food in case the mother cannot breastfeed for one reason or another. Especially when the mother is sick or likely to pass away, mixed feeding would easily allow one to compensate a meal of breast milk since the child is already accustomed (Fjeld et al. 2008). Mixed feeding

---

[5] Some private companies, particularly in the clothing industry, had already established workplace programmes by May 2006. Around 22 factories host a branch of the NGO Apparel Lesotho Alliance to Fight AIDS (ALAFA) and nine factories provided a health station. In the town of Mafeteng, the garment factory collaborates with private practitioners and the hospital for antenatal care.

In general, mothers who work in the clothing sector within a factory that provides counselling and care through a workplace programme additionally receive formula milk for their child, which assures a short duration of maternity leave. Three weeks after delivery the young mothers report back to work. ALAFA writes on their homepage that 38,000 women have access to testing, treatment and on-going care within the factories in Lesotho, and all children born to ALAFA members tested negative in 2010 (www.alafa.info).

therewith provides security for the child if anything happens to the mother, and sickness of the mother or child is a great concern due to the uncertain liminal state while women are "in between life and death". Moreover, a mixed diet allows other members of the household community, apart from the mother, to look after the child when the mother takes up her work chores again after her liminal phase. In fact, the introduction of additional food as part of a welcoming ceremony ends the liminal phase of mother and child.

Additional food intake besides breast milk can moreover prevent malnutrition in mother and baby where food shortages are evident such as in Lesotho. Perhaps more importantly than the nutritional aspects is a long-term parallel feeding practice including breast milk and water due to its social values. Firstly, the close physical contact it provides acts as a social bond between a mother and her child. Breastfeeding is rarely abandoned as it additionally pacifies the baby and gives emotional satisfaction and comfort to mother and child. In Mali, Dettwyler described that children are also nursed "if they are hurt, sick, tired, or frightened. This aspect of nursing is considered as important as nursing for nourishment" (1988). For Lesotho, Ashton adds that "consequently weaning, when it comes, probably creates a break of emotional rather than nutritional significance." (Ashton 1952: 34). Mothers who were not able to breastfeed their children regretted not fulfilling expectations of good mothering. As with Dettwyler (1988), breastfeeding in Desclaux and Taverne's study was also associated with comforting and nourishing the baby, to sooth it when scared and cosset when tired (Desclaux & Taverne 2000: 37).

Hence, in Lesotho, breastfeeding as a supplement to other nutrients will not usually cease until two to three years post-partum. Around that age a child will be physically and psychologically mature enough to be sent to relatives until it "forgets about the mother's breast" (Ashton 1952: 35).

7.2 Social (Re-)integration of Mother and Child

The end of liminality for the child is marked by its familial incorporation which starts with nutritional integration into the social sphere. The introduction of complementary (non-commercial) nutriments, for example, fulfils various acts such as welcoming, naming, social integration, spiritual testing, clan affiliation, when in emotional and physical discomfort and for practical reasons for the child minder. In many cases the purpose can hardly be classified as purely medical, magic-religious or social. It is difficult to distinguish between that which is considered a clan practice, a family practice or a coincidence and that which is considered general or individual knowledge about child-nutrition. Most definitely, though, elder female family members had a broad knowledge about necessary practices, which younger women did not know about but waited for assistance at the right time.

A complex rite of socialisation of mother and child commences with the child's first mouthful of food. As part of a rite of passage it integrates the child into the family and therewith welcomes mother and child as full members. Ashton describes a special meal, *lelomolo*, given to the baby almost immediately after birth and before being suckled. Comaroff reports sorghum-porridge to be a transitional food in a liminal stage followed by the consumption of meat as a ritualised way of marking the passage of male novices in initiation school after circumcision.

> Once circumcised, the novices were metaphorical infants in the domain of the social. The ritual was structured so that signifiers of social and physical development ran parallel, the former impressing their significance on the latter. The remainder of the liminal stage represented a condensed passage from birth through childhood and an accelerated growth into social maturity. Thus the newly circumcised boys were naked by day and slept at night on the bare floor of their huts – both signs of a condition minimally refined by human socialisation. For the first week after the operation, moreover, they ate only porridge, the diet of babies (Schapera 1971: 215 in: Comaroff 1985: 99).
>
> After the first week, meat was consumed in quantity, for the men of the settlement engaged in the uncommon practice of regular slaughter in order to foster a concentrated process of growth in the novices (Comaroff 1985: 92).

Ashton adds that within the first month after initiation, for neophytes, "the food is prepared at home by a *motsoetse* or other ritually pure woman" (Ashton 1952: 50). Certainly, porridge is associated with purity and passage into a new social status. Sechefo (n.d.: 15) similarly describes a rite whereby an old person, close to death, is served a last supper. A small piece of meat is stuffed between the teeth. The similarity of the rites of passage at the beginning of life, during initiation, when having delivered a child, and when approaching death, suggests a pattern. All four events mark important passages into a new social status which is accompanied by ritually prescribed meals and dishes of porridge served by a ritually pure person followed by meat. Despite this common ethnographic observation of rites of passage, as indicated before, study participants were not aware of these ritual explanations. They mainly referred to an enhancement of milk if a woman in childbed (Sesotho: *motsoetse*) ate copious amounts of porridge.

The Demographic and Health Survey of 2010 recognised that about one third of newborns get a prelacteral meal although it is less prevalent in the Southern Lowlands with about 27% (MoHSW et al. 2010: 137) and most prevalent in the Northern and Eastern region (36%). Regional differences in the diffusion of the practice, as the survey suggests, may be linked to differing clan practices which are also found among other Southern African people. In the Mafeteng District, where early introduction of breastfeeding during the first hour after delivery is most common, I observed that a practice called *lelomolo* takes place when naming or when the child arrives at the paternal family home aged three to four months. Other clans may perhaps give the ritual *lelomolo* bite at different times.

After three to four months of acclimatisation for the mother and child, the pair moves back to the husband where the mother fully resumes her household chores. The husband comes for the mother and takes her, analogous to the elopement prior to the wedding ceremony, to his place where she is again welcomed as a bride. This second elopement confirms the fully completed marital contract since this time she is accompanied by the couple's offspring. On the way there, mother and child pass through the "undifferentiated space" and "unmarked sociomoral universe" (Comaroff 1985: 55) for the first time. They had previously lived in the protected house and vestibule of their matrilateral home, and after the journey they find themselves in the paternal vestibule, where both will be socialised according to family custom. Their arrival is then celebrated with a meal of sheep to welcome the family members. The mother receives the wedding dish *koae* once more; for the child a *lelomolo* bite is reserved which an honourable person of excellent conduct pre-chews and feeds to the child (Field notes Kroeker: 05/12/2008).

> A young child ready to be given solid food, should be given it by a chosen man known to be of a good temper and morals. He gives a slice of meat, which the child sucks eagerly as if it were suckling into itself the good qualities of that man (Sechefo n.d.: 26-27).

Nowadays, not only a man, but equally a woman of good conduct may be elected to transmit her moral values to the fosterling when sharing a bite (Field notes Kroeker: 14: 04/12/2008; 10: 21/5/2009; cf. Maher 1992: 9-10).

Depending on the clan practices, welcoming the child also includes protecting the infant from witchcraft affliction. This first meal also serves as a test of the child's humanity. If refusing to take the porridge the child may be associated with witchcraft (Ashton 1952: 31). I did not get to hear about that, although in some clans a stigma of ash marked on the child's forehead or plant or animal parts worn by the child in the form of charms, prevented witchcraft affliction. Depending on clan culture, some children receive the same necklace the mother was wearing when she left her in-laws' house in her last trimester of pregnancy and which indicated her bond with that household. Others wear bands with seeds around the neck or beads around their abdomen to, on the one hand, show ancestral clan affiliation through the colour of the beads, and on the other, assist in measuring the child. Sargent (1989: 30) states that mothers in rural Benin gave their children waistbands or curing amulets as protection against folk diseases. Practically, the tightness of the band around the baby's hips will indicate whether the child had lost or gained weight. The mother therewith easily monitors the child's growth and extends the band whenever the need occurs. Also, as soon as the child manages to rip it off, parents will not replace the band but the child will be considered mature (Field notes Kroeker: 13/06/2008; 6: 18/11/2008).

Some families rather use it as a token and the symbolic value is what counts. Numerous children wear simple black bands, *khoetsa*, either cut from sheep cloak or simple cotton, around their neck. Ashton assumes that the leather band results from the sheep that was slaughtered at the child's welcoming ceremony and besides dentition it also facilitates the closing of the fontanelles (Ashton 1952: 29, 31), which is a great concern since witchcraft can easily harm a child while they have not fully closed over. Some mothers mentioned that the band particularly facilitates growth of the child in general or especially "growth of the teeth". Growing teeth additionally related to weaning. This time marks maturity and full social integration of a child, who will now be able to consume adult food. Comaroff's notion of teeth amongst closely related Tswana implies coming of age whereby teeth stand for maturity or manhood (Comaroff 1985: 98, 101) and therewith social status. The necklace bridges generations as the *lelomolo* meal did. The bite is handed down through generations of men to the child, while the necklace travelled from the hands of the mother-in-law to the expectant daughter-in-law and then to the child, which signifies, according to my interpretation, affiliation of the matrifocal group across three generations.

Whoever will be chosen, the child's ceremony involves patrilineal male relatives. In the event they are unavailable to host the ritual, funding is not yet available, or other important reasons, the ceremony may, however, be postponed to an undefined time (Field notes Kroeker 21: 05/12/2008). Rituals, such as welcoming a child, which are neglected for a long time cause displeasure of the ancestors. This manifests itself in misfortune or sickness, which then urges the family to inquire as to the cause and to make concerted efforts to host the feast (Gay 1980: 55). In many cases, ancestral punishment sanctions negligence of rites and hence enforces compliance with the elder's advice.

Whether the child's feast took place or not, the mother, for her part, takes up her household chores again upon their return to the matrimonial home and the group of women at the household shares the task of child minding. While in childbed at her maternal home the mother did not resume household chores during the first three to four months, but she now relies on others to watch over the child. Breastfeeding accompanies the whole transitional phase of a child until full social integration into the community and familiarisation with adult nutrients occurs slowly (Sechefo n.d.: 26-27; Gay 1980: 55; Field notes Kroeker: 04/12/2008). Female family members and children usually gather and socialise within the vestibule where food is processed, thus, children easily have contact with soft or pre-chewed morsels while the community of female next-of-kin prepare food. These nibbles allowed mothers to leave their babies for short periods of time in the vestibule, where other relatives or guests take care of them and the child gets used to the taste of an adult diet. In contrast to other African cultures (Dettwyler 1988), the Basotho disapprove of wet-nursing a child (Ashton 1952: 34; Desclaux & Alfieri 2009; Moland 2004; Field notes Kroeker: 05/07/2008), however, other women typically continue to feed water or bites to the baby (Ashton 1952: 34; Leshabari et al. 2007)[6]. Deploying a wet-nurse was however suggested by a hospital counsellor in Mafeteng when a mother passes away and a HIV-negative mother may be able to nurse the child (Field notes

[6] In my opinion, it would be wise to consider this option following medical and social research, since it could also replace expensive replacement feeding in areas with high HIV rates and maternal mortality. Some African cultures are also familiar with medication that induces lactation "medicaments mammifères", presumably those where wet-nurses are more common (Hartge 1986; Föllmer 1983).

Kroeker MaThloni: 4/3/2009). Nevertheless, nurses disapproved of it and clients did not feel very confident about the matter either.

Even though the architecture has changed and many women currently live in single rooms or rectangular houses without a backyard, the idea of joint supervision of a child and early acclimatisation with bites of adult food remains in practice. Exclusively breastfeeding women, who are obliged to carry the child with them at all times in order to avoid additional feeding, will also have to expose the child to the apparently unsafe periphery, while it would usually stay close to the house while the mother runs errands.

7.2.1 Harming Mother and Child

Urban living conditions with small household communities and thus minimal authoritative supervision increased the likelihood of missing crucial aspects of preventive rites which can show in bouts of misfortune and sickness. A traditional healer may therefore be consulted to mediate between the ancestors and inquire as to the reason for discontentment or whether jealousy from fellow living beings has caused affliction. Witchcraft, as a harmful condition that is sent by a present person, can be purposely used against the mother and child. Though, at times people, particularly those in a sensitive transitional state such as new mothers and young children, may be harmed collaterally by strong substances. I will now describe two frequently occurring pathologies which require timely treatment from an experienced traditional healer but not a biomedical doctor.

A baby may, for instance, cry and refuse to drink the mother's milk after it saw an animal, a vehicle for witchcraft, drinking from the mother's breasts in a dream revelation (Field notes Kroeker: 12/03/2009). The child's refusal or spitting out of the milk, if it drank a little due to hunger, can result in death. Symptoms suggest a Basotho disease sent via *Tokolosi,* evil human shaped spirits which transfer witchcraft and deploy animals as carriers. If a *Tokolosi* drank a mother's milk the breast typically becomes painful, hard, and may also change in colour unless she consults a traditional healer for recovery. The *ngaka* will mix an orally applied solution (*pitsa*) and an ointment for the mother including medicinal plants to treat the physical complaint and the malevolent powers spiritually. Sometimes healers will additionally advise the mother to bathe in the river and walk back without turning around and she will then receive the *pitsa* back home. After being relieved she may be able to breastfeed the child again (ATCBM Kroeker: 10/07/2008; 08/07/2008; Field notes Kroeker: 17/03/2009, 09/03/2009). In a situation of constant jealousy and greed a mother refrains from breastfeeding instead, such as in the aforementioned case of LeTharo (Chapter 6.5.1) and another study participant who weaned her child because of her in-laws with whom she does not seem to be on good terms. The woman argued that she had stopped breastfeeding because her relatives were greedy[7] (ATCBM Kroeker: 15/07/2008), a common term for being affected by witchcraft. Without further knowledge of the story, greed certainly refers in this context to a particular condition of people that wanted to limit her prosperity[8].

In hospital treatment, a mother with the symptoms mentioned above will be treated for mastitis and usually asked to wean completely and to start feeding the baby with formula milk. Notwithstanding, the treatment only provides relief from the physical afflictions but does not deal with the witchcraft causation. While hospital counsellors discourage approaching traditional healers and encourage seeing a biomedical nurse or doctor for any complaint, in the case of mastitis, respectively "*tokolosi* drinking from breast", a healer seems to be able to solve the problem, while securing further breastfeeding. The biomedical treatment cannot secure on-going safe nutrition of the child but urges mothers to change the feeding practice altogether and abruptly (Field notes Kroeker MaThloni: 06/2008).

The second ailment which is common in young infants is also caused by witches and enters a child through the fontanelle (cf. Sargent 1989: 28-30). In terms of the symptoms, the baby will show general weakness, the fontanelle will sink and may pulse. "Pulsing fontanelles" (*Puoana*) relates to various diseases suffered by children whose fontanelles are still soft and not completely closed. It urges a mother to seek speedy assistance from a traditional healer, since it is also mostly caused by witchcraft (cf. Scheper-Hughes & Stewart 1983: 882) and may have fatal consequences:

> Looking at traditional practitioners, one finds that their help is often sought for the treatment of sunken fontanelle (90% of the above cases). Western medicine considers it a symptom of dehydration. Most Basotho consider this to be a disease in itself and because it is often suspected to be caused by witchcraft, they seek help of [traditional practitioners] (Hall & Malahleha 1989: 26; cf. Sargent 1989: 28-30).

---

[7] "*Bane ba nyanya haholo*" (ATCBM Kroeker 15/07/2008).

[8] Well-being of an individual or a family collectively is somehow considered a zero-sum game in Lesotho. One person who succeeds and whose assets prosper achieves this at the cost of others who are left unwell and in a devastated condition.

The child contracts this affliction, either deliberately or accidentally, even while in the mother's womb, when the mother carelessly passes a gate where jealous people have applied powerful substances. *Tokolosi* will transmit it then to the child which will become sickly and cry. MaRobong, whose baby brother had died from *puona,* describes it:

> During the day you will think you see a child but during the night you see a doll[9]. My brother was so small and I was even scared of him. He was small and became ugly and his head started pulsing. Whenever the fontanelles are pulsing it is a sign that a healer is needed and *Tokolosis* are involved (Field notes Kroeker 29: 12/03/2009).

Her mother did not believe in a witchcraft cause and brought the baby to the hospital, instead of a traditional healer and the boy passed away after one month[10]. She assumes that the doctor did not treat the cause, which was witchcraft and family elders insisted that the child should have seen a traditional practitioner who would have mixed *pitsa.*

Even people who do not have much involvement with traditional explanations of disease know and fear *puona* in a child and take it to a healer so that it can be treated successfully. LeRobong's child also passed away of "pulsing fontanelles" aged four months. The baby was HIV-negative and was fed exclusively on replacement feed until then. Makhotso's baby, who was not exposed to HIV and weaned, still had pulsing fontanelles at one year old. The child was treated by a traditional healer, which Makhotso usually refuses to visit, but the child recovered quickly thereafter (Field notes Kroeker Makhotso: 20/04/2010). In biomedical terms, pulsing fontanelles is treated with water enriched with salt and sugar in addition to other commercial medication.

---

[9] Einarsdottir also describes a witchcraft affliction in children who look like a doll, a clear indication that they are bewitched. These children are suspected to be non-human, without a human soul, and considered to be a threat to the matrilineage for which reason the family may commit infanticide without the mother's consent (Einarsdottir 2005: 37).

[10] Often, if a child had passed away, a subsequent sibling will be given a bad name in order to warn off another episode of witchcraft "in the hope of lulling the sorcerer's vigilance" (Ashton 1952: 33). Naming the child with an unpleasant name remains a common practice, although urban mothers also choose names according to their individual taste and not as suggested by an elder. MaRobong's mother again did not listen to her elders and called her next child Lerato, meaning Love. This time she was again affected by an unfortunate event: her husband passed away shortly after the baby girl was born. Nowadays, she visits traditional healers which she did not trust earlier.

Alternative explanations and treatment methods also concern a disease known biomedically as malnutrition. As far back as the early 1990s, documented malnutrition was on the rise. The Mafeteng Government Hospital's Annual Report of 1993 reports a worrisome decrease in children's nutritional state. Malnutrition in children was a serious problem in the district then and the number of malnourished children showed an increase of 43.6% between 1992 and 1993. One reason might be that the number of households without land has increased by 20% during the last 20 years, another might be increasing poverty caused by reduced recruitment of miners (Mafeteng Government Hospital 1993). At present, it is estimated that about 39% of Basotho children under 5 years of age are stunted (height correlated with age) and this figure has increased in recent years (18% in 2000)[11]. 15% are severely stunted, whereas male children are more affected than females, and rural regions indicate higher numbers than urban regions (MoHSW et al. 2010: 132; cf. Romero-Daza & Himmelgreen 2004: 958).

In 2010, Nne's baby boy was sickly and thin like many other children. She approached the hospital and a counsellor diagnosed the child's malnourished state, but the hospital treatment did not help much. Nne also consulted her pastor for alternative treatment for the cause of the malnutrition. The pastor offered blessed water and food since she found the cause of the child's condition in the fact that "a rich person had touched the child" (Field notes Kroeker 4: 12/2009). Nne's baby had therefore suffered a loss of energy, from which a rich person who had touched the child had benefitted.

The death of a child before weaning will always be blamed on the greed of someone who had deployed witchcraft to profit. At that age no taboos apply for a baby and it can therefore not have caused ancestral discontent. However, some obstetric disorders, complications under delivery or during the time of breastfeeding the child, can therewith be traced back to the mother breaching taboos.

In any case, HIV-positive mothers are discouraged in hospital from visiting traditional healers and encouraged to adhere to biomedical counselling only. However, the reasons mentioned force mothers to combine treatment methods and to hide their usage of traditional medication.

---

[11] The Demographic and Health Survey 2009 indicates three measurements: Height-for-age (stunting), weight-for-height (wasting) and weight-for-age (underweight) (MoHSW et al. 2010: 133).

7.3 Biomedical Options for HIV-positive Mothers

The advent of HIV/AIDS and the realisation that the virus can be transmitted through breastfeeding (Cutting 1992; Lederman 1992) crucially altered the public health message surrounding breastfeeding. A new controversy concerned bottle versus breastfeeding. Especially in countries with a high prevalence of HIV and low quality drinking water "safe infant feeding" posed a dilemma to policy makers. The World Health Organization attempts to "balance the risk of infants acquiring HIV through breast milk with the higher risk of death from causes other than HIV, in particular malnutrition and serious illnesses such as diarrhoea among non-breastfed infants" (WHO 2001: 5; cf. GoL 2009 (a): 57). Recommendations were revised time and time again, since health benefits (i.e. immunological benefits, full nutrition, birth spacing), risks (i.e. transmission of HIV, side effects of the drugs, dependency on milk substitute), availability and affordability were not commensurate. IBFAN concludes that more children in Sub-Saharan Africa will die if not breastfed and diarrhoea will kill 14 times more children than the transmission of HIV through exclusive breastfeeding would (Kisanga 2000: 4, 7). The network states:

> IBFAN Africa is concerned that if formula or other artificial feeding replaces breastfeeding in poor families with meagre resources, the outcome might be marginal reduction of HIV transmission and much higher rates of morbidity, mortality and malnutrition. (...) Even in countries with high seroprevalence of HIV, (25% of women infected), fewer than 4% of infants will be affected through lengthy breastfeeding. (...) Recent research indicates that infants whose mothers are infected with HIV and exclusively breastfed, had a similar risk of acquiring the virus as those who were artificially fed, and this risk was significantly lower than for those who were mixed fed (Kisanga 2000: 5).

Furthermore, IBFAN Africa argues that the risk of vertical HIV transmission through breast milk has been overemphasised due to misinformation and the benefits of breastfeeding for mother and child must not be neglected (Kisanga 2000: 5, 14). In spite of this, to date, HIV-positive women in industrialised countries are advised to replace breast milk altogether, whereas in resource-constrained settings HIV-positive women shall breastfeed exclusively to prevent a vertical transmission of HIV. Desclaux and Taverne recognise diametrically opposing recommendations for HIV-positive mothers as "AIDS of the North" and "AIDS of the South" (Dexclaux & Taverne 2000:

8). Notwithstanding, women who know about their HIV-positive status, but do not receive any counselling on infant feeding, tend to disregard breastfeeding and therewith underestimate the beneficial effects due to fear of harming the child (Gottlieb et al. 2004). While mothers in Lesotho are told during counselling sessions that HIV can be transmitted through breast milk, counsellors also advise, at the same time, to feed this harmful nutrient. For the mothers it is confusing to hear how exclusive breastfeeding can reduce the HIV transmission while breast milk itself contains the virus (Desclaux & Alfieri 2009). Causation in many cases is not sufficiently explained or at least not in any comprehensive way. Reasons given in the national guidelines on PMTCT as of 2009 include the following:

Benefits of exclusive breastfeeding

- Breast milk provides complete nutrition for the infant for the first six months of life
- Colostrum, the milk produced during the first few days of the infant's life, is rich in vitamins, antibodies, and has other anti-infective properties
- Breast milk contains antibodies from the mother which are beneficial to the infant, as the infant's own immune system is not completely developed during the first few months of life
- Breast milk provides vital protection against deadly childhood illnesses such as diarrhoea and respiratory infections
- Breast milk is easily digested and its composition changes to meet the developmental needs of the growing infant
- Breast milk contains enzymes that help digestion of fat
- Breast milk is natural and does not add extra cost
- Breastfeeding promotes bonding between mothers and their babies
- Breastfeeding helps the uterus to contract after delivery and reduces postpartum bleeding
- Breast milk is always available and no special preparation is needed (GoL 2009 (a): 57).

The first national guidelines for Lesotho, which were published in 2004 by the Ministry of Health and Social Welfare, stipulated that health workers shall encourage expectant mothers to breastfeed exclusively for six months. Background information is not given in this document. Medical research, however, supports exclusive feeding methods with the following explanation: a mixed nutrition would dissolve the child's protective layer on the mucous membrane and raise the likelihood of allowing the virus to enter, whereas a healthy gut lining acts as a viral barrier (Coutsoudis et al. 1999: 471-476; Kisanga 2000: 16; Ng'andwe 2007).

As an alternative, the PMTCT guidelines suggested expressing milk from the breast and boiling it before giving it to the child. IBFAN considered "Heat-treatment of breast milk expressed by an HIV-positive mother kills the virus in the breast milk. Heat-treated breast milk is nutritionally better to other milks" (Kisanga 2000: 69; Piwoz et al. 2005: 935). Kisanga, Piwoz and colleagues, and Tomlinson and Madjarov (2002) have likewise suggested that pasteurising breast milk would be a far simpler and more practical solution than antiviral therapy for preventing HIV transmission through breastfeeding.

As a third alternative, mothers may opt for exclusive replacement feeding with commercial infant formula if considered "Acceptable Feasible Affordable Sustainable and Safe (AFASS)", however, healthcare workers were also encouraged to warn mothers about the stigma of not breastfeeding (WHO 2001; GoL 2004: 31; Desclaux & Taverne 2000; Desclaux & Alfieri 2009).

Benefits of replacement feeding with commercial infant formula

- There is no risk of HIV infection to the baby
- Commercial infant formula contains most of the nutrients an infant needs
- Other people (besides the mother) can feed the infant (GoL 2009 (a): 57).

Health counsellors shall assess the mother's situation individually to help identify the most suitable feeding option. However, Desclaux and Alfieri (2009) recognised that the assessment of the AFASS criterion by health counsellors predominantly hinges on solely economic concerns. Indeed, formula milk was extremely expensive and therefore no option for women who were unemployed or with unstable sources of income. Those who were dependent on family income needed to discuss the allocation of money for powdered milk.

Local appropriation and additional research on efficiency and effectiveness were factored into the guidelines which changed with respect to the eligibility criteria, length of feeding, time of weaning and preferred options. New guidelines came out in 2007 in a draft version following the 2006 WHO revision, and as full guidelines in 2009, and changes also took place in the meantime which nurses and counsellors were informed about during evaluations and in training sessions. At the start of 2011 new revisions were drafted and counsellors trained. In the guidelines, timeframes and methods of weaning were adjusted time and time again. Abrupt cessation of breastfeeding was firstly stipulated after four months of exclusive feeding and then later after six months, and weaning should take no longer than two to three days, which was also later revised and it can now take two to three weeks. The 2009 guidelines moreover banned the recommendation of heat-treated breastmilk but offered a feeding recommendation which applies for malnourished children only: up to two years of mixed feeding after six months of exclusive feeding. This recommendation concerns many mothers in Lesotho and corresponds surprisingly well with the advice from the breastfeeding campaigns of the 70s and 80s, an era before HIV. These changes added to the confusion among counsellors and mothers, since practices which were discouraged were changed and now applied in accordance with new guidelines.

7.3.1 Decisions on the Feeding Practice

My interviewees in Lesotho clearly point out that they were well aware of the feeding advice from hospital, and that these recommendations may interfere with other social obligations and behavioural expectations. Exclusive breastfeeding of children born to HIV-positive mothers proved difficult, as women might be advised differently by family elders and in many cases relatives would feed the child additionally, since counselled women avoided lecturing and controlling superiors and inverting an age hierarchy. The same challenges were evident in many African countries and apparently only a "disappointingly low" fraction of women were able to adhere to their feeding option "perhaps because of social norms and the complex decision making surrounding these practices" (Tavengwa et al. 2007: 103; cf. Bland et al. 2007; Liamputtong 2011). Evidently, the guidelines had focused solely on biomedical concerns of "safe infant nutrition" while neglecting the social ramifications of food, which imply security, support and integration of mother and child into their community.

In short, the biggest obstacle is posed by the term "exclusive feeding". In the guidelines it was defined as feeding the infant nothing other than either breast milk or formula milk and any prescribed medications for six months (GoL 2009 (a): 56). Mixing different nutrients, even giving water to the child, was discouraged in the guidelines and in the counselling sessions. For the mothers this advice proved difficult in practice since it meant that only full disclosure will allow one to engage in the exclusive feeding practice given that others will not be able to take care of the child while a mother works, for instance, as this would mean they would have to feed it additionally. Full disclosure is in fact not an easy decision for HIV-positive women in a precarious situation (cf. Desclaux & Alfieri 2009).

Generally speaking, exclusive feeding practices which are not normative indicate a disease, for instance a HIV infection, and women fear falling victim to stigma (Bland et al. 2007; Thairu et al. 2005; Desclaux & Alfieri 2009) as depicted in these two statements from nurses:

> Yes, it is (...) a stigma, because when [the mother] tells somebody that she does not breastfeed the baby, this person will enquire as to the reason and she will be suspected of being HIV-positive. For some it is difficult. Even when the baby is seven months old or one year, she will say, she has difficulties in weaning the baby, because [family members] will ask, why is she not breastfeeding? (Field notes Kroeker Mampho: 27/03/2007, cf. Moland 2004).

A second nurse explains the stigma women feel when opting for exclusive breastfeeding, a term which is generally associated with HIV-positive mothers only.

> So when she has to tell the family that she has to do exclusive breastfeeding that is going to be a problem because she will have the fear that (...) they might think that I'm HIV-positive. (…) Especially for the HIV-positive mothers we find that this mother will even be afraid to tell them "the nurse had said, that I should not give the water, I should not give anything, I should just give breast (…) they will know that I'm HIV-positive, oh, I can't tell them!" (Field notes Kroeker Mampho PMTCT: 22/03/2007).

In my quantitative survey including 161 women, by far the largest proportion chose mixed feeding as it is the cultural norm and even 10% of those who tested HIV-positive did so even if advised otherwise by medical staff. Of those who chose replacement feeding with formula milk, about two thirds were HIV-positive.

To my surprise the numbers of those who chose exclusive breastfeeding were not commensurate with those women who tested HIV-positive. This has two reasons: first of all, exclusive breastfeeding is nowadays generally recommended to all women who attend antenatal care. Nurses caution that some of them may be HIV-positive but the virus is not yet detectable or may contract the virus while pregnant, during delivery or while breastfeeding. Secondly, this reduces stigma for those who are HIV-positive. For more than ten years now exclusive breastfeeding has been promoted as the healthiest and cheapest option for mother and child. With this message even elder gen-

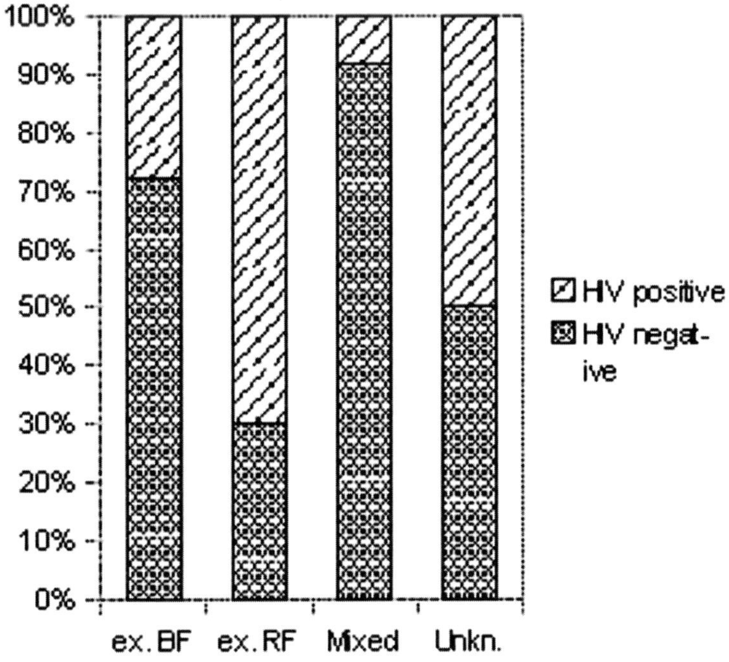

Infant Feeding Choice among HIV positive and HIV negative mothers (Source: ATCBM study Kroeker 2008)

erations were confronted and advised their young next-of-kin accordingly. However, generally speaking, clients of antenatal care units chose between rather practical and impractical recommendations and only incorporated those into their lives which proposed the greatest benefit while being the least difficult to apply (cf. Stuart-Macadam & Dettwyler 1997: 124).

I will now present three cases which illustrate decision-making on infant nutrition. In all cases decision-making was a long-term process over several months in which the women discarded plans and aligned their strategy. All thirty women received counselling on biomedical arguments during antenatal care and practical assistance from family members. MaMapeli decided on exclusive breastfeeding for six months. Leshome opted for exclusive replacement feeding, whereas Tselela decided to mix feed her baby.

7.4 MaMapeli's Socially Safe Practice: Exclusive Breastfeeding

MaMapeli lived with her mother, a brother and a younger sister in the backroom of their little shop. MaMapeli was 25 years old and pregnant for the third time, when I met her. She had already tested HIV-positive in 2006 after her second baby had passed away and she disclosed her status to her mother, *Nkhono*. Nkhono also went to the hospital and was tested positive in the presence of her daughter. They had a very comprehensible and understanding counsellor who made them aware that they may have been infected when caring for a sick brother who had died of AIDS without disclosing it. Further to this explanation, the counselling sessions helped mother and daughter to understand and accept their test results and MaMapeli now concludes that both her children must have died of the disease, which they had contracted through her.

MaMapeli did not get married when she fell pregnant for the first time aged 16 and again aged 21. Now, in 2008, MaMapeli fell in love again, but fears that her boyfriend will reject her if she discloses her HIV status to him. Since she had already tested positive he will blame her for bringing HIV into the relationship. She thus keeps silent about her infection and assumes that he will not accept her otherwise, since "he is not clear about these things". MaMapeli fears losing another important person in her life after earlier disappointments with her previous boyfriends and after having lost two children. Luckily, this one proposes to her, she accepts and soon falls pregnant again, however, MaMapeli had no idea how she was going to comply with PMTCT as she had not disclosed her status to her in-laws. Nevertheless, especially since she experienced difficulties with her previous babies, which now urge her to comply with PMTCT, she has plans to strictly breastfeed the baby exclusively for six months. Of course, she is worried that her mother-in-law may criticise her feeding practice and try to feed additional food to the infant, thwarting MaMapeli's plans. Nkhono and MaMapeli discussed the issue and agreed that the mother-in-law will, according to her role as teacher, advise MaMapeli on good infant care and nutrition, in fact, she has the right and duty to do so.

> MaMapeli blames herself for having lost the children and seeks ways to have a healthy child this time. This time, the personal conditions are much more favourable than during her previous pregnancies. MaMapeli recalls that during her first pregnancy she was working in the textile factory, which was stressful and physically exhausting.

> When she went to work the child was fed by a caretaker and she breastfed after work. After being sickly her baby boy passed away aged 14 months. From her present perspective she concludes that she must have been infected with HIV already, however, an HIV-test was not done in antenatal care at that time.
>
> In her second pregnancy she tried traditional herbs to treat complaints which she related to problems in conception or early pregnancy (I assume that she underwent a cleaning ritual which she had not done after the first baby's death, although she did not say so explicitly). Her family had no history in traditional medication but faith-based healing, but MaMapeli wanted to combine preventive measures. On her own MaMapeli bought herbs from a street vendor in town. The *pitsa* gave her unbearably strong but short labour pains and the baby was delivered prematurely in the 7th month of pregnancy[12]. The child died the following day and she reflects retrospectively, that traditional treatment gave even worse results than the hospital care with her first pregnancy.
>
> Now in her third pregnancy, one of her brothers sends income from South Africa and she no longer needs to work in the textile factory. She feels more relaxed helping out in her mother's tuck shop and the HIV-treatment has made her physically fitter. Moreover, family relations are settled since this time the child will be born within wedlock and her marriage makes her happy. At the same time the explanations from the counsellors gave her peace of mind about what happened with her previous children. Consequently, she trusted their advice.
>
> In her early pregnancy she had moved to her in-law's home in Mohale's Hoek after the wedding and now shifts again to her mother's house in her seventh month of pregnancy.

The fact that she moved to her mother's house, and that she feared so much interference from her mother-in-law, made me think that her in-laws did not know about her earlier pregnancies (cf. Kaufman et al. 2000: 2). Pregnancies out of wedlock as well as HIV suggest low moral values and I assume that she concealed this information, whereas being unwed without children at the age of 25 and working in a family-owned store, made for a much better reputation.

---

[12] This suggests that she received the *pitsa* which is usually given during labour and not the one for pregnancy (see Chapter 5).

> MaMapeli as well as her mother were shy and silent persons who bestirred themselves to please others and MaMapeli did not feel entitled to instruct her mother-in-law who, on the contrary, is meant to instruct MaMapeli on their clan practices. Under no circumstances does she intend to disobey her mother in law's authority and hence lose her support. Nkhono and MaMapeli eventually find a solution that avoids having uncomfortable discussions: MaMapeli will stay in Mafeteng for six months until she has weaned the child instead of moving back to her marital home after three to four months post-partum. The child will be able to eat adult food by the time they return to Mohale's Hoek.

I visited MaMapeli and her mother a few days after the delivery. Both complained that MaMapeli did not produce enough milk to breastfeed the baby. The baby was crying at night because it was hungry but milk was in short supply. She had experienced the same problem with her first child but supplemented the little milk with other nutrients, which the PMTCT counsellor had discouraged her from doing now.

> Nkhono and MaMapeli are frustrated and scared. Both fear that the child will starve since they are not allowed to give it prelacteral liquids. Nkhono prepares maize-porridge to make her daughter "strong and help to produce more milk", and eventually milk comes which relieves mother and daughter.
>
> In the meantime, MaMapeli manages to disclose her HIV-status to the in-laws. When the parents-in-law come for the naming ceremony after the umbilical cord falls off, Nkhono talks to them about HIV and asks them to let MaMapeli stay in Mafeteng for six months. Although it is not easy for her to tackle the issue, fortunately the in-laws react in an understanding and supportive way. MaMapeli also learns from them that there is another relative living with HIV and hence the family is used to the procedures already. Yet, her husband however has still not been tested (Field notes Kroeker: 19/11/2008-29/04/2009).

After having lost loved ones before, MaMapeli avoids situations that would push her family-in-law away, while she experiences loving support from her mother. She did not realise that the marriage she was so looking forward to could cause conflicts because it would be difficult to comply with her HIV treatment.

According to these considerations mothers may not dare to discuss their health and PMTCT advice since it would dismantle the family's social integrity. The fear of stigma in that case impedes an open discussion on the topic and any kind of support needed cannot be granted. Hence, it is not necessarily the woman counselled during antenatal care who decides based on the information given, but her social expectations and the environment with which she interacts.

HIV-positive people often avoid mentioning their status as this may lead to marital disputes and therewith they invoked others to speak on their behalf. "Passing" conflicts or sending mediators appears a common means used by HIV-positive mothers to avoid losing face. In the course of my study, a discussion among elders, as suggested by Nkhono to solve MaMapeli's dilemma, often proved a successful means of disclosing the information. Other women benefitted from a talk among elders as well, while they avoided direct confrontation. Thus, a mediator represents an opinion and uses own resources (arms, strategies, social position, power, etc.) to fuel the argument.

Leshome, the protagonist of the following case, enters into conflict, unlike MaMapeli. However, she also discovers difficulties with intergenerational roles, involves a mediator and "passes" in the end to settle the dispute.

7.5 Leshome's Informed Decision-Making: Exclusive Replacement Feeding

In Leshome's family there were also known cases of death due to AIDS and these family stories contributed to her attitude towards the whole issue. Accepting her family history, Leshome volunteered to train as a peer educator for HIV-positive colleagues at her workplace in the textile factory through which she learned more about the subject and encouraged other people to be tested[13].

> Leshome, 36 and in a long-distance relationship, is known in her neighbourhood to be an activist and even initiated a support group at her rented room. The support group helps her in two ways: She therewith brings women together to discuss challenges which accompany

[13] Support groups contribute to frank discussions on social and medical conflicts, decision-making, and exchanging successful strategies amongst people living with HIV (cf. Desclaux & Alfieri 2009).

the infection and, secondly, she combines these meetings with her small business of selling household goods. Leshome sees her open way of dealing with her infection as a way to avoid finger pointing and stigma. She concludes "it will be easier to accept it, if you are open".

After she had learned about PMTCT in her training she recognises the treatment as a chance for producing a healthy child (cf. Rethabile in Chapter 8.2). Being a role model for others she opts for the method she considers medically safest in order to prevent a vertical infection: A Caesarean Section and exclusive formula feeding. She will there-with schedule the time of delivery and go back to work after six weeks of maternity leave.

Leshome intends to take her mother to one of the antenatal care examinations in the hospital so that she can also be informed about PMTCT and assist her with the early infant care accordingly. Although Leshome had all the information, she flinches from entering a discussion with her most important supporter, thus, Leshome expects a counsellor to initiate the discussion about controversial practices of safe pregnancy, delivery and breastfeeding.

Leshome did not inform her mother about her delivery by sectio but when she visits her daughter after the delivery in the hospital she was told so. The mother admits that she was very worried about the "scissor-delivery" when she heard it and would never have opted for it herself. She had delivered eight healthy children normally and suggested that natural birth is the right way for mother and child whereas operations are highly uncertain. Leshome nevertheless opted for it to reduce the probability of infecting the child and additionally she trusted the nurses to be professional.

Leshome's mother now comes daily to visit mother and child in the hospital where Leshome stays for one week. The granny runs errands like washing the nappies, bringing food, clothes and baby products, changing the baby and looking after house and garden like a grandmother would do after a home delivery. However, she has to bring all equipment needed to the hospital, which is a burden for the old lady. Despite not using traditional medication herself, granny argues that it is unsafe to bath in the bowl used by everybody in the hospital. Often traditional healers gave powerful liquids as a bath additive and they may affect Leshome in her condition between life and death if using

> the same bowl and she therefore prefers to use her personal items. Bringing along these materials was considered a disadvantage of hospital deliveries.
> Leshome is hardly able to move during the first few days because of the stitches and discovers, in contradiction to her previous plans, breastfeeding more convenient than preparing artificial baby milk in the hospital. She can hardly get up since her scar hurts and the crying baby will wake the other babies in the post-delivery room. Leshome's mother supports her decision to breastfeed and advises her on the benefits of it. Granny assists moreover in holding the baby properly, advises to change the breasts several times and teaches Leshome on how to take care of the nipples. Leshome agrees to exclusive breastfeeding for 21 days until she has to report back to her employer in the textile factory where she will collect tins of milk formula. She finds this a practical compromise of medical and familial instructions.
> Granny explains to me later that only few women will not breastfeed at all because of health problems. Most will breastfeed like she breastfed all her children exclusively for nine months but when she had to leave the house others fed her infants with cow's milk. Leshome enters into the discussion and insists that she will have to set a certain time for complete weaning whenever she can no longer assure full breastfeeding on demand.

In the course of our discussion it turned out that mother and daughter had different definitions of "exclusiveness". While the grandmother referred in the discussion to the time of introducing solids, her daughter defined the term "weaning" as the time when nursing ceases.

The predominantly English terminology used in the biomedical setting seems to be a general challenge. Even if the new mother was able to tell her elder family members about her desire to exclusively breastfeed and gained their support, much confusion exists in the community over what exclusive breastfeeding entails. A nurse explains:

> We find usually the mothers-in-law giving water to the children, even if they are supportive of exclusive breastfeeding. They don't see water as a replacement food, they don't find it a problem." (Field notes Kroeker: 11/06/2008).

Often relatives do not distinguish between water and milk, since milk consists of water to a large extent. Leshome's mother likewise considers animal milk and water still part of an exclusive milk-based diet of an infant. Leshome understood from the hospital counselling sessions that exclusive breastfeeding does not allow water or dairy products. Despite this, exclusively-breastfed children are given antibiotics (cotrimoxazol) as prophylaxis while being exposed to HIV in the milk. Hence, this syrup could be easily misinterpreted as a supplement to breast milk, contradicting "exclusiveness". Vitamin K syrup, which a newborn receives instantly after delivery, would literally also fall under the definition of prelacteral or additional food, thus contradicting an exclusive feeding practice in a strict sense. However, neither traditional nor biomedical prelacteral food fulfils a nutritional purpose but a medical one. Both are meant to prevent some hypothetical deficiency in the baby's body. The definition would either prohibit both practices or neither of them, depending on interpretation. An additional challenge is the *lelomolo* bite as part of the ceremony when a mother returns home to her marital household after her seclusion at her paternal house:

> Leshome and her mother also discuss the child's naming and welcoming ceremony. According to their clan two feasts have to take place, one when the child is a few days old and another some months later when the child receives the first *Lelomolo*-bite. Being sick and a first time mother, Leshome finds herself dependent on a supportive family network including favourable ancestral conditions. Therefore Leshome considers this family integration a crucial rite she will not miss out on. However, Leshome and her mother arrange that it will take place a little later when the child is old enough and weaned already. It was not possible to fulfil other clan practices due to practical reasons: Actually, the baby is also supposed to wear a necklace of wildcat tail, but since these animals are almost extinct, her family decides to neglect this rite.

Several women in the study faced the same difficulty as Leshome when attempting to combine exclusive breastfeeding and the welcoming ceremony. Like Leshome, both LeNne and LeMeli decided to delay the *Lelomolo* ceremony until the child no longer suckles (Field notes Kroeker: 04/12/2008; 12: 13/01/2009).

In summary, even though Leshome was well-informed and made her mind up about her safe feeding practice, she discovered difficulties in following her conviction. She nevertheless managed to combine medical and cultural demands as she appropriated advice as best suited her respective situation. On the one hand, she was well-informed about biomedical advice through her work as a peer counsellor and had strong support on a familial basis for those arguments through her family history. On the other hand, both her boyfriend and her mother supported her, but the geographical distance leaves decisions up to her. The only thing she did not manage, despite great efforts, was to teach her baby to drink from a cup. Eventually she gave up trying, as the baby spilled the milk and she bought a baby bottle although the nurse complained when she saw it. Thereafter, in hospital counselling sessions she would not use the bottle but try to feed using a cup, although at home and in the crèche this feeding practice was just not feasible. Despite the disapproval of the nurse who refers to the guidelines, a counsellor also admits that feeding a baby with a cup is just impossible. She therefore counsels the mothers according to the guidelines but did not comply with this advice herself. In her opinion, especially at night, it would take a long time to prepare and feed, while the milk would be spilled over the bed, clothes and the child, whereas a bottle can be readily prepared before going to sleep. In her opinion, mothers should be taught how to keep the bottles in a hygienic condition instead of banning their use. Nevertheless, she has to counsel the women on the basis of the guidelines, which prohibit bottle feeding (Field notes Kroeker MaThloni: 02/04/2009).

7.6 Tselela's Struggle with Tradition, HIV and Infant Feeding

Four young women under study were single and pregnant when I met them. All of them had attended secondary school but lacked life prospects such as a job or other occupation. This resulted in dissatisfaction with their situation and left them lonely, insecure and lacking confidence. They eagerly sought love, attention and support from their social environment and while three girls expected to find a constant partner and get married after falling pregnant, one sought attention from her father. This unsatisfied demand for someone to care and love for them rendered them somewhat short of options and decision-making power.

Four older, married women, amongst them Tselela, also shared this characteristic of lacking in prospects. Those women had children already but were not living with them since they grew up with relatives while these four older women stayed in single rented rooms in town for various reasons: some were looking for work which left them frustrated, others had lost their employment and had not yet moved back to their relatives, while others assumed urban life to be more exciting than village life and did not want to stay with their families, and, thus, also did not want to move back there after having experienced urban life. Some older women, in particular, had only attended primary school and therewith had little chance of being employed in town but depended fully on a partner in labour migration, whereas the younger girls may also have intended to find a boyfriend or husband. In conclusion, all eight women, for different reasons, found their occupation in caring for a child.

Besides these structural difficulties of their livelihood, all of them found it extremely hard to accept their HIV-positive status after being tested in antenatal care. Due to denial of the test result, disclosing to their partner as well as accepting treatment was more or less impossible. When comparing the cases and looking for similarities, I also learned that all eight women frequently missed check-up appointments and were not accustomed to structuring their day. The households were in poor condition and they had no idea how to pass their time and keep themselves busy. Maybe a larger household community and living and working in a group of female next-of-kin who share household chores would have helped them, however, on their own they felt highly vulnerable and lonely. I assume that anxiety about caring for a child well and a lack of collaboration with familiar community members, who support mother and child during the post-partum period, added to that (cf. Avishai 2011: 28-30). Furthermore, they all had low self-esteem and on their own without any company, guidance and duties, their strategy concerning pregnancy and child-care appeared somewhat irrational and confused as they tried to orient themselves, as shown in Tselela's case:

> Tselela aged 32 lived on her own in a single rented room. Her two children, 11 and 8 years, remained with her relatives when she had moved to town two years ago. Despite little education she found employment in the garment sector, however, she is currently no longer working there and completely relies on her husband's remittances from abroad. She speaks of him in a bad way, telling that he is not making money, hence does not care for his wife and children sufficiently.

I found Tselela to be lonely, as well as craving attention and a means to keep herself occupied. While trying to keep a stiff upper lip, she was shocked to test HIV-positive in antenatal care and she doubted the result to be true. She tried to convince herself that nothing had changed and avoided telling anyone about the test. In manifold creative ways she tried hard to hide the stigmatising information, whereas in hospital she presented herself as a compliant and understanding client. In front of the counsellor she stated that she had disclosed to her husband, her two sisters, one of whom is living just next door in the same terraced house, and that she was well supported by her relatives. In short, Tselela produced answers which she thought would please the counsellor in hospital, her family and last, but not least, me. Further questions and participant observation during my home visits, however, revealed that she rarely had a clear understanding and became entangled in contradictions while making up stories.

> In the counselling session Tselela agrees to deliver in hospital just like she did with her previous children and opts for exclusive breastfeeding for six months. The counsellors were satisfied with her compliance not knowing that she keeps on changing her medical book in an attempt to behave as good client, whereas during home visits she indicates doubts about the practices she agreed upon in the hospital.

In a subsequent visit Tselela told me that the third child was born in a home delivery assisted by her relatives. She is breastfeeding the child, but she complains that she does not produce sufficient milk to satisfy it. With her previous children she also had problems providing milk but at that time she introduced complementary foods at an early age to solve this problem. Like MaMapeli, Tselela, as well as many other mothers, doubted that breast milk was enough to satisfy their baby's hunger. However, counsellors insisted frequently that they were not trying hard enough and milk will eventually come in ample amount, if they would only keep on trying. In contrast, mothers felt that they were malnourishing their child if they did not add supplementary drinks.

> Aged six weeks the baby weighed a meagre 3.6 kg and it had only gained a further 0.9 kg by 13 weeks old. Moreover, the baby failed to thrive and developed dark stains on its tiny, pale body. Regardless of whether Tselela was not providing sufficient milk or she introduced complementary food too early and therewith inhibited a sufficient milk production, just as a counsellor suggested, Tselela opted for mix feeding. I shall add here that an increasing number of women indeed have difficulties to breastfeed sufficiently, like Tselela. For an increasing number, a lack of financial means create food shortages and hence malnutrition affects the milk production and thus the national guide-

lines on PMTCT foresee mixed feeding as an emergency plan for malnourished mothers and children (cf. Kroeker & Beckwith 2011).

In Lesotho, food insecurity often results in malnourished women who lack milk for feeding their babies, according to a nutritionist at Roma University in Lesotho. Due to scarce resources and high levels of malnutrition women may not provide enough milk to feed the baby solely on breast milk, hence the time for introducing additional foods also depends on this factor (cf. Maher 1992: 8). Especially during the first couple of days after delivery, young mothers were usually served with maize porridge by their caretakers such as that received by neophytes in various rites of passage. A common Basotho belief emphasises the need to serve young mothers with maize porridge as "the more they eat, the more milk they are going to provide" (Field notes Kroeker 7: 25/11/2008; 29: 30/11/2008; Kroeker: 04/12/2008), and also in the biomedical discourse maize porridge is known to enhance lactation (Bianccuzzo 2005: 31, 55). Despite attempts to enhance milk production, in many cases around age four to six months supplementary foods need to be introduced to prevent additional health constraints of the infant (Field notes Kroeker: 05/07/2008; cf. Gottlieb et al. 2004). I cannot say whether Tselela was actually malnourished and therefore lacked milk, if she lacked milk due to other reasons, or whether she merely thought she lacked milk. Maybe she also said this to justify a mixed feeding practice.

In any event, there is a close connection between nutritional intake and immune function as physicians warn against a devastating cycle of malnutrition for HIV-positive people and in particular HIV-positive breastfeeding mothers. Nutrition and HIV are intimately linked, with malnutrition having deleterious effects on the health of people living with HIV/AIDS. Malnutrition exacerbates the weakening of the immune system, which is already compromised by HIV. The effects of malnutrition on the immune system are, according to Piwoz and colleagues, much like the damaging effects of the virus itself (Piwoz et al. 2005: 934). For this reason, the WHO recommends increased macronutrient intake for people living with HIV, including the need for an increase in 20-30% of energy requirements during symptomatic HIV (WHO 2003: 4). A breastfeeding mother consumes about 2700 kcal a day compared to 2200 when not pregnant or breastfeeding. Consuming less than 1500 kcal a day is discouraged at any time in pregnancy or while nursing a child (Biacuzzo 2005: 87, 89). According to the Food and Agriculture Organization of the United Nations, the average dietary energy requirement in Lesotho for 2004-2006 was 2,200 kcal per day and the minimum was

1,770 kcal per day (FAO 2010: 1). However, anthropologists Romero-Daza and Himmelgreen advise against assuming that calorific intake is sufficient for assessing nutrition among the Basotho (Romero-Daza et al. 2009: 26). Diets too heavily reliant on carbohydrates, which comprise over 76% of the dietary energy supply in Lesotho, lack essential macro and micronutrients, which are needed for healthy immune functioning. A low immunological condition of the mother, which correlates with a high viral load, makes a transmission from mother to child more likely. Once again, bearing these arguments in mind, the value of breast milk over replacement food for children who are exposed to HIV can be questioned from a biomedical point of view.

Despite the dilemmas which exclusive feeding practices entail, various cultures suggest, based on local medical notions, that breast milk is not healthy for the child in particular situations and warn against breastfeeding. Stuart-Macadam and Dettwyler as well as Maher present ideas whereby under certain circumstances such as tension, stress and tiredness, mothers in North Tunisia must not breastfeed since the milk would be "bad" due to their own "hot" condition (Maher 1992; cf. Liamputtong 2011). Stuart-Macadam and Dettwyler mention that stress reduces the amount of milk, since it constricts the blood vessels around the areola and hence inhibits milk ejection. This stressful and tense situation may affect milk production in a psychosomatic way as Quandt (1995) points out – actually this is a good reason why various cultures prescribe that mothers should stay at their maternal home where less social tension and good care helps with relaxing after a delivery. Tselela obviously finds herself in a tense situation as she struggles to keep up an impression of financial, social and personal security. In those circumstances, mixed infant nutrition seemed to be the most "Acceptable, Feasible, Affordable, Sustainable and Safe" option for her.

> After the child was unwell a counsellor authorised the feeding practice Tselela had followed out of her own experience. A counsellor explains: "Nowadays, there are so many malnourished women! That's why we say, they should continue breastfeeding if they can't afford to [wean and] introduce other foods. They should mix feed nowadays despite HIV. Malnutrition is the one killing the child" (Field notes Kroeker MaThloni: 27/01/2010). The counsellor furthermore states "[We] can give treatment to handle HIV somehow. However, if the baby dies of malnutrition it is better to mix feed it before that" (Field notes Kroeker MaThloni: 26/01/2009).

As in this example, and shown by the counsellor's comments on feeding practices, medical guidelines solely concern the health of the child, not the situation of the mother. In her precarious situation of dependency and little agency she did not want to be bothered with information about her deteriorated health and a sickly baby. Tselela basically relied on the practice she was already used to, her bodily feeling, and tried to secure her livelihood.

> While Tselela attends the under-5-check-ups in hospital, Tselela avoids the HIV-counselling sessions. She again pretends not to be HIV-positive which her new medical book also indicates. This (however wrong) information allows her to mix feed the baby. Complementary feeding also proves more convenient for her since it allows her to search for a job and leave the baby in the care of her sister.

I suppose that her desire to find a job and be ready to leave the baby with a caretaker factored into her decision (on the correlation of work and feeding practice cf. Liamputtong 2011), which must be respected against all odds.

7.7 A Quest for Order

While the traditional system granted social security, it lacked medical prevention of disorders that were detected in antenatal care. In a contrasting perspective, biomedicine offered assistance to prevent high blood pressure or HIV for example, hence diseases of the biomedical classification, but neglected disorders known by traditional healers. Women thus tried to combine advantages of both medical schools as far as possible (Sargent 1989: 46). Moland, who assessed the situation of HIV-positive women and their infant feeding choice, argues

> that it is the rural, economically poor and socially disadvantaged women that are least likely to practise what, by the health authorities, have been defined as safe feeding options, including replacement feeding of animal milk or infant formula, or exclusive breastfeeding. But this effect cannot be explained in terms of disbelief or distrust of medical knowledge and expertise. HIV positive women who breastfeed tend to do so because the alternative is worse and involves a great risk of losing status as a social person (Moland 2004: n.p.)

Since this statement, which concerns Tanzania, the situation has somewhat changed in terms of the guidelines, but not much when it comes to the social aspects. I disagree, however, that the rural, economically poor and socially disadvantaged find it hard to comply with biomedical directives. MaMapeli as well as Tselela found themselves in economically poor situations, however their limited options led to quite different choices. MaMapeli found herself in a socially safer and protected situation. Tselela, on the other hand, was in need of social support since she lacked stability. Her precarious situation and her insecure moves are proof of her struggle for order and security. She, hence, turned towards what seemed to be safest to her. For others, a traditional frame of reference gives orientation, while sorting life out. While other women who lived on their own in town, which also meant without close familial support, exchange, and supervision, were more often employed and hence at least economically independent in their decisions, Tselela stumbled in this respect.

After this last visit I tried to reflect on her situation. Tselela as well as the seven other study participants denied their HIV-positive status altogether. Their unsatisfactory financial, social and marital situation was unlikely to change any time soon. A baby would at least keep them busy. The HIV-positive test added a defective health prospective to their situation of social insecurity. In this insecure and precarious situation these women were in search of guiding principles as a means of security. The hospital situation, in contrast, caused additional discomfort, even more so if the medical book and counselling officially labelled them as HIV-positive. To avoid the stigma, they avoided situations, places and people that would remind them of their "spoiled identity" (Goffman 1963). Hence, non-adherence to biomedical advice appeared as the socially safest way to cover up the HIV-infection since adherence may confirm acceptance of their status. Tired of the repetitive conversations with the counsellor, Tselela changed her strategy of hiding and interrupts the counsellor's talk.

> T.: If a person is not willing to do what you tell her, why don't you just let the person die?
>
> C.: Because I am caring for the child. You can take care of the child, but the child can't take care of itself.
>
> T.: If I die, my sisters will take care of my children or you can take the child. If someone is dying it is the will of God.
>
> C.: God likes seeing you helping yourself.
>
> The counsellor suggests then that she would like to talk to Tselela's husband whenever he is around.

> T.: If he is here he might kick your ass when you are coming!
>
> In a silent almost sobbing voice she then says after a while:
>
> T.: It's just that you make me worried every time [when being counselled] and I don't like that (Field notes Kroeker: 30/10/2008-01/04/2009).

While the biomedical facility reminded Tselela of stigma and shame, she decided on a traditional delivery and traditional feeding practice which were socially safe and "HIV free". Expectations were served to the fullest and, even more than that, in order to avoid any attention by nurses or counsellors. Meanwhile, they argued in favour of traditional advice which they had not followed with earlier pregnancies, but which now gave them some control and behavioural instructions. Eventually Tharo, MaSupa and Tselela delivered at home, which they had not considered in earlier pregnancies. As with Peli, who had argued that her husband makes the decisions on her health (see 5.4), following a patriarchal family picture, for instance, they denied any agency to make decisions and decided to relinquish responsibility from their hands into the hands of elders and superiors guiding them which promised to keep them grounded. Insecurity impacted on a quest for order which they found in a partly neo-conservative turn of lifestyle. Insecurity, however, increased since someone may find out about their secret, a tainted identity.

For others, strictly complying with biomedical protocols gave some guidance. Urban women may not be confronted with traditional explanations as much as they are with biomedical information as they mostly live in small household communities and biomedical institutions, technologies and staff assured them constantly that they are doing what is best for their child. However, even here women were sometimes disappointed because recommendations changed time and again and therewith lacked reliability. Here the same was true for what Browner and Press described in US hospitals:

> Women also were sceptical about the validity of biomedical information because of the speed with which biomedical advice to pregnant women has changed. Although most said they believed the advice they themselves were receiving was more correct than that given their mothers, that it was often so different gave some pause.(…) Finally, many multiparous women had received prenatal care from a different physician for each pregnancy, and had received conflicting advice

> from each, providing further evidence that they could not simply accept what doctors said (Browner & Press 1997: 118).

First and foremost, constant changes in the guidelines and updates trickled down from the ministerial to the counsellor's level. While counsellors in the hospital received training on shifts and changes in the policy, counsellors in the health centres had not yet been updated but acquired new information during their monitoring instruments. Procedures therefore differed from one site to another, between medical hierarchies, and perhaps even in the same facility (Field notes Kroeker: 15/01/2009). Secondly, criteria for starting treatment of mother and child also changed time and again. While one client received syrup to give to the baby as prophylaxis during the first week of life, others did not receive it since prophylaxis was already administered to the infant through the mother's milk, while she took her tablets. As a result, one of the counsellors complained that there is no stability and continuity concerning information on which the counsellor and the women can rely: "This thing of HIV makes child-bearing difficult" (Field notes Kroeker Violet: 21/05/2009).

Resetting the Reproductive Cycle

For those like Tselela who lived in town on their own without any occupation, relationships, such as extramarital affairs, entailed attention, sexual desire and material presents from the lover. In all these cases I will impute loneliness, lack of attention, no or little occupation, inadequate financial means and marital dissatisfaction. To make myself clear, I do not see a general correlation between unemployment and extramarital affairs. Some cases in my sample rather suggested that a lack of familial community, supervision and care made sexual relations a pass-time (cf. Gronemeyer 2006 (a), 2006 (b)). For women, relationships also bring along material gifts, thus, for someone in need perhaps this also matters. Moreover, gifts carry values of appreciation (Mauss 1968) and are signs of love, both of which these women lacked. Even though Tselela and Tharo, who I will present in Chapter 9, were longing for some occupation both had difficulties accepting the child when it was born, presumably, the *corpus delicti* of an affair, but who knows.

Getting pregnant by a husband in labour migration was sometimes difficult. Spouses usually came home monthly after payday for one weekend - always at the same time of the female cycle. Even when neglecting contraception it would prove difficult for the women to fall pregnant by their husband, which they would have appreciated to keep them occupied. Some women additionally intended to mend a relationship by getting pregnant particularly after some upset and quarrels. For others, a boyfriend or a casual fling may have been welcome in an economic, sexual and entertaining respect.

Before the introduction of modern contraception, family planning concerns contributed to encouragement of long-term breastfeeding which can be brought down to two reasons: physical health of mother and child as well as ritual re-integration.

Time-gaps between deliveries are widely regarded as important to women's health while still recovering from an earlier delivery whereas early weaning is criticised because it is associated with short spacing between pregnancies (Stuart-Macadam & Dettwyler 1995: 25; Bledsoe 2002). Accordingly, hospital files recording births in patients, particularly women with a high number of births show regular birth intervals which suggests that traditional methods of child spacing were followed. The Basotho spaced their children without contraceptives by practising long-term breastfeeding and sexual abstinence at the same time (Hall & Malahleha 1989: 53, 59;

Stuart-Macadam & Dettwyler 1995: 125; Field notes Kroeker: 20/03/2009). While a couple continues to have intercourse during pregnancy and the father therewith "feeds" the child in the mother's womb, a taboo forbade intercourse while the mother lactated. Hence, the average time between births spans three years - two years of intensive childcare followed by nine months of a subsequent pregnancy (Field notes 3/2007; Ashton 1967: 34). Usually, birth intervals were shorter (27 months) if the preceding sibling had died (MoHSW 2005: 55).

For the mother, sexual abstinence not only has a medical but also a ritual connotation. Turner (2005: 102-103) describes abstinence as being part of the indifferent asexual character of a person in a transitional state (Ngubane 1976: 282; Gausset 1998, 2002). Commencing sexual activity correlates with re-integration as a complete adult member of the society. Meanwhile, birth spacing is not only beneficiary for the mother but also for the baby which may be harmed if weaned too early. By the age of two the baby is considered to be physically and psychologically mature enough to be independent from the mother.

Similar taboos prescribing combinations of breastfeeding and a postpartum sex taboo are reported across cultures in many communities around the world:

> According to communities of the South Pacific like the Maisin and Kaliai (...) semen are believed to contaminate the breast milk and make a child sick. The aim of postpartum abstinence is to preserve the health of the child, and some groups like the Akan of Ghana practice it due to the belief in the negative impact of closely spaced pregnancies, and a woman's ability to care for her children (Bleek 1990 in: Yovsi 2003: 22).

Likewise Bledsoe notes for the rural population in the Gambia:

> There are two distinct types of concerns with respect to overlap: those surrounding the resumption of sex while breastfeeding and those surrounding the possibility of becoming pregnant while breastfeeding. With respect to the former, a significant worry is that male fluids may dilute the breast milk, exposing a breastfeeding baby to nutritional risk. As a result, the baby may become "dry" (thin) and weak from fever and diarrhea. As it gets older and begins food supplementation, the dangers posed by dilution recede and increasing the frequency of sexual contact is considered to be safer (Bledsoe 2002: 103).

In Basotho people's local discourse the taboo likewise implies the idea that ejaculate affects the milk and therewith harms a suckling baby (cf. Maher 1992: 6; Field notes Kroeker: 15/03/2009; 08/04/2009; 17/03/2009) and Sechefo describes that a break in this sexual taboo will leave a baby malnourished (Sechefo n.d.: 26; Hall & Malahleha 1989: 53; Romero-Daza & Himmelgreen 2004: 961). Romero-Daza further explains the consequences of breaking the post-partum sex taboo among the Basotho:

> there is a strict taboo against sexual relations during the post-partum period and especially during the breast-feeding period, which may extend for up to two years. Engaging in sexual activity during the lactation period is believed to result in the contamination of the breast milk by the semen, which causes serious health problems to the infant. "Senyeha" as the disease is called, is characterized by rapid weight loss, severe diarrhoea, loss of appetite, and failure to thrive, and may be fatal to the infant (Romero-Daza & Himmelgreen 2004: 961).

According to Ashton, the same belief relates to replacement or mixed fed children. Cow's milk as infant nutriment is only safe if the cow has not been covered since calving (Ashton 1952: 32). Covering will also affect a cow's milk which is therefore not safe for a baby to drink.

Contrasting this notion, a traditional healer explained that it is not the ejaculate that harms the child, but the violation of the taboo. The husband's contact with other women for sexual gratification at that time may transfer afflictions and bring them along to the marital home. Therefore it is in fact adultery which is harmful for the child and the mother's abstinence shall protect it (Field notes Kroeker: 27/03/2009). Therefore the taboo is meant to prevent sexually transmitted diseases.

Notwithstanding, the taboo on sexual abstinence while the baby is still small did not apply to men. In European countries in the 16th-18th century a post-partum sex taboo was also the norm and sexual intercourse in this context was likewise believed to "spoil the milk". However, husbands preferred to prevent their wives from breastfeeding than forego their sexual privilege (Maher 1992: 6). In other societies a long post-partum sex taboo was discussed in correlation with polygynous societies. Bretschneider (1995), however, cannot confirm a correlation of a post-partum sex taboo and polygyny. While one wife was breastfeeding a husband would resume a sexual relationship with another wife or look for another one to marry. The long taboo in Lesotho, hence, seemingly relates to the earlier marriage system from a time before the missionaries had promoted monogamous marriages. Polygamy was the norm in pre-colonial times, while today very few marriages are polygynous. In consequence, the prohibition of this marriage type by missionaries resulted promptly in extramarital relationships since the change in the marriage form did not affect the existence of the taboo and elder women usually encourage young mothers to continue nursing the child and to abstain from sexual activity.

With respect to men's sexual activity and women's prescribed unavailability to their husbands, a social worker of a private clinic also points at the effects of sexually transmitted diseases. To shorten the time of prescribed abstinence would therefore curtail the risky extramarital affairs of the men:

> [The husbands] have their extra-marital relationships at that time. The husbands therefore don't mind [the post-partum sex taboo] very much. The exclusive breastfeeding for six months (like HIV-positive women are advised to, L.K.) will therefore also prevent many relationships and risks of the husbands at that time, since they would be allowed to sleep with their wife again (Field notes Kroeker: 17/06/2008).

Even before HIV/AIDS was a concern, Hall and Malahleha reported that some mothers "reluctantly had sex during this period because they were afraid that their husbands would seek sexual gratification elsewhere if they did not." (Hall & Malahleha 1989: 59). In order to prevent extramarital affairs, men, for their part, may have prolonged the taboo for their wives in their absence. If the husband is gone due to labour migration the taboo may be placed upon their wife for an even longer time and thereby forbid women from having sex for the sake of her child's health:

> Weaning marks an important change in conjugal relations by returning the *mosoetse* to a state of sexual availability. Some women said that although both they and their mothers-in-law felt their child was old enough for weaning, their absent husbands would not permit it until they came home on leave, for they feared their wives would commit adultery in their absence. Since only the husband has the right to decide about fosterage arrangements and takes the initiative in sexual relations, a wife fears to give the baby to a grandmother for weaning without his approval (Gay 1980: 56).

Consequently, the partner had an influence on the time for weaning in order to resume sexual activity and when it was also considered time for resetting the reproductive cycle. Following this line of argumentation, an interviewee argued that she weaned "because my husband wanted to have a second child" (ATCBM Kroeker: 14/07/2009; Field notes Kroeker: 09/03/2009; cf. Fjeld et al. 2008). Thus, in many cases the fathers indicated the time for weaning, and a weaning ceremony will mark the end of the period of infancy and relieve the taboo.

While elders focussed on the combination of breastfeeding which reduces fertility and abstinence at the same time, young women in Mafeteng town did not support sexual abstinence while lactating (Field notes Kroeker: 09/03/2009). Young urban women argued for neglecting the post-partum sex taboo since they were used to other family planning methods to space their pregnancies. Nevertheless, elders will remind their breastfeeding next-of-kin that they must not engage in sexual contact too early. Counsellor Sylvia adds "if elders in the family find out [that we engage earlier in intercourse], they would tell us that we must not do anything" (Field notes Kroeker Sylvia: 02/07/2008) and others confirmed the existence of the post-natal sex taboo but denied it to be practised nowadays. Meanwhile, young mothers were encouraged by their family elders to continue breastfeeding for periods longer than six months for the baby's sake, while in the hospital's counselling sessions women were encouraged to use modern contraceptives for their birth spacing.

In practice, the taboo puts women in a position to take care of reproductive health concerns and to balance the interests of their own health, their baby's healthy development and their husband's sexual gratification.

8.1 Contraception and HIV

In biomedical care, traditional care as well as in formal employment, the critical phase that requires special protection of a pregnant women and her unborn child starts with the 28th week of pregnancy. The end of this critical state, however, differs according to biomedical, traditional and work notions. It relates to changes in the child's nutrition (from six months up to two years after delivery), laws on maternity leave (in Lesotho: six weeks post-partum) as well as the resumption of sexual activity. According to a traditional notion, the latter would perhaps take place two years after giving birth and therewith reset the reproductive cycle. Modern contraception and the PMTCT protocol follow a much shorter time frame of six to eight weeks after delivery until a woman is ready to conceive again, however, it is in the interest of policy makers not to reset the reproductive cycle.

In the hospital, women who come for the six-week check-up of their babies receive counselling on family planning options. Breastfeeding, also called Lactational Amenorrhoea Method (LAM), is only considered as a temporary method for less than six months after giving birth, according to the PMTCT guidelines, and women should be advised to choose alternative ways of preventing conception (GoL, 2009 (a): 10). The counselling session for mothers in childbed therefore involves a pregnancy test unless the woman proves otherwise that she has not yet conceived again.

Although not specifically mentioned in the national treatment guidelines of Lesotho or in the HIV testing and counselling training courses for staff, in many cases women were advised to prevent subsequent pregnancies altogether and were discouraged from notions of large families (Field notes 17/6/2008; cf. Desclaux et al. 2009: 804). Among policy makers worldwide, HIV/AIDS was considered a serious enough threat to public health which justified discouraging pregnancies of women living with the virus and thereby limiting the chances of infecting a (yet unborn) person (Field notes: PMTCT counsellor 3/06/2008). Although there is no direct reference in the HIV policy or in the counsellor training books and Lesotho's guidelines in writing merely argue that knowledge of their HIV status enables women to make informed choices about future pregnancies and future fertility, in practice, counsellors emphasised that HIV-positive women must take contraceptives. Hence, the basic message received by HIV-positive mothers in counselling sessions was *not* to get pregnant (cf. Du Plessis 2003: 84; cf. Bennett et al. 1996: 185).

On the level of policy makers within Lesotho's Ministry of Health and Social Welfare it was argued, that "efforts to decrease the level of MTCT can also focus on reducing fertility among HIV-positive women" and strategies need to be identified to target the unmet need for contraception (Adair 2007: 1). In spite of this, family planning shall prevent mother-to-child transmission at the earliest possible stage, which is before conception, as a means to avoid HIV-infections in children (Thornton et al. 2004; Adair 2007; Warren et al. 2008) — a strategy which was not yet mentioned in the 2004 PMTCT guidelines.

Various aims are followed when family planning and care for people living with HIV/AIDS are interlinked and the new strategy was based on the assumption that the reduction of unintended pregnancies among HIV-positive women could prevent equal or higher numbers of paediatric HIV than the pharmaceutical prophylaxis within the PMTCT programme (GoL 2009 (b): 73). Adair, an Australian demographer and consultant, states that an increased use of contraception and an integration of family planning into HIV services was so far an undervalued and little-used way to reduce mother-to-child transmission of HIV in Lesotho (2007: 2). Warren and colleagues (2008: ii) point out, that there was no consequent follow up of HIV-positive mothers after having delivered a baby and, following this logic, in the 2009 guidelines future family planning was made a cornerstone of the new strategy. Policy makers had identified antenatal clinics as valuable entry points since many women learn about their HIV-positive status while attending antenatal care (Adair 2007: 2). HIV-positive mothers shall be informed about family planning options when coming for antenatal check-ups, before leaving the hospital after confinement, and during check-ups for their baby. Moreover, besides the reduction of paediatric HIV, USAID [United States Agency for International Development] argued with reference to the cost-effectiveness of the medical interventions:

> Family planning can have a significant and cost-effective impact on HIV/AIDS prevention efforts. A number of models and USAID-funded analyses indicate that family planning services in sub-Saharan Africa are preventing HIV infection in more infants than programs that promote and provide nevirapine to HIV-positive mothers (…) For the same cost, family planning services can avert nearly 30 percent more HIV-positive births than the antiretroviral drug nevirapine. A model presented at a high-level consultation convened by WHO in 2004 indicated that an expenditure of US$45,000 for contraceptive services would prevent 88 HIV-positive births, while the same expenditure to promote and provide nevirapine in antenatal care would prevent 68 such births (USAID 2006).

No other organisation is as candid when mentioning this economic dimension of family planning for the purposes of HIV prevention, however, economic reasons seem to underpin the arguments made by Adair, Lesotho's Ministry of Health and the National AIDS Commission, too.

Notwithstanding, the new policy intrudes on culturally inherited responsibilities as attitudes towards child birth entail diverse social aspects, yet, in practice, some family planning facilities approve of this policy in a strict way. Observing counselling sessions, I learned that counsellors were pushed to discourage HIV-positive women from getting pregnant in their counselling sessions (Field notes Kroeker: 12/07/2008). Likewise, the National AIDS Commission (NAC) also mentioned in one of its documents that they "regretted" that in 2009 24.4% of the women who already knew about their HIV positive status still got pregnant (MoHSW & NAC 2009: 42). This suggests again that, for the policy makers, it is undesirable for someone to fall pregnant despite knowing about a hereditary disease such as HIV. Other counsellors, however, stressed a woman's right to have children, despite her HIV status.

8.2 Rethabile's Desire

While mothers see reproduction as their right and a necessity for marital well-being, the National AIDS Commission views pregnancies of HIV-positive women critically and as problematic. However, some HIV-positive women, in contrast to the Ministry's notion, recognised the PMTCT programme as an opportunity and utilised family planning in a more strategic way as treatment will enable HIV-positive women to produce healthy offspring. Since the PMTCT programme has been in place for three years, which is a usual birth interval, some women are now beginning to return for a second treatment.

The next story shall indicate the dilemma of a HIV-positive mother, who is also a counsellor on HIV. Discussing with her these issues of family planning and HIV from a personal perspective as well as from a professional stance provided some ambiguous insights:

> Rethabile, aged 32, finds herself at the intersection of two antagonising notions. As a counsellor in an HIV-treatment-site she insists that positive clients must prevent pregnancies. When discussing HIV and fertility Rethabile tells me her "professional opinion": HIV-positive couples, like herself and her husband, should use condoms every time to prevent cross-infections and pregnancies.
>
> Personally, she feels however an unmet desire for a baby. After being widowed she now entered a second marriage with an HIV-positive man and the couple would like to bless their love with a child. When Rethabile fell pregnant, she discloses to me and adds that I should not tell her fellow counsellors since she fears mockery due to her non-compliance with the "official" opinion. The doctor who confirmed her pregnancy and the counsellor to whom she was referred both told her,

> as she had already expected, that they were not comfortable with her pregnancy. Her colleague lectured her that as a counsellor she should know better. Rethabile on her part knows from her training and her daily work about the good chances of having a healthy baby if she receives PMTCT. Few weeks later, Rethabile approached me again to tell me that she had "a heavy period"[1], meaning that she had lost the child (Field notes Kroeker: 09/01/2009).

Due to awareness of her own health condition Rethabile had decided to give it a chance. Hence, she and her husband used family planning in a more strategic way and stopped using contraception when Rethabile's health condition was monitored and considered to be fairly good.

As the case of Rethabile illustrates, her desire to bear children, counselling practices and strategic government aims do not seem easy to reconcile. Rethabile was over-proportionally well equipped with information on HIV prevention and had known about her infections for a long time when she made up her mind to have a baby. As demographers note in accordance with my anthropological data, desire for a child did not correspond with HIV infections. In quantitative surveys in various African countries planning a baby rather depended on the state of a relationship, health of the mother and of other relatives, money and housing conditions (Timaeus & Moultrie 2008). The social standing of a woman with child remains and an affirmative overall situation, such as being in a new stable partnership, drove the desire to have a baby. In accordance with Caldwell (2005), I would like to point out that family planning is a matter of time and space. The situation of the above mentioned couple was conducive to having a baby. More precisely, a baby confirmed a serious partnership with the blessing of offspring. Counselling, however, did not consider these social factors of a new social situation. The counselling is merely based on medical concerns.

Moreover, they avoided consulting health workers on it since they feared the confrontation. Consulting a doctor was a critical issue since the decision may be influenced by medical staff's preferences. The counselling would presumably not have led to the desired result and Rethabile feared that they would have to defend her right and desire to have a child.

---

[1] In many cases "a heavy period" actually sometimes indicates an abortion. In Lesotho, termination of a risky, mistimed or unwanted pregnancy is an unavailable option, at least legally. In this case, I am not sure whether Rethabile induced an abortion or she miscarried naturally. However, I assume it to be the latter.

8.3 Making Clients Comply

Monitoring the client's compliance with biomedical treatment, as assigned in the policy, was the remit of the nurses and counsellors. High numbers of compliant clients indicated success of the nurse's work. From my observations, time constraints, heavy workload and various administrative responsibilities in addition to the examinations, prevented time-consuming discussions between nurse and an unconvinced client. Of course, staff may attempt to reduce the workload, shift tasks around and limit the time which is spent on patient-staff interaction. Non-compliance of clients, in contrast, was more often seen by staff as a disappointment and non-appreciation of biomedical advice. An overworked and understaffed facility as well as a lack of commitment or motivation may affect the work flow within the facility which renders staff prone to disappointment, which was then blamed on non-compliant clients. To tackle this problem of over-worked and understaffed health facilities, counsellors were introduced into the hospital hierarchy to fill a gap in the communication between nurses and patients.

The dropout rates decreased when counsellors facilitated the communication. Notwithstanding, counsellors needed to meet their targets of high compliance with biomedical treatment and they often found creative ways to make clients comply. For instance, counsellors had to make sure HIV-positive women had not yet conceived again. In one of the governmental hospitals it was common practice that women only received their child's HIV test result if they had attended family planning counselling. At the family planning unit they either had to take a pregnancy test or present a bloody sanitary towel to the nurse to prove that they have not yet conceived (Field notes Kroeker: 26/01/2009). The pregnancy test was thereby indirectly made compulsory, while the PMTCT guidelines merely recommend putting HIV-positive mothers on modern methods of contraception (GoL 2009 (a): 10) as part of the post-partum protocol.

Some private HIV clinics even combine antiretroviral treatment with family planning provision in order to prevent offspring (Field notes Kroeker: 17/06/2008) and thereby to follow the protocol. In some of the clinics, Depo-Provera injections were administered to HIV-positive women every time they came to collect their packages of medication, explained a nurse:

> It is true, that in many other places contraception is given with ARV. They force the women to have contraception like the *depo*. They force

> them, but the decision should actually be with the individual (Field notes Kroeker: 19/06/2008).

While nurses were bound to follow ethical guidelines (which they sometimes ignored), counsellors were not part of the medical staff but usually employed by NGOs. Most of the counselling was therefore outsourced to them. In an interview a doctor (F) denied any conflict of reproductive rights and this current practice in the clinic.

> F.: The women agree to have an injection.
>
> L.: Do they feel pressurized by medical staff to agree to it?
>
> F.: They have to agree every three months and usually the women are coming back to get another injection. But I agree, medical staff seems to advise from a higher hierarchical point of view that might force women to consent on it. (Field notes Kroeker: 17/06/2008)

The debate on ARV provision in conjunction with contraception demonstrates the extent to which a government policy impedes upon social demands, such as the desire to have children and the way in which this problem was bypassed by introducing counsellors. Mothers, for their part, see reproduction as their right and a necessity for marital well-being. PMTCT is regarded in a more positive way than by policy makers and medical staff. PMTCT provides an opportunity to have a HIV-negative child despite the mother's condition. Meanwhile, this attitude did not correspond with the work targets of health workers.

Theoretical Optic: Uncertainty, Innovation and a Quest for Order

My empirical data shows that both dominant fields, the family and medical field, give advice on behaviour to expectant and young mothers. On the one hand, either frame of reference poses advantages, of which the mothers are usually well aware. On the other hand, in many cases, these recommendations contradict each other and cause confusion. For example, when a woman is requested to teach family elders about a hospital delivery and request money for that, while the family would prefer a home delivery assisted by a known and trustworthy local person without the need to travel through the wilderness. Or family elders recommend traditional medication to prevent spiritual harm, while the hospital staff prohibits traditional medication due to the interference with HIV medication. Meanwhile some of the mothers struggled to give the *lelomolo* bite and therefore welcome their baby into the family due to exclusive feeding options, while others walked barefoot but feared falling victim to ill health as a consequence. They were neither able to fulfil all expectations nor ignore them; they were caught between a rock and a hard place.

These situations plagued their thoughts while women tried to come to terms with their dilemma. Due to the consequences, which in the worst case may be fatal for mother or child in a social or physical sense, it is justifiable to call the whole situation a crisis. The situation in which HIV-positive and expectant or childbearing women found themselves was a situation of uncertainty and a quest to disarm potential harms. Not only did the contingency result from conflicting demands in their current situation, but the overall social situation in Lesotho is in turmoil. The changes in the economic realm since the 1980s impacted on family life, reproductive life and gender roles. Women took over previously male tasks and men were pushed to the side. Old guiding principles, such as patriarchal family structures with male dominance and gerontocratic orders no longer fitted the new social arrangements and a vacuum of guiding principles appeared. Women gained autonomy while simultaneously losing normative guidelines. It was during this period of social upheaval that HIV/AIDS also entered the social arena and led to new social challenges.

In times of permanent or temporary crisis, Jenkins and colleagues conclude that people "struggle for actual or immediate control" (Jenkins et al. 2005: 10). Sickness, as one of the very existential causations of uncertainty, raises questions of by what means the situation can be effectively improved.

> During crises we look for reasons and explanations, and possible strategies and plans are mediated by and through the meanings and knowledge we share with others. Substances, artefacts and techniques - medicines and technologies, or rituals and magic - offer various means by which we attempt to cope with or control illness and misfortune. With respect to all of these, there are generally alternatives available, which in themselves encourage further uncertainty about which is the correct response to a particular problem. (Jenkins et al. 2005: 11)

The previous chapters have presented numerous cases of women in uncertain situations. Most of them came up with ideas on how to cope with the situation, not knowing if they would work out or not. Thus, uncertainty had caused them to develop ways of controlling the situation which again caused uncertainty about achieving the desired outcome. Control and uncertainty were not diametrical opposites but two sides of the same coin. Moreover, uncertainty did not vanish since it is an integral part of life, however, the social turmoil left people confused about how to tackle it. Sometimes the way forward was not to fight uncertainties, but merely to avoid adding new ones. Those women who experienced high stress rates at least tried to avoid conflicts or to evade behavioural monitoring. Avoidance of supervision somehow opened up, on the other hand, new pathways.

This chapter will serve as a theoretical background to the struggle these women had to confront. However, before analysing Tharo's attempts to resolve her highly uncertain situation, the terminology for doing so, as used by other authors, needs to be clarified.

9.1 Managing, Juggling, Transcribing or Navigating

Various terms have been suggested in order to grasp the way people cope with alternative means of controlling information in order to mitigate the effects of uncertainty. Goffman determines the "management of a spoiled identity" (1963). All individuals he describes in his study carry a visible or invisible characteristic, namely a stigma, which they try to hide in order to appear as "normal" as possible. The stigmatised individuals develop various strategies to disguise the stigma or make an unintended publication of it look like a minor accident, something that others would not comprehend as part of an abnormality. The management of the stigma, hence, ways of hiding a characteristic, may include verbal and non-verbal interaction as well as "wise" people who know about the stigma and help to conceal it from those who do not. As a result, all strategies are either aimed at the stigmatising characteristic itself or are meant to manipulate those with whom the stigmatised person interacts. Unfortunately, Goffman fails to provide a clearer definition that would elaborate on "management of the spoiled identity" but suffices to mention various kinds of stigma rather than ways of managing these. In the cases I described, shifts and changes in the management of a discrediting piece of information, here either HIV/AIDS or disobedience, are in focus.

Sargent (1989) does not speak about stigma but of obstetric choices of women in Benin. She described ideals and narratives on how and where to deliver a child and uses the term "juggling" to describe a decision-making process. In her study, Beninoise women tried to combine various behavioural expectations such as status aspiration, religious aspects, familial approaches and the like, thus, diverse aspects, which they had to meet simultaneously. However, Sargent focuses merely on external pressures that need to be weighed against each other, thus, "juggling" interests. However, similar to Goffman, she does not define her terminology of juggling. Despite the lack of a definition, conceptually, juggling implies a servitude to orders. As we do not have any hints from her work, she may however argue that others make the plans and the respective mother waits for guiding principles and directions from her family decision-makers and nurses. Notwithstanding, all ideals are dealt with at the same time and seem to carry the same value. The balance between the expectations (or objects that are juggled) has to be found and it appears as if the person is reacting rather than reflecting and drawing conclusions. Sargent's study participants therefore lack agency. My study, in contrast, suggests that women have agency and are active and creative in dealing with external as well as internal pressures. Study participants rather combined fragments of two frames of reference and their own preferences instead of accepting the "objects" the way they are. The women tended to let objects fall to the floor, or they deformed or merged them in a pragmatic way.

Regarding material and immaterial tokens that are passed between people or institutions, Latour (1986) offered some thoughtful ideas by presenting two models - transfer by "diffusion" and remodelling by means of "translation". While Latour intended to explain power relations between stakeholders, his models also help us to understand how information and technology trickles down to the user. His model of diffusion concerns the spreading of technology over time and space, while the token itself is not modified. This model is less relevant to the scope of my work. Alternatively, Latour presents a model of translation. Here, a token passes between people or institutions along certain patterns, but, in contrast to the former model, every actor modifies it according to his/her own interests (1986: 268). "Translation" conceptualises the circulation and thus the transformation of something by handing it on from one group to another. This seems to be more applicable for my work than Sargent's unchangeable objects. Sargent would seem to neglect that pregnant women have their own ideas about how to achieve control over their situation. Goffman tends to focus on how information is hidden and only transferred unintentionally. Adding to the knowledge transfer, Latour brings power relations into the picture. All these aspects can be found in the works of political anthropologist, James Scott. In his works material and immaterial goods are deformed, merged and passed on to parties in a context of unequal power relations.

Scott (1990) speaks of hidden or public transcripts for coping in hierarchical systems such as peasant communities. Subordinates are expected by the dominant party, here land owners, to obey orders to which subordinates do not necessarily subscribe. Therefore, subordinates, as well as superiors, develop "hidden transcripts" among themselves, which translate into "public transcripts" if they are interacting with the other party. Subordinate groups in this social constellation therefore try to evade orders or to fulfil them with the aim of minimal disadvantage for themselves. Scott adds that putting the hidden plan into practice more often fails and the result does not meet the expectations. The terminology of "transcript" seems appropriate for the plans and the attempt to make it work, although nevertheless it also carries the connotation of being fixed, determined and inflexible. For the public interface, transcript seems to hold in the case of HIV-positive women who are pregnant. The biomedical field as well as the theoretical norm of behaviour that applies within Basotho society can be called a transcript, whereas the *realpolitik* of these women does not quite correspond with the idea of a transcript. Besides planning and efforts to make a transcript work, adjustment of the preliminary idea was evidently an important part of the life trajectory of my study participants. Scott's terminology, therefore, does not quite grasp this need for spontaneous shifts, flexibility, and adjustments, although his case studies do show flexibility. Thus the terminology of a transcript is somewhat confusing. Unfortunately, Scott does not specify, whether "hidden transcripts" can be applied by individuals or only by groups of people. In his earlier book on "Weapons of the Weak" (1985) he specifically cites examples of individual peasants and their everyday forms of resisting the orders of the dominants. The strategies peasants use in boycotting orders from someone in authority can, nonetheless, be easily compared with those pregnant HIV-positive women adopt to avoid supervision and behavioural expectations that are not compatible with their interests. Thus, the underlying idea of different strategies of interaction perfectly matches examples from my study.

For the path taken by HIV pregnant women in Lesotho, I prefer to use the term "navigation" following Christiansen, Utas and Vigh (2006), respectively "social navigation" (Vigh 2009). Having appropriated the term from a geographic disciplinary background, Vigh conceptualises navigation as an analytical model to describe an individual's actions in an uncertain environment. The comparison with a nautical situation suggests a volatile, changing situation to which humans adjust their moves. Vigh (2006: 51) tried to capture the way young people are "muddling though", which they call "*se débrouiller*" in Francophone Africa or "*doubria*" in the Lusophone regions.

The authors of "Navigating Youth" (Christiansen et al. 2006) mention navigation as an attempt to "make the best of meagre life chances and navigate their lives towards better positions and possibilities" (2006: 12), which suggests flexibility and short-term tactics when dealing with obstacles. An uncertain, insecure and rapidly changing situation causes individuals to steer around obstacles and currents with a view to keeping their heads above water pragmatically.

Implicit to this analytical framework is a "dialogue between agency and social forces" (Vigh 2009) and an interaction of people "with each other *and* the field" in contrast to Goffman's "management of identity" (1963), which merely focuses on interaction of people *in* a field of a rather predictable nature. Navigation also suggests a compromise between Scott's collective "transcripts" and Sargent's individual "juggling" in terms of agency, rationality and interaction. Yet, Vigh's analytical perspective suggests the idea that interrelated individual agency as people and their environment are in constant flux. Vigh therewith rejects a simplistic explanation of push and pull factors that affect a person's trajectory and stresses the interaction between people and their environment. Moreover, the concept of social navigation entails a time component, a life trajectory between "being" and "becoming". Vigh notes:

> Social navigation (…) encompasses both the assessment of the dangers and possibilities of one's present position as well as the process of plotting and attempting to actualize routes into an uncertain and changeable future. (Vigh 2009: 425)

Thus, individuals struggle in the immediate real time as they make decisions on a day-to-day basis, as well as making decisions for an imagined future.

Social navigation captures the image of a zigzag course as a means to avoid obstacles on an *ad-hoc* basis, which I therefore consider adequate for analysing the detours study participants made when dealing with conflicting demands in the hospital or with their family members. The hospital, including information, staff and technology, changes rapidly and unpredictably. Suddenly, one recommended practice no longer applies due to a change in guidelines, staff rotate and medication runs out of stock, to mention only a few parameters. On the other hand, the client of the health facility copes with a new personal and family situation, general living and working conditions, acceptance of health information, fear of harm, and keeping face. My informants navigated through the dangers of their obstetric condition *between life and death* as well as their physically and psychologically insecure health prospective due to HIV, stigma and their need for familial and medical care.

9.2 Tharo's Uncertain Situation and the Struggle for Love

While in all previously presented cases women manoeuvred through troubled waters, I will now present the case of Tharo whose ship capsized in the end.

Tharo, a woman from the rural hinterland of Mafeteng District, was 26 years old, married and had two children aged ten and seven, when she experienced a highly uncertain situation that she failed to secure. Struggling with her personal situation as well as her social environment, she had difficulties finding the correct response and various attempts brought her deeper into the dilemma. I present Tharo's case here because this story took a lot of twists and turns during the six months under study. Discovering her ideas, shifts and changes, as well as authoritative knowledge, taught me a great deal about how to analyse many other cases. Furthermore, she taught me about resistance, fear of disclosure and the social changes which disclosure entailed. Tharo also offered a framework of interpretation for other biographies. I need to add, however, that her case is not typical due to the numerous obstacles she had to face, which interfered with each other and thus added to her volatile situation. Owing again to the analogy of navigating in troubled waters, interference either cancels out or doubles the amount of waves, which also fits with Tharo's difficulties. Poor Tharo combined all typical problems at once, such as:

- social and geographic distance to husband,
- social and geographic distance to family and in-laws,
- lack of own financial resources,
- bad physical condition due to sickness,
- no occupation whatsoever,
- discordant couple (wife HIV-positive, husband HIV-negative),
- extramarital relationship,
- no trust in biomedical staff,
- limited social interaction resulting from her inverted and extremely careless character.

This is the story of Tharo:

> Tharo had attended school up to Standard 7 and did not seek employment to generate her own income. Instead, she fully relied on her husband's remittances from the mines, while her maternal as well as her marital family remained in the rural area with her elder children. At that time we met, Tharo was seven months pregnant and in the counselling session she mentioned that she had fallen severely sick earlier that year, was bedridden and about to die. She was admitted into hospital and recovered, but due to her weak health she then decided to move closer to the hospital and rented a room in Mafeteng town.

Usually, a patient who has experienced a severe bout of sickness and recovered complies well with the kind of medical advice that provides relief, as highlighted in several other cases. On the whole, the history of a deteriorated health status positively correlates with (either traditional or biomedical) drug adherence. Thus, the counsellor in antenatal care, who assessed her personal situation after the HIV-positive test result, did not envisage any difficulties with the client and the PMTCT medication. The treatment history would rather consolidate the client's uncertain situation as life-long treatment should give her certainty about the absence of physical weakness. Pharmaceuticals therefore act as means of control, administering these as prescribed is part of a patient's plan to disarm disease and add some routine, confidence and trust to their life.

> The counsellor also asked her about the most crucial part of HIV-positive life: disclosing the test-result and being supported. Tharo explained that her husband had visited her the previous month and she had disclosed her status to him at that time. His reaction was as if he accepted the result, "he was OK, but I didn't know how he really felt in his heart". She had not disclosed to anyone else up to now. Since no other person was living in her household the counsellor also did not expect any conflicts in terms of taking the drugs, for example, and no fear of stigma.
>
> Assessing her attitude towards "safe" delivery practice, the counsellor found out that both Tharo's children were born in the hospital in Mafeteng so for the current baby she had also opted for a hospital delivery. Regarding HIV transmission through breastfeeding, Tharo agreed to short-term exclusive breastfeeding and also did not consider anything to be different from her earlier pregnancies.
>
> Tharo denied having a history of traditional medication and already knew that pitsa may cause side effects with the biomedical treatment which she had already agreed to take following her bout of sickness in July 2008, although her supply had now run out. Following on, the counsellor interpreted the recent test results as stated in the obstetric record. Tharo had tested HIV-positive in antenatal care and her immunological status was considered very low which meant she should start a life-long drug regime with antiretroviral treatment. Therefore the counsellor accompanied her to the HIV clinic to put her on the system, so she could receive adherence counselling and the drugs. Tharo instantly agreed on taking treatment and, moreover, to participate in my study.
>
> After the counselling, the counsellor concluded that Tharo showed herself to be an uncomplicated and understanding client.

It turned out that my translator, who had previously worked as a volunteer in the HIV counselling testing site, remembered Tharo. Tharo had been among her first clients who tested positive and was in need of lengthy counselling since she did not believe the result. Denying it to be true she did not come back, yet, Tharo did not seem to remember MaKhotso. MaKhotso's memory had not failed her and Tharo's old file which MaKhotso had opened for her in the HIV clinic was still available. It revealed that Tharo had already tested positive in 2007, the test was confirmed in May 2008 with MaKhotso, she was then tested again in July 2008 when she was severely sick, and now in October 2008 when pregnant.

MaKhotso and I went on a home visit to Tharo's lodgings shortly after our meeting in the antenatal clinic. During this visit I became aware that all the information Tharo had given during the counselling session was in fact wrong.

The way she had presented her marital situation allowed the counsellor to assume that she had good support at home. However, this was only the case on a placid surface.

> Tharo lived on her own without family members. While family members take special care of *primagravida*, she had given birth to two children already and was therefore not the focus of familial guidance and did not intend to move to her maternal home. Notwithstanding, due to her general health condition, which worried her, she experienced this pregnancy differently from her previous ones. Therefore, Tharo had approached traditional health practitioners, about which, of course, she lied to biomedical staff. Nevertheless, she came for another voluntary HIV test (I do not know her reasons for a further test, but I assume she wanted to reassure herself) and enrolled in the HIV treatment in a biomedical facility too. However, she did not take the tablets or come to the clinic for her repeat prescription.

Tharo described her conjugal relationship in accordance with the dynamics of traditional gender relations. Her husband only came to visit her one weekend a month to bring money for her and the children, nevertheless, she undoubtedly considered him as head of the household, domineering and with a short temper. Tharo, for her part, played the loving and caring wife by pampering him and defining herself as his inferior at all times. Being dependent on his good will and money, she shielded him from conflicts to keep peace in the house. Despite her first HIV-positive test taking place two years ago she had kept this secret to herself for a long time since she did not want to spoil the little time they spent together with quarrels.

> While living in town on her own, she had engaged in an extramarital affair, mainly triggered by distance, loneliness and boredom. When her husband, Ntate, found out they argued and, as a consequence, their marriage went through a rough spell. Thereafter she did not want to inform him about her HIV status and feared Ntate might become violent and blame her for having an extramarital affair, which was the

> cause of the disease. During intercourse the husband had used condoms and she concluded from that that he may have been unsure about his own HIV status and assumed that he had engaged in an affair while abroad as well. Tharo concluded that he was infected with HIV and therefore had used condoms to protect his wife. Since things went her own way she kept quiet for the time being.

However, as she knew that all this information would label her as a "bad" client she had made up information which would please the counsellor and make her appear as a "good" compliant patient. Therewith, she chose to avoid conflicts and further counselling sessions. She decided on "good" information rather than "true" information, or as Goffman puts it: "A conflict between candor and seemliness will often be resolved in favour of the latter" (Goffman 1963: 75). Tharo aptly navigated around obstacles and found successful ways which posed the least disadvantage for her, including the least stigma.

9.2.1 Avoidance and Ways of Doing So

Why did Tharo conceal the "real" story and decide to lie in the counselling session? Why did she withhold crucial information from her husband, Ntate? Two characteristics ran through Tharo's manoeuvres as well as through those pathways most other study participants followed: firstly, their manoeuvres implied a trend to avoid conflicts and develop elaborate secret arguments. Secondly, their strategies changed quickly time and time again and thereby adjusted to a new situation.

Study participants instead attempted to create a situation of love, care, well-being and support aiming in the long run at a holistic notion of safety. Therefore, as Christiansen, Utas and Vigh suggest, in their above-mentioned statement, navigation captures immediate adjustments and an abstract objective. In my reading of social navigation, this analytical optic works well as the framework of conflict avoidance and hidden actions.

> The counsellor had asked Tharo about her last CD4 count and Tharo made the excuse that she could not remember the result and had also left her medical book in the hospital's waiting hall. With this answer she intended to hide her situation, since any other information would shed a negative light on her and stigmatise her as a "bad patient". She feigned carelessness when leaving her book outside, while, in reality, she wanted to hide the information it contained. She pretended not to

> know what day she went for the last check-up – feigning false ignorance. The counsellor changes the topic and asks her about the adoption of safer sex practices and Tharo explains that her husband also went for HIV testing, but he had not given her any affirmative answer on that. She, therefore, had argued for using condoms and he had agreed, extricating herself from the situation.
>
> After the counselling session the counsellor accompanied her to the HIV clinic to enrol in life-long therapy, not knowing that it was already for the third time. Due to other commitments the counsellor left Tharo in the waiting hall and Tharo took the opportunity to abscond from this baleful place. She managed to escape the counsellor's supervision and therewith physically avoided an uncomfortable situation.

Taking this example of a counselling session to a more abstract level, I would like to refer to the literature on avoidance (*Meidung*) as one way of conflict management. Avoidance as a conflict mode was previously addressed in sociology and political anthropology, yet, I found it to be a common way among HIV-positive pregnant women in Lesotho in their interaction with hospital staff and family elders. Avoidance provides a non-violent strategy which does not require involvement of institutions or third parties to resolve a conflict.

In sociology, strategic manoeuvres of avoidance have been described since the 1960s. Again referring to Goffman (2009), people interact with another "on stage" but reflect and plan their moves shielded by "a curtain" from gazing eyes. Behind the curtain and invisible to others a person figures out how he or she would best negotiate their own interests and avoid discrediting oneself in front of others. In particular Goffman's thoughts on tainted identity (1963) include descriptions of individuals who carry a stigma that they want to hide from others which were widely quoted in medical anthropological studies on HIV/AIDS (cf. Jacoby 1994; Kipp 2007; Simbayi et al. 2007). As mentioned above, he did not offer a typology of ways to avoid conflicts.

Brown and Levinson (2006) discussed communicative strategies of avoidance. The authors described ways whereby interactional partners avoid Face Threatening Acts (FTA) and therefore keep face, a term they adopted from Goffman. They figured out that gender and power relations reflected on communicative acts and FTAs were used by the dominant party (Brown & Levinson 2006: 30f). Social psychology speaks of avoidance behaviour (cf. Sachse et al. 2011), which can be caused by imagined reasons. In game theory as debated by economists, mathematicians and in law, decision-making and evasive manoeuvres are key concerns (cf. Rieck 1993). However, these theoretical approaches shall not be discussed any further within the scope of this study.

Scott's work also refers to power relations although, in contrast to Brown and Levinson's example, they are long-term. He builds his theoretical approach on the historian Hobsbawm's thoughts on social rebels (1962) and their resistance to domination. Rebels avoid overturning the social hierarchy by causing major conflicts. Scott argues that subordinates not only acted rationally but also negotiated among themselves how to undercut the dominant party without questioning the relationship as such. This situation is comparable to the situation of young pregnant women and their family elders as well as their relation to hospital staff. Whereas Goffman establishes an onstage-offstage relationship of conflict parties, Scott describes a more flexible front line which is capable of negotiations.

In social scientific texts avoidance is often understood as physical avoidance such as flight (Hirschman 1974; Elwert 2004; Inhetveen 2006). Subordinates escape from the dominant party or the consequences of its usage of power (Inhetveen 2006). Most prominently, Hirschman (1974, 2010) discussed exit, voice and loyalty as three ways of sanctioning unacceptable behaviour. He distinguishes the relationship between unsatisfied customers and companies whereby the former employ voice and exit strategies. Loss in sales, which he calls "exit", will show indirectly that customers were dissatisfied and the invisible hand of the market indicates that a product needs to be improved in order to convince buyers again (1974: 13, 19). Moreover, open criticism, which he calls "voice strategy", in contrast, shows dissatisfaction directly. These bipolar ways of protest, exit and voice, were analysed for economic enterprises but also for political relations. Yet, Hirschman did not apply his ideas to individuals and their interaction but only for groups.

Elwert (2004) analysed different forms of dealing with conflicts and established, like Hirschman, an indirect mode of conflict management, namely avoidance. Generally, situations of conflict leave a choice to the parties involved and offer therefore possibilities to change from one mode to another as the conflict escalates. Hence, a conflict which was avoided in the beginning may be solved later when institutions get involved (2004: 31). Avoidance as a strategy is characterised as little or no compliance to rules, minimal social embedding and negligible institutionalisation (Eckert 2004: 15). Alber (2004), who analysed avoidance among the Baatombou in Benin, proposed a definition of avoidance and determined two types. Avoidance hence includes:

> those social actions, which rest on a perception of incompatible interests or intentions of involved people or parties and who, yet, try to camouflage or evade those. With this strategy of avoidance which a conflict party applies, she intends to avoid the conflict as such, ignores it or lets it gain no traction by means of not reacting. Or the party uses strategies of avoidance to shield her actual interests from the other conflict party. Between both types we find intermediate stages and gradations, which also rely on diverse gradations of intentionality of actions (Alber 2004: 177)[1].

The application of avoidance depends crucially on the social and geographic space and the nature of the problem: permanent or temporary. With regard to peasant communities in Benin, Alber assumes that avoidance becomes a valid strategy due to the fact that means of production are not necessarily shared in the community and therefore individuals or groups may choose to separate from the community of origin and therewith avoid conflicts through geographic distance, similarly to Hirschman's exit strategy. Splinter groups then found a new village to avoid constant disputes and therewith collaboration with the rest of the group ceases. Generally, avoidance is often shorthanded and informally organised without involvement of socially accepted institutions and most useful if the dominant party has no means to control a side step (2004: 169-185).

In Häberlein's study, Mongolian pastoralists are dependent on each other which makes avoidance a useful tool of conflict management, as she argues in contrast to Alber. Häberlein (2007) describes cases where conflict parties depend on cooperation in the long run to sustain their livelihood. Excluding someone from the cooperation for a given time indicates a conflict. Afterwards the parties will work together again which is indispensable

---

[1] Meidungsstrategien sind jene soziale Handlungen, die auf der Wahrnehmung von teilweise inkompatiblen Interessen oder Intentionen der beteiligten Personen oder Personengruppen beruhen, diese jedoch zu verschleiern oder zu umgehen versuchen. Dabei versucht die die Meidungsstrategie anwendende Konfliktpartei entweder, den Konflikt als solchen zu umgehen oder zu ignorieren und ihn durch Nicht-Handeln ins Leere laufen zu lassen. Oder sie setzt Meidungsstrategien ein, um ihre eigentlichen Interessen möglichst vor dem Konfliktpartner zu verbergen. Zwischen beiden Typen gibt es Zwischenformen und Abstufungen, die auch auf unterschiedlichen Graden der Intentionalität der Handlungen beruhten" (Alber 2004: 177, translation mine).

for the community as a whole. Avoiding a dispute by excluding someone is thus not only a matter of geographic and social distance but of juridical problem solving (2007: 310). I agree with Häberlein that avoidance applies successfully particularly in cases of long-term relations that require collaboration and therefore shall not be disturbed by open disputes but the interaction is instead paused. Basotho families were in many cases already separated geographically, albeit without any intention to disconnect socially. The women in my study were highly dependent on their family network due to both sickness and child-bearing, and therefore chose to avoid open disputes and thereby kept social ties intact. Owing to this crucial connection, avoidance seemed an acceptable strategy since an open conflict would break the relationship. Avoiding a dispute, on the contrary, implies disagreement but also peace and was used in long-term relationships of dependency which would also be of crucial need at an unpredictable time. As in Scott's descriptions, due to power relations relationships were antagonistic as well as collaborative (1985: 205).

With the exception of Goffman all examples involved social groups rather than individuals. With my examples, however, I intend to show that avoidance is even more useful in close, individual relationships which are marked by unequal power distribution and long-term collaborative interests.

9.2.2 Tharo’s Manoeuvres

Coming back to my example of Tharo, one finds that being with child as well as knowing about her sickness made Tharo and others dependent on their family network, as well as for love, care, and resources. Tharo finds herself, however, in a difficult situation and tries to find some balance and control without losing face. However, her manoeuvres built on lies had not yet led to more control over the situation, but conversely to more insecurity since she now has to manage her lies, her public transcript, as well.

The counselling about protecting the baby from HIV increasingly worries Tharo. She wants to protect the baby from contracting the virus but every step she would take in that regard would also force her to disclose her HIV status. How can she justify PMTCT treatment when the husband was around when she had told him that she had tested negative? Tharo fears stigma related to the biomedical advice of short-term breastfeeding, which she considers at odds with the practices she had used with her previous children who were breastfed for two years.

> After Tharo's baby was born around the festive season, she comes to the hospital for a baby check-up in February. She is now scared that the same counsellor might remember her name and that she had left the clinic that day without having received any treatment. Therefore, Tharo uses her maiden name and disguises any association with her married name[2], which she had used last time (cf.: Goffman 1963: 92). Her old *Bukana ea Bophelo* had an entry that referred her to the HIV Clinic, where she of course did not receive a following entry, which could indicate that she missed out on the examination. She also brings a new booklet with blank pages and without indication of her HIV status and the spoiled name. Tharo presents herself as a new client in the Under 5s Clinic for a baby check-up of a baby who had been delivered in a rural clinic. However, Tharo underestimates the tools of biomedical control: the counsellor doubts her information and asks her about the baby's vaccination scar, which was nowhere to be found and Tharo almost loses countenance. Tharo has to admit remorsefully that the baby boy was not vaccinated since she had not delivered in a biomedical facility.

Her disguise has blown up in her face. The baby's missing body inscription conveys the message that she is not "a good patient", and she was subsequently confronted with her "bad behaviour".

> When I visit Tharo's place she is not at home (or at least does not want to open the door). Her neighbour, who washes her laundry outside tells me that she had to assist in Tharo's delivery. Notwithstanding, the woman is younger than Tharo and had never assisted in a delivery before nor were they on close terms, the neighbour tells me, as she is still quite overwhelmed from the ordeal. She cannot understand why Tharo called her and had not prepared for a delivery at her rural home or in hospital. Moreover, Tharo had only called her at the last minute, while in severe labour and still at home alone and said that the baby came so fast that she could not make it to hospital in time. I ask the neighbour if she has thought about HIV when assisting in a delivery. The neighbour answers that she had no time to consider these things, she could not just leave Tharo alone in severe pain in the middle of the night. Tharo later explains to me that she had delivered at home since

[2] Basotho women change first and last names when getting married and often their neighbours and relatives only know them by one of these names.

> she did not want to go to hospital, but could not stop dithering about where else to go. Additionally, she had not told her birth assistant about HIV, since they were not on close terms.

Shortly thereafter, Tharo falls severely ill and is again admitted to hospital. Her mother had taken her there against her will and Tharo needs a new hidden transcript to break free of her mother's and the hospital staff's authority:

> Tharo does not want to take medication and refuses to bathe so that the doctor refuses to examine her. Tharo appears ashamed and depressed while becoming physically weaker before my very eyes. I meet her mother by her bed and get to talk to her. The mother takes care of the baby boy and it turns out that the mother also knows about Tharo's HIV-positive status and that her other daughter had also tested positive. Whereas Tharo is in denial, Tharo's sister is in fact an active member of a support group and open about her status. Tharo's mother suggests that Tharo should also join the support group to overcome her denial. More surprisingly, the mother also knows about the mother-to-child-prevention programme and supports short-term breastfeeding. The mother then suggests in a joint counselling session that she will approach Tharo's husband next time he is in town to discuss HIV, treatment and feeding options for the baby.
>
> Tharo's many attempts to control the situation included various strategies: she avoided visiting a place she disliked, she lied to the counsellor, and disturbed the expected procedure of a delivery – to have well known, experienced and trusted people around her - and followed her mother to the hospital against her will.

All these manoeuvres were necessary to avoid open disputes with hospital staff or her family supporters and I will now go on to differentiate between four ways of overcoming a conflict.

9.3 Avoidance of Conflicts

The analysis of Tharo's case, as well as other cases in earlier chapters, suggested four ways of navigating. Study participants generally navigated around open disputes and conflicts wherever members of different gender and generations met and when confronted with affiliates of institutions on which someone is dependent, such as medical staff. Thus, these strategies, which also matched usual ways of problem solving in (family-) politics and of approaching superiors, allow the subordinate to keep face, since an open discussion will be avoided.

Strategies of avoidance included four pathways of avoidance:

- Simple adherence to dominant's orders. Compliance may, though, include grudging compliance enforced by supervision.
- Secondly, physical avoidance of a conflict until tension has eased.
- Thirdly, women found excuses which enforced or justified a certain form of behaviour, although the actual arguments were not revealed. An excuse is merely a rhetorical trick.
- Additionally, a standard procedure may be disturbed, as Scott suggested as part of the 'Weapons of the Weak'. The procedure will fail to reach its goal.
- As a fifth option, some informants involved a mediator, who would speak verbally and openly on their behalf. Involving a mediator is a usual strategy of conflict resolution in Basotho culture. This pathway includes an institutionalised social medium for addressing a person one cannot speak openly to otherwise.
- The sixth option actually concerns that which is avoided at all costs: a break in protocol with an open confrontation which is what happened to Tharo after she was not able to present the baby's vaccination scar.

Below I will present those points in detail and with reference to examples from earlier chapters.

9.4 Grudging Compliance: Feigning Agreement under Supervision

Overall, my informants finally complied with advice given by family elders due to their hierarchical relationship even if they disagreed with the content of this advice. However, whenever there was no monitoring of their observance they neglected to do whatever they were told. In the case of disagreement the willingness to obey abated, too. Scott already considered this grudging compliance as part of a subordinate's resistance to a dominant party. Provided there was no way to avoid control, open disputes were hence avoided by feigning agreement. This kind of behaviour moreover allowed one to keep face towards to dominants but behind the scenes subordinates discussed their disapproval and negotiated their reactions towards it (Scott 1985: 302).

Scott may overstress the terms of protest and resistance in that case, however, a dispute is indeed avoided while both parties have opposing interests. Hence, I would count grudging compliance, as Scott does, as a way to avoid breaking protocols. Generally, in my observed interactions as well as in Scott's descriptions, subordinates were aware of their unequal power relations and agreed to collaborate with the dominant party even if they disagreed with their behavioural expectations.

Like many other pregnant women in Lesotho, LeRobong was advised by her mother not to sleep during the day even if she was tired (see also 4.7). Her mother had told her that she will have a difficult birth because her laziness during pregnancy will affect the baby during delivery. Due to the baby's laziness it will get stuck in the birth canal and thereby cause a difficult and long labour. Hence, an expectant mother should abstain from napping during daylight hours. LeRobong disapproved of this advice and the given explanation but resisted the urge to lie down when her mother was around in the house. Whenever her mother had left the house LeRobong took the chance to get some rest. However, she complained to me "[this advice] is only meant to scare expectant women!" (Field notes Kroeker 19: 01/04/2009).

An old woman explained to me, expectant woman who sleep during the day find it difficult to sleep at night. Sleeping during daylight may result in bad dreams, sorrows and worries, which affect the mother in such a way that she becomes afraid of pregnancy or delivery. Stress and anxiety in the mother will therefore harm the baby's development. Moreover, insomnia and nightmares can also become pathological and indicate witchcraft afflictions, which then need to be treated by a traditional healer (Field notes Kroeker 4: 12/01/2009; Dilger 2005: 290). Usually, however, these explanations are not given to pregnant women, the old woman described to me. Young women will understand the value of the advice not to sleep during the day in due course when they take care of pregnant daughters or daughters-in-law, she added. The current youngsters may, thus, play out their dominance once they become elders and can take revenge on a younger generation.

As another example, many women who had decided to bottle feed their baby with a baby bottle at home used a cup or spoon, as the nurse insisted due to hygiene, when in the hospital for a check-up. Dummies were likewise only used at home as in the hospital the nurses and counsellors confiscated them (see Chapter 7.1.1). Hence, mothers comply with nurses' advice depending on the place.

Behind the scenes and in absence of family elders, young women complained about this advice, as LeRobong did (see 9.4). When in the company of their peers they exchanged opinions and vented their displeasure. To the person giving the advice they rather refrained from answering back for the sake of peace and quiet. Their grudging compliance was therefore paired with resistance behind the curtain on a day-to-day basis. HIV-positive pregnant women showed this kind of behaviour equally towards sources of authoritative knowledge such as family elders or hospital personnel if they felt dependent on an ongoing undisturbed relationship with them.

Scott adds that despite discomfort, these kinds of relations can be kept up over a long time especially if in the long run subordinates may come into the position of dominants, such as in generational relations (Scott 1990: 4).

9.5 The Sidestep: Leaving the Battlefield of Interaction

Physical avoidance has been described in the anthropological literature on migration as well as in the literature on domestic conflicts as a cause for migration (for Lesotho see Rosenberg et al. 2004: 401; Böhm 2006). Few authors, however, have discussed migration in relation to conflict avoidance. Among these few, Alber (2004) mentions that the Baatombu people of North Benin utilised physical avoidance to set up negotiations. The avoidance of conflict by leaving the compound and postponing return was a non-verbal means of initiating conflict mechanisms. Comaroff (1985: 71) suggested as well for Tswana women that they may leave the marital compound in the case of conflicts and conflict parties will be summoned in the *thakaneng* (cf. Rosenberg et al. 2004: 399; Gay 1980: 270), the court for female affairs. In Alber's example, Baatombu women instead of returning to the matrimonial home after a visit to "the real home", overstay with their relatives. The husband notices his wife is missing and inquires as to the reasons for the wife's undue disappearance. Hence, the husband will request her return and ask for forgiveness (Alber 2004: 180) which sets up a negotiation process.

This is very similar to when women in Lesotho avoid direct verbal disputes as Tharo did when she absconded from the waiting hall of the HIV clinic after the counsellor of the antenatal clinic had taken her there (see 9.2). As soon as possible, she fled that place again and therewith avoided (her third) enrolment into the antiretroviral treatment programme. Thereafter, she avoided the hospital for her delivery. Other examples have already been mentioned in earlier chapters:

- MaRobeli, who was already introduced in 6.4.2, decided to take residence in the waiting mother shelters until her delivery and thereafter to stay with her maternal family until she weaned the child. She had told her in-laws that her high blood pressure needs to be monitored in hospital. MaRobeli came from a remote village close to the South African border and while her husband worked in the South African mines she spent time at her marital home with her mother-in-law. Yet, mother-in-law and daughter-in-law did not get along very well. MaRobeli recalled that their difficulties were due to her first pregnancy not long after getting married in 2007. The pregnancy ended in a miscarriage in her seventh month after she had not felt the baby move for some days. The mother-in-law accused her of being a witch and of having induced an abortion. She took MaRobeli to a traditional healer who cut her chest several times (*matebele*) and inserted pharmaceuticals to cleanse her of the miscarriage and from witchcraft afflictions (cf. Gausset 1998: 646). Aside from MaRobeli's disapproval of traditional medicine, which her maternal family did not use, the relationship with her mother-in-law became very tense thereafter. Now, in her second pregnancy and with hypertension and HIV, she doubted her mother-in-law would understand her preference for biomedical treatment and her discomfort when staying at the conjugal home in the absence of her husband. Hence MaRobeli avoided entering a debate with her mother-in-law and, consequently, presented an excuse (see 9.6) about her need for medical assistance in the hospital, before shifting places.

Others likewise made efforts to leave a place when they expected trouble with their relatives or hospital staff:

- MaMapeli (see 7.4), who did not intend to return to her in-laws' house to avoid interference from her husband's elders, chose physical absence as a means to relax before an upcoming conflict. She stayed with her mother who knew about her HIV infection and her history of having had two miscarriages before presumably due to an undetected HIV infection. Her absence resulted in a proceeding strategy since she involved her mother as a messenger.
- Nne (see Prologue) shifted households from her maternal to her paternal grandmother whenever she felt pressurised.

- Tselela (see 7.6) avoided a conflict with the nurses by moving to her family home for the delivery. Since she did not consider herself as HIV-positive and therefore did not intend to take any treatment during delivery, she went for a "HIV free" home delivery. She later combined physical avoidance with a verbal avoidance strategy: she gave the excuse of having to attend a funeral which prevented her from getting to a biomedical unit. Additionally, Tselela pointed at traditional gender relations when she argued that her husband has to take decisions on the baby's treatment even though she was living on her own.
- Leshome (see 7.5), Robong, LeTselela, and others chose to stay in town and not to share a household with either a partner or their family. They therewith avoided gender and generational expectations.

For Lesotho, physical absence was not an uncommon way of managing conflicts. The fact that many women move permanently to the towns in the low land belt as labour migrants is proof of this and was discussed earlier (see Chapter 4). However, in many cases of conjugal conflicts or conflicts with elders the absence from the homestead was on a temporary basis and the women moved back to their usual homestead whenever the cause for disagreement abated.

9.6 The Excuse: A Rhetorical Trick

If discussions or explanations were unavoidable, excuses often became a useful tool to avoid stigma. Excuses were used by dominants and subordinates likewise. However, dominants spoke from their position of authoritative knowledge and therefore there was rarely a situation in which young pregnant women answered back and questioned any of their excuses.

Dominants enforced excuses by way of phrases or taboos, such as not sleeping during the day, not lingering at harmful places such as the doorway, prohibition of certain foods and eating proteins, or dress code and applications with spiritual connotations. The reasons that are given to the subordinate party, in this case the pregnant woman, mostly imply harm that will come upon her, her child or her family. For boys and underaged men, violation of taboos may result in harm to themselves or their agricultural resources, hence, family wealth.

Bledsoe (2002) mentions several excuses of women who were not interested in having sex with their husbands or wanted to avoid a pregnancy.

Since they accepted a man's dominance in sexual matters they used arguments such as prolonged breastfeeding, care of close relatives in a distant village or a ritually impure condition due to menstruation or sickness to refrain from intercourse (2002: 116)

As in the aforementioned story of LeRobong (see 4.7) who was not told why she must not sleep during the day, her mother avoided discussions by saying that LeRobong will have a difficult birth because of her laziness, which is obviously not true. As part of her public transcript, LeRobong's mother has obviously used an excuse and not presented her actual reasons why she does not want LeRobong to sleep. This argument remained her hidden transcript. LeRobong, for her part, reacted with feigned compliance (see 9.4). MaRobeli argued, as indicated earlier in 6.4.2, that she needed to stay in the waiting mother shelters because of the severity of her condition. In fact, her condition was not as severe as she claimed but fulfilled her aim of staying away from her mother-in-law's house. She, thus, applied two types of avoidance: an excuse and a sidestep (see 8.4.2).

While dominants did not need a good explanation to enforce a particular order, subordinates compensated their lack of power with arguments that appeared more credible that their actual reasons. Strong arguments tended to include a lack of economic means, unavailable transport, family obligations and formal employment. Arguments of this nature usually convinced others (see 6.1). Family obligations are valued more highly than individual interests and having to attend a family meeting carried a lot of weight when neglecting other expectations. In reality, a young person who takes family obligations seriously rather enhances his or her credit[3]. Excuses consequently justify a behavioural strategy without getting into a discussion about her actual motives:

- LeRobong (4.7) was asked in the post-natal room why she was not breastfeeding the child and was advised by elder relatives that she should do so. She responded that her job in the textile factory prevents her from breastfeeding the child on demand and therefore she needed to introduce formula milk. Likewise, LeTselela's mother also argues: "She brought formula milk with her and started replacement feeding straight away. She decided to give only formula milk to the baby, and she did not breastfeed even after the delivery because of

[3] Maybe it also adds to an elder person's credit to give orders. At least if subordinates follow suit. However, this is an empirical question which requires some further investigation.

work". Apparently, LeTselela presented her choice of formula feeding to her that way, since LeTselela had not disclosed her HIV infection to her mother and neither did LeRobong want to reveal her HIV status when explaining her feeding choice.

- Tselela (see 7.6) justified her home delivery in front of the counsellors with having to attend a funeral, which did not allow her to come to hospital. A funeral appears as a rather more convincing argument than her choice of a home delivery.
- Counsellors, who knew the situation of HIV expectant mothers from experience, sometimes provided women with excuses if a confrontation could not be avoided. Some mothers, who had not yet disclosed their status and feared that someone may ask why they are taking tablets, should answer according to the counsellor: "These tablets are Vitamin A which I need in pregnancy or when breastfeeding", while they were actually antiretroviral treatment drugs. Hiding the tablets would in many cases lead to non-compliance with the treatment programme. Having prepared an answer, in contrast, shall enable patients to take the tablets regularly and at the right time. On the other hand, taking the tablets without fear and arguing that they are vitamin supplements avoided stigma. If young pregnant women had said that these tablets were part of an antiretroviral therapy they would have also engaged in a debate on how they got infected with HIV.
- Secondly, counsellors sometimes told mothers, who feared that a mother-in-law may interfere with additional food while the mother was supposed to comply with exclusive breastfeeding, to say: "I had mastitis, therefore I needed to wean the child already". This excuse subsequently allowed them to feed the child exclusively with replacement food and therefore to comply with biomedical guidelines for the prevention of HIV transmission. Notwithstanding, some traditional healers may have treated mastitis without having to wean the child (see 7.2.1), however, once the milk dried up elders had to accept it.

Consequently, excuses are arguments which are more effective than a discussion on actual reasons would be. Interestingly enough, while uncomfortable situations are bypassed, the rhetorical device of presenting an excuse often resulted in empathy, support and respect. Thus, an uncertain situation in various cases even improved. Excuses are therefore a means to an end and help to conceal stigmatising news.

9.7 Disturbance: Sabotage of the Normal Procedure

All examples in this section include incorrect or incomplete fulfilment of orders. Besides physical avoidance of conflict, Comaroff mentions the disturbance of a normal procedure as one means of protest which Tswana women deployed in marital quarrels. If a husband did not comply with normatively defined responsibilities, a wife could withhold her sexuality and labour (Comaroff 1985: 71). If a woman was married by force she may have hoped that her failure to produce a child resulted in being send back home (Bledsoe 2002: 84). The secret use of Depo-Provera injections and her consequent failure to get pregnant was interpreted as sterility, describes Bledsoe, which led to an annulment of the marriage. This form of protest is based on the mutual knowledge of both parties concerning what the correct and complete way forward would be. Thus, altering the standard procedure can be recognised as non-verbal protest against it. As Alber shows, for instance, disruption to the normal procedure may already signify a conflict even before or instead of a physical and geographical escape from the dominant force.

Secondly, the secret use of contraceptives also interferes with the normal procedure. Women have allowed men to play out their masculinity when it comes to sexuality, but have taken decisions concerning family planning and household composition into their own hands. The most commonly given method of family planning are Depo-Provera injections for three month periods followed by the pill (MoHSW et al. 2010: 56; cf. Bledsoe 2002: 84). Even schoolgirls preferred injections since they would go unnoticed by their parents (Tuoane et al. 2003)[4] at a time when their parents would expect them to not yet be sexually active. Nonetheless, ethnography reveals that the secret use of contraceptives by women is widespread and women drive decisions on family planning by stopping contraception, spacing or postponing pregnancies (Bledsoe et al. 1998: 45, 50; Bledsoe 2002; Timaeus & Moultrie 2008; Moultrie et al. 2012: 241). The use of contraception behind the partner's back first and foremost deprived him of having offspring and allowed a woman to have informal relationships, just like men do. As a public transcript, the relationship remains fruitless, without any offspring, and may

[4] Before 1994, the pill was requested more than injectable contraceptives, apparently also because it was discreet (Tuoane et al. 2004; Lucas 1992).

therefore be unnoticed by family elders. As a hidden transcript a couple may nonetheless consummate their relationship.

The relationship with the male partner may be casual until his girlfriend surreptitiously disturbs the normal procedure by secretly withdrawing contraceptives. By getting pregnant she may intend to expedite the path to marriage and propose love, which is not foreseen in the common gender arrangement. So the boyfriend may be trapped by the *fait accompli*.

Other ways of disturbing the procedure were:

- Changing booklets and names to disguise identity or leaving booklets lying around for family members to find out about one's HIV status "by surprise", as with MaMeli (see 3.2) and Robong (see 5.3).
- Introduction of exclusive replacement food before elders may have access to feeding the child, just as MaMapeli did (see 7.4).
- Tharo was told by a doctor that he will not examine her if she does not bathe. Since she detested biomedical treatment and wanted to avoid interaction with the doctor, she refused to bathe (see 9.4.6).
- Tharo, in addition, had to agree to take treatment while hospitalised. The nurses brought her a cup with tablets and she always returned the empty cup. However, when Tharo was discharged and the bed lining was removed, all the tablets were found under the mattress.

In summary, a change in the normal procedure did not happen as part of an exchange of arguments but by changing the practical implications. An expected outcome was not reached for one or the other reason and actions gained no traction. This happened mostly in connection with an excuse. Attention was thereby drawn to a different subject and a space was opened to follow hidden interests. Particularly unavoidable aspects were still staged and others neglected for practical reasons, as Browner summarises:

> It would be unrealistic and impractical to adopt all prenatal recommendations, [the patient] selected those she could incorporate into her life with the least difficulty and to the greatest positive effect. (Browner & Press 1997: 124)

Pragmatics, thus, helped to adapt particular aspects and neglect others with the aim of minimal disadvantage.

9.8 The Institutionalised Option: Involving a Mediator

In addition to avoiding conflict, a more institutionalised but non-violent strategy must be added: *proceeding* (*Verfahren*) (Elwert 1999). Proceeding involves a third party which serves as a mediator for the stigmatised and subordinated person's interest. The mediator arrived at legitimacy through access to one or more of the following resources: money, social status, control over supernatural forces (Eckert 2004: 20) or, in our case of Lesotho, support due to age as well as the dominant medical system. Goffman (1963: 28, 31) calls these intermediaries "the wise" and therewith refers to a person who knows about a stigmatised identity, but the individual does not feel shame or a need to control the stigma in front of that wise person. Bailey speaks of a "middleman" who is able to facilitate communication between members of hierarchical social structures. A middleman effects a compromise between conflicting parties (1969: 167-169). Bailey furthermore distinguishes between a "messenger", who simply transmits information whereas a "broker" follows own (economic) interests. A "mediator", in contrast, seeks to settle differences in conflict situations, which comes closest to the social function I describe. A mediator mitigates and discusses how to proceed with a situation, however, this person does not need to be an expert in the field under debate but holds a socially valuable position based on trust. In several situations above mediators were used:

- MaMeli (see 3.2) let her mother-in-law explain to the doctor what had happened to her baby. The mother-in-law however had not been there at the time but dared to enter a discussion with doctor and midwife. For MaMeli it would have been disrespectful to talk back to her mother-in-law or the doctor.
- Leshome (see 7.5) took her mother to a hospital counselling session and therewith asked the counsellor to speak to her mother. She expected a counsellor with the backing of a biomedical health institution to be an authoritative figure. Therewith, Leshome intended to strengthen her point of view and convince her mother without entering a dispute from her subordinate position to her mother. Despite her knowledge she lacked authority, while a counsellor would be in a knowledgeable and authoritative position.
- Tharo (see 9.2) requested that a counsellor and I helped her to disclose her HIV status to her husband and her mother. She feared getting into a fight if she talked to her husband by herself. Tharo con-

vinced the counsellor to help her by saying that her husband is a violent man and would beat her up. Thus, she used an excuse to make the counsellor help her out. Despite a counsellor's medical confidentiality the counsellor arranged the joint HIV test and therewith took the lead to enlighten mother and husband about Tharo's health condition. During the talk the counsellor left it to Tharo to announce her test result. Thereby the counsellor did not violate her professional code of ethics.

- Robong (see 5.4) also asked MaThloni and I to help her in disclosing her HIV status to her mother, although she did not turn up for the meeting herself. The counsellor disclosed the information and counselled the mother since it was explicitly Robong's wish. Robong had already attempted to notify her mother about the test result by leaving her medical book lying around. However, her mother did not understand the encrypted medical language. Robong later called MaThloni to hear how the talk between us went and whether she could now expect her mother to factor HIV into her advice.
- Nne (see Prologue) did not manage to disclose her status to her grandmother until she was in the presence of a friend and a counsellor. She then expected her grandmother to inform her other grandmother, so she would not have to repeat the process of disclosure. Likewise Peli (see 5.4) waited for a situation when she would be accompanied by someone in authority who would assist her in raising the topic. The counsellor paved the way and prepared the mother for the positive test result, but then insisted that Peli was the one who told her what the test result was. The counsellor thereafter took over again for post-test counselling. Nne and Peli both felt a weight had been lifted after the revelation of their status and when their elders had promised the counsellor that they would support them.
- After MaMapeli (see 7.4) had decided to enter a conflict by not returning to her mother-in-law, she also sought to settle the conflict at an early stage, which was before the actual day scheduled for her return. Her mother, as a high ranking social individual, spoke to her in-laws on MaMapeli's behalf and hence set out her concerns and motives. Her early integration as a mediator allowed ample time for all parties to reflect on the situation before an actual outbreak of conflict would considerably affect relations.

- Robeli (see 5.1.5) sought help from MaKhotso and I since her husband denied that HIV existed. He refused to allocate any money for transport, counselling and treatment and disagreed with using protection. After a discussion which involved MaKhotso, Robeli, her husband and me, in which the husband repeated his statement, Robeli left the marital home and did not return to him.

In the course of the study and while learning more and more about the women's condition, worries and strategies, I was approached time and again by the study participants to discuss their situation with household decision-makers. Study participants requested me to speak to superiors on their behalf. In order to explain my decision regarding this request, we firstly need to focus on the women's motives for coming up with this idea.

The strategy of involving a mediator applies not only on a macro-political level but also within the family and can therefore be considered a culturally founded conflict strategy. Mediators evolve in an institutionalised way in marriage negotiations, since *malome*, a particular maternal uncle, may be approached to speak on behalf of a man who feels ready to enter marriage. Women tended to use ways of distancing themselves from their marital home or disturbing a procedure before they turned to a relative or friend for help and assistance in mediating. The trusted person was usually of the same sex and, depending on the addressee of the information, of the same age set, holding symbolic power (Eckert 2004: 20) or a professional position of authority. HIV-positive expectant women preferred, in some cases, for a hospital counsellor to speak on their behalf despite the fact that many women do not live with the family at all times. Hence, the Mothers2Mothers counsellors, who were also trained rhetorically, sometimes took over this function on request.

Despite knowledge about particular advice given in PMTCT counselling sessions, the mothers found it difficult to instruct others on why they would have to follow this advice in order to protect their baby from HIV. It would not have been easy to explain the medical language and complex ideas to an untrained family member who would then convincingly transfer the information to elders. Clients accepted the orders but did not feel that they were capable of convincing superiors with their reasons.

Mothers frequently asked my interpreter and me to assist as mediators as they gained trust and confidence in us. They expected us to be knowledgeable as well as convincing. Moreover, we had looked into the family situation and knew a great deal about conflicts and relationships. In addition, we already knew some of the household members through our home visits and interviews[5].

A mediator would need to have a good reputation, high social standing as well as being a trustworthy friend of the subordinated conflict party, thus, client and mediator would devise a strategy of talking in front of elders or the partners. In cases where women did not find an adequate mediator they would rather carry on with a strategy of avoidance or indirect conversation (i.e. through the *Bukana*, leaving evidence for someone to uncover, etc). Last but not least, matters would be adjourned until a later, more promising date.

9.9 All Strategies Fail: Entering Open Conflicts

Tharo had tried all the above mentioned strategies of avoidance. However, her plan to navigate around situations that may have revealed the secret about her HIV status became a difficult endeavour. The high levels of stress and uncertainty led to the decision to open up and disclose her HIV status to her husband, in an attempt to gain some control over the situation and to receive his support. Thus, reviewing manoeuvres, or rather avoiding new obstacles, created more insecurity on whether the new manoeuvres would work out. Under pressure she admitted to me that it was true, she had been in denial about her HIV status for a long time, but she now needed to talk to her husband about it. "It is difficult to live with someone who doesn't understand at all", she says, and "while trying to do the best, you completely mess up" (Field notes Kroeker 3: 11/02/2009).

Tharo devised a plan that would solve her dilemma: if the couple could get tested together both spouses will turn out positive and thereafter comply with biomedical treatment for the baby's sake. Neither of the spouses would need to disclose first which would avoid blaming the one who had brought the virus into the relationship. In the best case scenario, the test could break the ice so that they could talk about their status, be open about health recommendations and re-gain the faith in the relationship which she had already lost. A counsellor would help her to get the message across and she would again avoid having the uncomfortable conversation with her husband on her own.

---

[5] Reference is made to Spittler (2001: 1-25) who argues in favour of a *thick participation*, beyond the scope of participant observation, in order to gain access to certain interactional methods. This interference with the field of study shall be determined as intentional and part of the methodology.

Scott assumes that hidden transcripts usually stay hidden for a long time, as is the case with Tharo (although she took longer than average to disclose her situation). Conflicting ideas are dealt with by disguise, avoidance or a lie rather than with direct confrontation, in the interest of safety (Scott 1990: 86). An open confrontation will require a good dose of courage, the right moment and preparation. It implies insecurity and uncertainty on the way to address the situation adequately as well as successfully.

> Any public refusal, in the teeth[6] of power, to produce the words, gestures, and other signs of normative compliance is typically construed – and typically intended – as an act of defiance. Here the crucial distinction is between a *practical failure* to comply and a *declared refusal* to comply. The former does not necessarily breach the normative order of domination; the latter almost always does. (1990: 203)

As an example, there is a distinct difference between telling a mother-in-law about replacement feeding because of work commitments and because of a risk of transmitting HIV to the baby, which will definitely entail significant consequences of one sort or the other since it triggers further questions. It may easily harm the reputation of the individual but also that of other family members who were expected to instruct the person; to teach moral behaviour. Aside from being infected with a non-curable disease which significantly kills family and friends in Southern Africa, the sexual connotations often related to prostitution, promiscuity and immorality affect the self-esteem of the person involved. The effect of transferring a good reputation, as it is transferred to a child with the *lelomolo*, also works in a reverse negative way: a bad reputation can also be transferred to acquaintances who must stay away from stigmatised people in order to keep face.

> In general, the tendency for a stigma to spread from the stigmatized individual to his close connections provides a reason why such relations tend either to be avoided or to be terminated, where existing (Goffman 1963: 30)[7].

---

[6] It is interesting to note, that Scott uses the phrase "in the teeth of power" while teeth stand for masculinity, age and authority in Basotho culture. Thus, the *koetsa* band is meant to facilitate growth of the teeth in children as mentioned in Chapter 7 on early infant care.

[7] Sechefo describes that in the Basotho understanding of health, even a stigmatised person entering the room may affect someone in a liminal condition, such as a sick person: "Instantly when the [stigmatised] party enters the room, the sick person is depressed and attacked by

People living with HIV may thus avoid having the conversation in order to keep peace because a transfer of stigma would spoil the partner's and the family's identity. However, at a certain point, people living with HIV may dare to breach the normative order not only with a practical failure to comply, but with an open declaration of refusal, like Tharo plans, when the pressure becomes unbearable. Nevertheless, disclosure marks the most crucial and fearful part of being HIV-positive and many clients delayed having the discussion and women mainly disclosed when the situation became "unsafe" due to their fear of physical harm. Notwithstanding, disclosure of a hidden stigma is an irreversible step to take. Furthermore, the problem is that if someone else knows about it the person loses their grip on the information and has no control over where it is spread. Social sanctions may be a consequence for the individual or even kinsmen. At a certain point they found the time and words to confront others with a wisely selected piece of information.

The reactions from dominants after learning about unpleasant news can range from ignorance to violence. Dominants may, for instance, elect to ignore the piece of information and pretend they did not see or hear anything (but may take it into consideration and include it in their hidden transcript). Secondly, challengers may be accused of being deranged and their act will be deprived of its significance. The addressee may be shocked, thrilled or infuriated. Sanctions may apply, some of which may grant social-reintegration ("I'll overlook this infraction providing that…") (Scott 1990: 205). A person may moreover be labelled as deviant or sick and a medicalised interpretation may have the person institutionalised (see 2.1). On the other end of the scale, a challenger's act may be stigmatised in order to make a public example.

All these reactions take place in the arena of open interaction, however, the violation may significantly affect the uncertain situation. In the end, the situation may become worse due to the insubordination and following reprisal. The small rhetorical space available to subordinates could become even narrower and sanctions may follow. On the other hand: the complaint may be accepted, the situation could improve, and a sustainable change may be initiated at that point. An escalation of conflict may even enhance loyalty to the dominant due to the trust and responsibility transferred. All parties

---

visible signs of the "melikane" i.e. fits and sweating such that might cause rapid death." (Sechefo n.d.: 20).

gained status, power and freedom from such conflict resolutions which are usually avoided. All this is part of the uncertainty.

By the end of February Tharo took the bull by the horns: the couple underwent a joint HIV test and counselling. To the surprise of all of us the couple's test results were discordant and left Tharo astonished. Her plan, however, that was meant to consolidate her situation, did not work out as planned; her best-case scenario had completely failed. She was more uncertain than ever as it again shed light on unexpected difficulties that she had not factored into the equation. Uncertainty had resulted from an attempt to resolve the situation, however, the situation had once again turned into one of uncertainty in a downward spiral.

In the counselling session, the husband, Ntate, easily agreed upon condom use and his medical book showed he had been tested the previous month and several times before and was extraordinarily well informed about HIV, transmission and the prevention of mother-to-child programme. Ntate, moreover, did not seem at all surprised about his negative status and his wife's positive test result. He took it with quiescence and agreed instantly to an adapted feeding practice for the child according to biomedical PMTCT guidelines.

To understand this awkward situation, I interviewed him as well. Ntate mentioned that he had guessed about Tharo's status already, since she was so sick last year. He also remarked that he "did not expect this child to be born alive". I was not sure whether he had assumed his wife to be HIV-positive or had found out about it through her medical booklet, or perhaps someone had given the game away in hospital during her severe bout of anaemia in 2008. However, he explained to me that it was his suggestion that she should stay closer to town and therewith closer to the clinic and he therefore found her a room in town. As he expected (or knew) about the outcome of the test already, for him nothing much had changed, he added. He said that he would proceed to support her regardless of her HIV status[8]. Ntate, Tharo's husband, also remembered that he asked her about her HIV test in pregnancy, but she denied that she had tested positive, which he had then assumed to be a lie. Now he learned that he was right. The counsellor asks him whether he will support wife and child. Ntate agrees instantly and adds: "I want my parents

[8] One may assume that Ntate only reacted so calmly because the counsellor and I were present, while he may have reacted furiously if he and Tharo had been alone, as she expected. However, Ntate did not give the impression of someone who was very surprised or shocked during the counselling and testing procedure.

to support me, therefore I will do the same for my child" (Field notes Kroeker: 21/02/2009).

Tharo and the baby received a lot of attention following disclosure to the husband. Her mother had learned about her HIV infection when she was in hospital during her sickness and she had promised the nurses to look after her daughter. Now, the mother regularly talked to Tharo about HIV, a fact Tharo did not want to be reminded of, and also discussed her case in her absence, acting as Tharo's unauthorised mediator. This reaction was not at all what Tharo wanted. She had expected an aggressive reaction resulting in silent agreement and no further talk about the whole dilemma. She wanted some more freedom to combine crucial aspects of familial and medical protocols after having had the discussion and to independently enact her plans with regard to the child without justifying her behaviour. Now everybody knew and talked about her. The public transcript changed considerably into the opposite or as Scott puts it: "many acts that almost any reasonable observer would call acts of resistance may backfire and produce the very opposite of what was intended" according to "the law of unintended consequences" (1985: 295; cf. Whyte 1997: 22). While navigating around one obstacle another one appeared and when Tharo reacted, her environment had also already changed, hence, a situation of "Motion in motion", as Vigh used to describe people's ways of adjusting in contexts of an unstable social nature (2009) or "multidimensional practice", which is:

> the non-sequentialized relationship between movement related to immediately encountered change, movement toward an imagined position and the constantly sought dialogue between the immediate and the imagined, that is, what is envisioned as coming after the next wave, the next weather front, next current and so on, which can be pondered but of which we can never be certain as it is dependent on the interplay between forces, and hence outcomes, that are too numerous to predict. (Vigh 2009: 430)

While individuals try to control uncertainty, the constant struggle is contested by new elements of uncertainty. A strategy of navigation fails since its grounds have shifted in the meantime.

While Tharo's basic assumptions about her relationship to her husband, mother and biomedical practitioners failed, she feared the next upcoming obstacle. Up to that point no-one had paid any attention to her extramarital relationship and the doubts about whether the baby boy was her husband's child. The whole situation confused her and she wished things could be undone. Tharo blamed herself for her mistakes and I got the strong impression that she punished herself for her dilemma. She felt stigmatised, which was real for her, and she behaved accordingly. However, the stigma was not commensurate with an enacted stigma (Jacoby 1994). Numerous HIV-positive people put themselves in a minor position as acts of self-punishment for immoral or wrong behaviour in the way Lipp describes (1975). The stigma one feels goes hand in hand with familial punishment, however in some cases a punishment did not actually take place, merely the expectation of comeuppance led to devote repentance (Kroeker: forthcoming a). The issue concerning her extramarital affair appeared as a new challenge on the horizon.

Tharo from that time onwards avoided all kinds of attention, both medical and familial. Moreover, she again obtained a new medical booklet which did not contain any information about HIV. Hence, she did not receive medication. Her Hb fell from 3.6 to 1.6 and when her condition further deteriorated the nurse ordered blood transfusions from Maseru and sent the doctor time and time again to look after Tharo. Frustrated, the nurse told me "that she was hiding her status from them and she also refused the treatment. If she continues like that then she should go home and die there. She won't get any treatment here anymore". While staff lost patience with their client due to her refusal to cooperate, Tharo eventually agreed to the treatment. She promised to be well behaved and a "good" patient, again in order to be discharged from the hospital sooner, a new manoeuvre Tharo tried as an instrument of control. Therewith she planned to deploy physical absence as a strategy of avoidance after all minor strategies had already failed.

9.9.1 A Walk of Shame

Having in mind that Steffen (2005) analysed life-long treatment for chronic stigmatising disorders in a threefold sense, I passed by Tharo's house and she admitted that she had frequently thrown up after taking the tablets. Steffen considered that patients using medication as a response to addiction may see this treatment as cure to the problem, or maintenance of an incurable condition. Thirdly, the treatment moreover disciplines a person's drinking habits as part of self-punishment (Steffen 2005)[9]. Tharo, for whatsoever

[9] Reference is also made to Foucault who understands social sanctions in institutions that correct deviant behaviour as "moral orthopaedic" (Foucault 1991). However, in contrast to the stories I analysed in an African context, Foucault has a linear model of lifetime. In Lesotho,

reason, did not take her tablets and refused to go back to hospital when her condition deteriorated again. Only a few days later, on the 18th of April 2009, she finally passed away.

Why exactly she stopped accepting treatment time and again never came to light completely, although it fits into Lipp's conception of self-stigmatisation (*Selbststigmatisierung*). According to Lipp, stigma is not only constructed through interaction but merely reproduced actively by the deviant individual who takes responsibility as an indication of moral subordination. Lipp resumes that stigma does not primarily relate to power relations and authority, but to subordination as the person does penance (Lipp 1975: n.p.). Hence, social conditions of stigma will be re-defined by the stigmatised person and serve as motivation for deviant behaviour in a moral reading.

> In situations of crisis, when the paths traced out in front of us become too difficult and uncertainty threatens to be a dominant feature of quotidian life, we must act as human beings. So we try to change the world or the circumstances under which we live, in order to make things more tolerable. (Jenkins et al. 2005: 27)

As Tharo's case shows, someone eagerly tries to control uncertainty with clumsy uncertain steps. A just punishment would have guaranteed something reliable and some kind of order. She therefore expected her husband to be furious and beat her up when disclosing her status, however, she could not even rely on that. After she had once again failed to interpret the situation correctly and the dominant powers did not punish her, as she rightfully expected, she punished herself for her lies, her immoral behaviour, her mistakes and violations. She re-invents a system of order and morals to guide her. Would rituals have helped to overcome Tharo's struggles for prosperity, safety and gender? Perhaps, but her social environment pushed her in another direction and time was not on her side. Did anyone ever ask what she wanted? Counsellors should have.

---

and probably most of Africa, a concentric model applies, which includes ancestors and not yet born offspring. Punishment can result from the ancestors' discontent with moral wrong-doing. Severe wrong-doing can however prevent someone from becoming an ancestor. In Foucault's works punishment is restricted to earthly institutions and contemporary social life, yet this discussion cannot be elaborated on here.

In our last meeting Tharo cried that she did "everything wrong and wanted to make it right", but her assumed social death is followed by a physical death, which likewise surprises medical staff and family.

Being in a liminal state between life and death due to HIV and in childbed, Tharo took death as an option. Her depressed state, her social isolation and refusal of medical assistance suggested that she gave up on herself. One would have assumed that a mother like Tharo would fight for the sake of her baby. Quite in contrast, for her this child reminded her of her mistakes on a daily basis, which she found unbearable and had put her in this uncertain situation. Children should be the fruit of love whereas Tharo's baby was instead a product of mistakes that brought her into an adverse situation. Eventually, Tharo must have considered this a *walk of shame*[10]. Having lost her aim, a revitalised relationship of supportive spouses, she manoeuvred towards an option of no return.

---

[10] The walk of shame refers to a phenomenon in which a person must walk alone past strangers or peers, who are aware of the reason behind the embarrassing situation, before reaching a place of privacy.

"This thing of HIV makes child bearing difficult"

This comment from a HIV-positive mother and lay counsellor referred to the angst mothers have of harming their child and losing love and support. It was meant in a physical, as well as in a social and psychological sense. Her rhetoric of calling HIV a thing did not only refer to the virus itself, but the concurrent disadvantageous conditions, hence, the whole complex situation. Childbearing, which should be one of the most normal activities in African societies, turns out to be impeded. The transition into the new social status of being a mother brings along uncertainty anyway, however, the condition of carrying a virus destroys norms and orders and altogether affects the grammar of social life. In this book, I intended to describe arguments that guided women during an uncertain period of their life and it ended with the story of Tharo who was not only confused by contradicting principles but no guidelines at all. She had nothing to hold on to. In a rapidly shifting social situation in Lesotho in general, as well as a rapidly changing personal situation of pregnant women who are living with HIV, most individuals managed to find ways that attribute some order to their social situation and they sailed around disputes in crucial long-term relations. As the examples also showed, uncertainty produces control which produces uncertainty again, since control and uncertainty were two sides of the same coin.

10.1 Changing Living Conditions

The foundations on which Basotho people in general, and HIV-positive pregnant women in particular, act are shaking. In the last thirty years, socio-economic changes due to the involvement of women in formal employment and the retrenchment of men from labour migration challenged family life. Marital careers and gender relations were under scrutiny since they no longer promised economic and familial safety. The retrenchment of international labour migrants in South Africa reduced male participation which, added to the down-scaled agrarian production and deteriorated health situation of family members in the most productive segment of society, resulted in less family income, a reduced ability to produce cheaply (e.g. agricultural products, food, handicrafts), and higher costs for goods that could not be produced (i.e. medication, clothing, building material and school equipment). While losing stability from institutions of marriage and family networks, women in the urban areas had gained access to economic means and therewith independence and decision-making power. New employment opportunities for women caused a significant increase in female economic participation. An increased number of women involved in local politics, the educational landscape, a major shift in household-economy, and the need for women as primary caregivers for the sick made women indispensable members of public life as opposed to their predominant role in private life in precolonial times. Men did not gain additional roles due to these changes but lost social standing which led to frustration.

Besides, fertility rates dropped due to the introduction of modern methods of contraception in the late 1970s. Women no longer accepted only being appreciated for obedience and fertility but adopted many other previously male roles in addition. Producing offspring retained its high value for family life, but the number of children per woman decreased. Obedience to men and elder community members, on the other hand, remained key in the social interaction: men defended their authority over sexual life as inherent to masculinity, and elders defended their right to authoritative knowledge. Women have allowed men to play out their masculinity when it comes to sexuality, but have taken decisions concerning family planning and household composition into their own hands in the wake of male absence. Thereby, the influence of authoritative knowledge also dispersed.

As a second conclusion, such data suggests that women quickly adjusted to social change as they took over as family breadwinners to meet the increasing demands of family networks. The gender and generational contracts remained, however, unscathed as soon as their spheres merged again and women had no general interest (or means?) to overturn these. Compact urban housing conditions resulted in geographically divided families causing a mother with children or a childless couple to reside in town. Some women thus preferred to remain independent by not getting married or keeping households separate, albeit with a strong interlinkage with next-of-kin. While gender and generational relations remained somewhat manifest, women therewith were geographically distant, which allowed for individual decision-making on everyday life.

In my opinion, traditional roles were not contested by young women. Men as well as elders retained authority over media that would be needed to initiate sustainable social change. Young women rather looked forward to marriage and intergenerational family life, in which reproductive activities and marital status in theory were strongly interlinked and social hierarchies remained in place. Hence, spouses accepted time-tested models of gender and generational arrangements, even if they could no longer secure care and psychosocial support in times of need such as in "between life and death", respectively times of rapid change. That arrangement granted order, security and guidance. With this I do not mean particular sets of actions and consequences that are fixed norms, but a security which allows pragmatic solutions to be implemented for the purpose of security. A change of gender roles would relate to religious and micro-political transformations in authoritative family politics: subordinates, in this case young women, did not question familial roles *per se*, but merely broadened their personal freedom. Besides strategies of avoiding conflicts, these women also actively established pathways that circumvented their sphere of influence which compare to Scott's "everyday forms of resistance". Women in urban Mafeteng preferred ways of avoiding directives and duties as well as supervision. A lack of familial togetherness created space for individual decisions but also resulted in a dearth of adequate guidance.

10.2 Matters of Sexuality and Communication

A more individualised lifestyle in town also gave rise to a more individualised sex life dissociated from reproduction, which is also reflected in the high uptake of contraception amongst Basotho women. Young women engage in relationships with or without any intention of marriage, and if marriage is intended many young women actively engaged in decision-making: pregnancy initiated marriage negotiations between the two families. Hence, women drive decisions on spacing, postponing and even aborting children and thereby engineered partnerships. However, these hidden plans which women devised as a means to the end of marriage ended in some of them being left in the rather insecure and uncertain situation of being a celibate single mother. While sexuality had turned into a personal matter, offspring remained a crucial part of family and generational well-being and is thus beyond women's decision-making. It involved traditional authorities, their knowledge and supervision.

When HIV/AIDS entered the social arena in the mid 1980s a new open and proactive communication was promoted by policy makers and awareness-raising campaigns. Moreover, HIV testing and counselling in Lesotho was not a right but a duty and disclosure of the health status to sexual partners was highly recommended. By means of biomedical counselling sessions at HIV testing sites, awareness-raising campaigns, on the radio, TV and on billboards, Basotho people were encouraged to speak openly about topics such as sexuality and reproduction with their elders and partners. Reproductive health was expected to be a public topic. In contrast, etiquette and local norms of communication in the grip of power follow unchanged interactional patterns. In a local sense, health communication on maturity, conjugal rights and duties, contraception, pregnancy, delivery and early infant care were rather a matter of non-verbal communication. In contrast to this, in the biomedical discourse, all these topics were no longer part of private life but of the medicalised and, thus, institutionalised public domain.

The public health approach has targeted women as gatekeepers to reproductive health – a position young women were not (yet) able to fulfil due to the predominant gender and generational structure. Moreover, biomedical counselling as opposed to the interaction across gender and generations followed a very different approach: within the families enlightenment about certain topics did not take place in a preventive way, but when the need occurred as shown in the education on delivery and infant feeding procedures. Preventive measures, however, played an important role with respect to local afflictions due to witchcraft, ancestral content and familial well-being in general. The idea of prevention in a local context rather included prevention of a behaviour and therewith an indirect prevention of the actual risk (i.e. expectant mothers must not expose themselves to risky places, instead of actually preventing witchcraft in this place). Prevention related to actions rather than verbal education. Quite in contrast, in the hospital counselling sessions there are talks about potential risks and behavioural options to educate the women in advance. The topics relied on western, evidence-based principles and natural scientific laws, although this rarely formed part of the medical discourse with the clients in a hospital. The counselling rather proposed options to the women and demanded that they make rational decisions based on few parameters. Notwithstanding, the counselling was supposed to be non-directive and free from coercion, which was seldom the case due to the work targets of medical staff. Nevertheless, clients were asked to opt for one or the other feeding practice or contraception. Those decisions clients made in the counselling sessions were, however, not necessarily applicable in practice. Moreover, after biomedical counselling those women did not necessarily receive practical assistance when the need arose. Expectant women were, for instance, expected to administer medication by themselves when in confinement.

Whenever knowledge was transferred from the biomedical realm to family members, and subsequently upwards within the generational hierarchy, HIV-positive pregnant women rather chose to avoid the communication and, hence, to avoid conflicts. Employing mediators, as a way to avoid conflict, had proved a powerful tool, both throughout the political history as well as in family problem solving.

Communication from the family domain towards the health facility, on the other hand, was rather open as long as it did not concern personal matters. Women discussed familial concerns and directives in order to receive second opinions on certain topics (i.e. sleeping during the day, nutritional prescription and restrictions, taking *pitsa* medication, wearing a *selapa* shirt). Nevertheless, authority and authoritative knowledge within the family as well as within the biomedical facility merely resulted in decisions about supervision, control and avoidance of both. Therefore, informants engaged strategies such as physical avoidance, excuses, involving mediators, or grudging compliance to influence the outcome of decisions that were made for them.

10.3 Conflicting Demands

In a family setting having offspring assured a full social position and secured the social support system. Having at least one child confirmed or initiated a marriage and social well-being. From a public health perspective, HIV-positive women should refrain from having offspring or at least plan it well in consultation with a health practitioner in order to secure their own physical well-being as well as that of their child. Generally speaking, a health facility follows a rather scientific-technological approach to pregnancy and HIV whereas the client and her family mostly see a spiritual and social-emotional side to the situation. Due to these differing perspectives safety in a biomedical sense merely focuses on physical health and particularly on ways of preventing HIV transmission, such as sexual abstinence, the use of condoms, counselling and testing of the general population, and timely enrolment in treatment programmes. Medicalisation of procreation has had significant effects while prevention and care consequently relate solely to physical disorders despite invisible symptoms. The absence of symptoms may nevertheless result in the treatment of an individual body. Meanwhile, this individual approach of biomedicine ignores all but physical risks to well-being, the correlation between social factors and health, and therewith exposes the need for a broader approach. Biomedical health care was backed by the

World Health Organization guidelines, which Lesotho's government health structures copied with only minor changes to the cultural context[1].

In contrast, a holistic, in many cases collective, approach to local health care does not exclude biomedical tools but works in conjunction with doctor-priests as a provider of certainty rather than health. Clients may thus use knowledge systems for prevention and care in pregnancy and delivery complementarily, which means traditional as well as biomedical means of preventing misfortune. Traditional practitioners, in contrast to biomedical practitioners, did not limit their clients to certain tools and meanwhile traditional and biomedical medicine had undergone an amalgamation which has made both somewhat inseparable (i.e. the use of sugar and salt solutions, the usage of rubber gloves and disposable knives) in any case. Biomedical practitioners, however, did restrict clients to biomedicine and viewed traditional medicine as harmful and abdicable and hindering the success of biomedical treatment. Biomedical medicine was moreover regarded as of higher value than traditional medicine and, as a consequence, physical factors were deemed to be more important than social factors. The biomedical and the traditional medical system clashed with respect to length of the liminal phase, the kind of medication given in pregnancy and during delivery, the kind of support needed in labour, technology needed during delivery, length of exclusive feeding practices and composition of baby's diet, the kind of harms that can affect an infant and how to treat them. Moreover, the health systems differed in the teaching approach (preventive or when need occurs) and whether decisions were made individually or by decision-makers.

The health systems did not differ with respect to authoritative knowledge. In both systems, special places are considered suitable for deliveries and particular persons are authorised to attend a delivery.

HIV-positive pregnant women considered the biomedical field, their own embodied knowledge as well as local sources of knowledge equally important when learning about pregnancy, delivery, infant feeding practices and the management of disorders. The biomedical system gained acceptance through the use of technology and the hegemony of the global biomedical discourse. A biomedical delivery largely provides a notion of security due to the equipment available, trained medical staff and the power of medical technology. Here, in contrast to home deliveries and traditional birth facili-

---

[1] Copying here means no or minor attempts to adapt something to a local context, whereas appropriation includes new ideas which contribute (Beck 2009: 151-173). In this case copying seems appropriate.

ties, birth assistants kept a professional distance. The traditional medical system, however, was important because it was delivered by trustworthy and familiar people and referred to local particularities and culture-bound diseases. Since the birth process does not only consist of biological functions and bodily reactions as biomedicine would suggest, the social environment of trust and care also plays an integral part when deciding on the place of birth, particularly as many women fear maltreatment by medical staff during confinement. With respect to diseases which were discovered in biomedical antenatal care, such as HIV/AIDS or pregnancy induced hypertension, the hospital as a birth facility was favoured because of medical technology for the prevention of harm to the child. Tharo's delivery in her rented accommodation with an inexperienced neighbour as birth assistant was therefore extremely risky in all respects.

The emphasis on physical safety for mother and child versus the social integration of mother and child in a larger family network seems to result from antagonising notions. I come to the conclusion that, within the family, my study participants were primarily considered pregnant and, if the family knew about it, their HIV-positive status was regarded as a secondary factor. Quite in contrast, in the biomedical facility my informants were HIV-positive in the long-term, and temporarily pregnant as a supplementary condition. Hence, this justifies the reasoning why HIV-positive women must not get pregnant again but care for their own well-being first.

As a consequence of the latter, PMTCT technology in a biomedical setting is generally considered as an emergency option to prevent the infection of a child of a HIV-positive mother, although the mothers may view PMTCT rather more positively. PMTCT provides a chance to have a HIV-negative child irrespective of the mother's condition.

10.4 Uncertainty

Conflicting demands as well as an insecure and uncertain general life situation rendered the study participants highly vulnerable and in need of direction and practical guidance. In order to find this, some oriented towards global biomedical norms and others towards local practices. Yet, the majority managed to combine important aspects in a way that offered the best personal as well as social well-being. For this pragmatic application, social support and the level of uncertainty someone felt played a crucial part. Participant observation, meetings and interviews over several months made it somewhat possible to evaluate decision-making processes, arguments that were considered valuable, hopes and fears. All these criteria were subsumed to uncertainty. Uncertainty in that realm implied a realistic evaluation of present and prospective challenges, ideas on how to face them, as well as the ability to adapt the course pragmatically.

The assessment of certainty and uncertainty in the life situation is depicted in the diagram below. This diagram is of course highly speculative and according to my estimations of uncertainty. It shall nevertheless depict degrees of uncertainty and represent the relative situations of my interviewees. In order to illustrate degrees of uncertainty in relation to one another it does not require a scale. Moreover, it only included informants from the qualitative study and the numbers correlate with the numbers in the annexed list of participants. It needs to be noted, however, that the examples from the previous chapters only mentioned particular aspects of the informants' life trajectory, while this diagram evaluates the overall situation, including uncertainties not necessarily mentioned earlier. Content-wise, it is based on the following factors:

- Lacking a social network, particularly in the households.
- Lack of financial means or lack of access to resources which would allow for individual decisions without having to ask for financial support. Moland argued that the economically deprived and socially marginalised mostly tended to neglect biomedical advice due to the high social costs of losing face (2004: 96).
- Conjugal situation, whereby a functional and loving relationship was considered certain and a situation of quarrels, long distance relationships or a woman's attempt to be loved (such as an attempt to force a man into marriage or seeking familial attention) were considered uncertain.
- Physical or spiritual unwell-being.
- Malnutrition of mother or child.
- Denial of the HIV-positive test result.
- Heightened fear of stigma that greatly affected the lifestyle.
- Familial pressure and disputes, i.e. extramarital affairs or conflicts with in-laws.
- Very low self-esteem, perhaps in relation to self-stigmatisation.
- Having failed to comply with behavioural expectations and being under special control either at home or in the biomedical facility for that reason.

- Being entrapped in a web of secrets, lies and excuses.

For the women who were confronted with behavioural expectations at home through experienced elder clan members and perhaps through traditional practitioners as well as in the health facility, any of these forms to sort out individual perceptions of uncertainty were included in the scheme. They are comparable to Whyte's classification of misfortune including failure of health, failure of prosperity, failure of gender and failure of safety (Whyte 1997). Local advice in the graphic entails rites and familial notions of preventing or controlling these uncertainties. Biomedical advice in contrast implies biomedical technology, pharmaceuticals and equipment, which likewise aim at controlling failure of health, but with different presumptions.

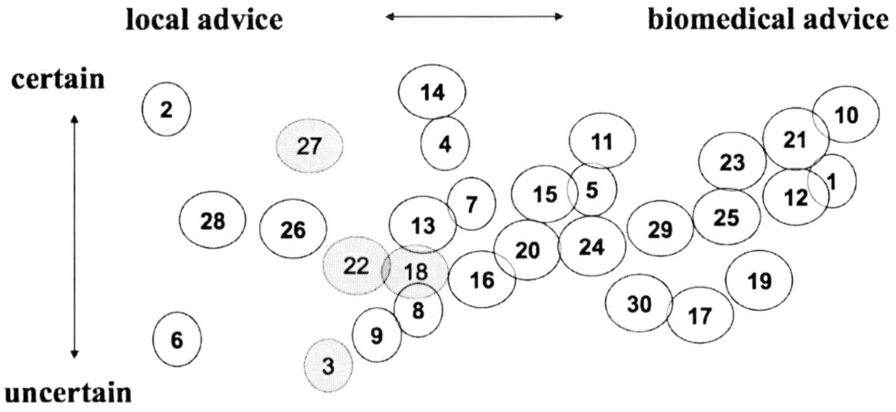

Leshome (in diagram number 10; see also annexed list of participants), for instance, was well aware of the challenges, made conscious decisions, combined local and biomedical advice and added some flexibility. Being financially independent, living on her own but maintaining a close and supportive network of personal relations with her boyfriend as well as her mother made her situation rather stable. Moreover, she had tested HIV-positive some time ago and was well equipped with information due to her occupation as peer educator in the textile factory and her support group for people living with HIV. Tharo (number 3 in the diagram), like many others, found herself interacting with a volatile environment. She was in poor health, lacked financial resources or any occupation that would keep her busy and was not able to make conscious decisions. Her extramarital affair had made her vulnerable and devoted to her husband. Her lies and excuses were no longer under control and she feared being confronted with her disobedient behaviour by people she obviously depended on.

Tselela (number 6 in the diagram), as with Tharo, was without economic means, in an insecure conjugal situation, and under a lot of pressure. Moreover, both feared great stigma. While they tried to manage their outward impression, they found themselves enmeshed in a network of lies and fears. Insecurity limited their options. Thus, they navigated in an uncertain zigzag course. Yet, it was uncertainty that paralysed any attempt to make a decision.

Last but not least, some numbers in the scheme are shaded. These numbers refer to the life stories of women which ended fatally in the state between life and death: LeRobeli (18) had a miscarriage, MaMeli's (22; see also Chapter 3.2) baby passed away one day after the delivery, MaSupa (27) delivered a stillborn child. Tharo (3) passed away leaving a six-week-old infant, a ten-year-old and a seven-year-old. All four cases with a fatal outcome happened in the highly uncertain time span which was metaphorically assigned as "in-between life and death".

10.5 Detours of Minimal Disadvantage

HIV-positive pregnant and child-bearing women navigated thoughtfully and rationally in order to combine the most important aspects of either medical system. At the same time their manoeuvres helped to bring their ideas (or *hidden transcript* as Scott (1985) calls it) forward. Notwithstanding, women were reluctant to openly contradict the expected behaviour and aimed in the long run for ongoing love, care and support and, hence, safety for mother and child. Patients in Africa usually depend on their family's social and financial support and mothers may, for this reason, avoid raising a controversial issue openly. Thus, in the case of disagreement, the women used grudging compliance with advice if they could not avoid being supervised. Besides, I found four other ways of avoiding conflicts: In my typology I labelled those types of avoidances as:

- Sidestep: Physical distance from certain people to avoid their supervision or to avoid disadvantages related to a particular place.
- Excuses: Finding arguments which are more likely to be accepted. Often the hidden argument entailed some stigmatising or otherwise discrediting information.
- Disturbances: The normal process was sabotaged so that intended aims or consequences failed to meet their target.

- Mediator: A mediator of high social rank was involved to mitigate between parties or to transmit information.

These types of avoidance were used in creative ways and depended on the changing environment or personal availability. Obvious aspects of certain standardised procedures were staged while less obvious ones were neglected, aspects were modified and people included or excluded as and when it served a certain purpose. Moreover, ways of dealing with conflict situations were deployed in a complementary or alternative way and frequently the strategy changed when a mode no longer looked promising.

On a more abstract level, time played a major part. Detours in social interaction were thought to be most useful when the problem was solved in a certain time frame. Hence avoidance strategies only needed to be deployed to bridge a time gap. For instance, mixed feeding is only problematic until the child is weaned after six months. Thereafter, the mother would meet her relatives again without concerns of them feeding the child additionally or asking questions on stigmatising exclusive feeding practices. In conclusion, there was a high chance of getting away with excuses or physical absence for some days, weeks or months until the social relations returned to normal. Likewise, medical procedures can only be applied during certain time frames. Visiting a healer for spiritual protection against witchcraft during pregnancy would not be a topic once the child was delivered. Taking medication to prevent mother-to-child transmission of HIV was also not a topic after confinement.

Besides time, avoidance is a useful means depending on social constellations. As I have demonstrated, in long-term relations of dependency with unequal power distribution various types of avoidance are in use, all with the aim of keeping these relations intact. In the small body of literature on the matter, avoidance was described for social relations of groups (with the exception of Goffman 1963), whereas I describe avoidance for individual, close social relations[2].

Only in highly uncertain situations were open confrontations taken into consideration, however, in some cases negative consequences were already anticipated, as in Tharo's case.

---

[2] It remains an open, empirical question, whether the types of avoidance I established are also found in social relations of groups.

10.6 Means of Gaining Control over an Uncertain Situation

Two terms seem to be undefined but crucial in the whole debate surrounding uncertainty: safety and rationality.

As international public health experts equivocate over how best to prevent HIV transmission and contradict the former guidelines based on new research findings, the Lesotho Government follows suit and health counsellors and patients on the ground struggle to adapt. Young mothers attempt to integrate what they learned in PMTCT counselling about "safe" feeding practices into their challenging lives. In the context of HIV/AIDS, what does "safety" actually mean? I cannot provide a clear definition, however, the abstract aim the mothers wanted to achieve definitely orients towards control of the physical, psychological and spiritual well-being of mother, child and the household community. Uncertainty about forthcoming misfortune, in contrast to safety, was never completely eliminated but rather a part of everyday life. This translates into the attempt to avoid conflicts and an approximate value of certainty. Whyte considers "In the process you may never achieve certainty, though you may gain some degree of security. Sometimes you simply have to accept uncertainty and live with it or try to ignore it" (Whyte 1997: 224).

The fusion of traditional and biomedical advice, hence, the appropriation of conflicting notions, resulted in an inseparable local custom. The expectant mother shelters at Mafeteng Hospital frequently house young women dressed in pink *selapa* shirts and wearing protective charms. While these girls and their families found the hospital "safe" for their delivery, other spiritual protection nevertheless applies and it also gives some peace of mind and therefore a feeling of certainty. Neglecting traditional practices is considered to be hazardous for mother and child and, hence, a child may develop abnormally. In the traditional clinic, Maluela, the healer, appropriated biomedical practices and therewith combined treatment methods. Hospital outreach programmes addressed birth attendants from time to time for training, of course, only registered traditional birth attendants participate unlike many elder women who casually oversee the deliveries of relatives and neighbours.

Consequently, local understanding of harm and its prevention did not dissipate; on the contrary, relevance continued as hospital care was added. Differing roles and therewith norms of adequate behaviour became apparent along with time, place, personnel, and social environment. Due to conflicting demands certain norms consequently needed to be broken as they could not be met by the mothers.

In my understanding, these mothers acted strategically and very rationally when staging their public transcript. Minimising uncertainties was achieved through the application of well chosen aspects of local or biomedical frames of reference that were meant to guide women. As a third frame besides local and biomedical protocols there is that of individual feasibility (I agree, however, that this separation of the three frames of reference is very artificial). Suffice to say, the zigzag courses were part of an attempt to control the personal situation beyond predominantly family driven and biomedical interests. In most cases the ideas behind any changes were based on rational, intentional, creative thoughts. In the ethnographic literature on uncertainty and social navigation it is debated whether these changes are rationally planned.

It would have been highly uncertain to neglect practices that provided certainty and thus to tempt fate. Thus, combinations of arguments from various frames of reference were the norm rather than the exception, yet, these combinations were far from arbitrary. At least in the individual biographies I followed I presume rationality, since the women were able to explain why and how they adjusted their course. I am, however, not able to tell if they followed a short-term tactic, a long-term strategy or whether these categories make sense at all in this study. In any case, the combinations made sense for the individual.

Annex: List of Abbreviations

3TC: Lamivudin

AFASS: "Acceptable Feasible Affordable Sustainable and Safe"

AIDS: Acquired Immune Deficiency Syndrome

ALAFA: Apparel Lesotho Alliance to Fight AIDS, Maseru, Lesotho

ANC: Antenatal Care / Antenatal Clinic

ART: Antiretroviral Therapy

ARV: Antiretroviral Drugs

ATCBM: Attitudes towards Childbirth in Mafeteng Study

AZT: Zidovudin

CD4: White blood cells that are an essential part of the human immune system, their number indicates the condition of the immune system

DHMT: District Health Management Team, Mafeteng, Lesotho

FAO: Food and Agriculture Organization of the United Nations

GGGI: Global Gender Gap Index

GoL: Government of Lesotho, Maseru, Lesotho

HAART: Highly Active Anti-Retroviral Therapy

Hb: Haemoglobin

HIV: Human Immune Deficiency Virus

HTC: HIV Testing and Counselling

IBFAN: International Baby Food Action Network

ICAP: International Center for AIDS Care and Treatment Programs at Columbia University's Mailman School of Public Health, USA

ILO: International Labour Office

INFACT: Infant Formula Action Coalition

INSTRAW: United Nations Entity for Gender Equality and the Empowerment of Women

IOM: International Organisation for Migration

IUD: Intra-uterine Device

KYS: Know Your Status Campaign

L.K.: Lena Kroeker

LENA: Lesotho News Agency, Maseru, Lesotho

LLLI: La Leche League International, Schaumburg, USA

LPPA: Lesotho Planned Parenthood Association, Maseru, Lesotho

MDG: Millennium Development Goals

MoHSW: Ministry of Health and Social Welfare, Maseru, Lesotho

MSF: Médecins sans Frontières

MTCT: Mother-to-Child Transmission of HIV

NAC: National AIDS Commission, Maseru, Lesotho

NAS: National AIDS Secretariat, Maseru, Lesotho

NGO: Non-Governmental Organization

NVP: Nevirapine

PEMS: Paris Evangelic Mission Society, Roma, Lesotho

PLHIV: People Living with HIV and AIDS

PMTCT: Prevention of Mother-to-Child Transmission of HIV

TBA: Traditional Birth Attendant

TT: Tetanus Toxoid Vaccination

UNDP: United Nations Development Programme

UNICEF: United Nations International Children's Emergency Fund

VCT: Voluntary Counselling and Testing

VDRL: Venereal Disease Research Laboratory Test

WHO: World Health Organization, Geneva, Switzerland

Annex: Glossary of Sesotho Terminology

Balimo (Pl.): ancestor spirits, spirits of the dead (Ashton 1952: 317).

Ba robetseng: literally: those who sleep, dead people.

Bohali / lebola: marriage, family or home of one's husband (Morija 1998: 80); bride wealth payment, both terms, bohali and lebola, are used synonymously in Sesotho, lebola derives from isiZulu.

Bukana ea Bophelo: Personal medical booklet that contains information about visits to a health facility, anamnesis and treatment.

Chobeliso: Elopement as part of the traditional process of marriage initiation (Rosenberg et al. 2004: 56).

Karabong: literally: the place of the answer (Karabo), name of the HIV site at Mafeteng Government Hospital named after the present Queen Karabo, who opened the site.

Khoetsa: black necklace of cotton or leather a child receives.

Khotla: Male dominated spiritual and political centre of a settlement, place of public gatherings, juridical court (Ashton 1952: 317).

Koae: dish of mutton which is served to a bride before she can eat other food from this new family.

Kraal: enclosure for cattle or other livestock (Ashton 1952: 322).

Lebese la Litlobo: colostrum, first yellowish milk a mother produces. In biomedical terms colostrum provides manifold values for the newborn, in various ethnic groups lactation is stimulated already before the delivery and colostrum must not be fed to the baby (Ashton 1952: 28-29; Stuart-Macadam & Dettwyler 1995: 9; Fjeld 2008).

Lefetoa: spinster (derogative) (Morija 1998: 102).

Lesheleshele: soft porridge from either maize or sorghum flour.

Letsoku: ochre, initiates wear red or white letsoku over face, torso or over the whole body as part of their ritual outward appearance.

Lifaqane: time of war between various clans between about 1840 and 1870. (Coplan 2003: 977-993).

Malaene: "single roomed dwelling units attached to each other in a linear form and in clusters of tenements" (Mapetla 2005: 131-152).

Mali: blood (Morija 1998: 108), ejaculate.

Malome: mother's brother / mother's brother's wife (Ashton 1952: Appendix I); the relationships implies a social connotation. Malome describes a guardian and mediator between Ego and family elders, particularly the parents.

Matlala: Sesotho disease which can kill a person instantly without signs of sickness. It is caused by a strong *muthi* that was applied at the door to someone's house or to some person and affected the afflicted person by accident.

Matebele: cuts in which a healer rubs plant parts or ashes thereof as part of treatment. Visible scars remain from these insertions.

Moato: cattle, livestock, (wealth).

Mokhachane (Sg.) / **bakhachane** (Pl.): pregnant woman / pregnant women.

Morena: chief of a village. (Morija 1998: 113).

Motsoetse (Sg.) / **bo-motsoetse** (Pl.): "woman who has recently given birth (...) such women are supposed to eschew sexual intercourse and so are ritually pure" (Ashton 1952: 318).

Muthi: strong medication which prevents or attributes witchcraft.

Nakeli: rodent animal (wildcat?), claws, fur or tail are used for necklaces in some clans.

Ngaka (Sg.) / **Bo-ngaka** (Pl.): Traditional Healer, the different terms refer to certain schools of healing, however, laymen in Basotho use both terms interchangeably. The Sesotho term *mathuela* rarely applies, though.

Ngoetsi: daughter-in-law (Morija 1998: 115).

Nkhono: grandmother (Morija 1998: 116).

Ntate: adult male person, father.

Nyopa: barren or childless woman (derogative) (Morija 1998: 117).

Pitsa (Sg.) / **Lipitsa** (Pl.): literally: pot, but also a collective term for traditional medication in the form of water-based infusions including herbal or animal parts.

Phuoana: fontanelles of an infant, mostly used referring to a Sesotho disease which manifests in pulsing fontanelles.

Rondavel: traditional round clay or stone-brick houses with thatched roof.

Seotlo: vestibule, reed-fenced place surrounding the entrance of the kitchen and female residential house, threshing-floor (Morija 1998: 127).

Selapa: pink piece of garment pregnant women receive from their elders.

Senyeha: to become spoiled, damaged (Morija 1998: 127), Sesotho-disease that affects children which suffer rapid weight loss, severe diarrhoea, loss of appetite, and failure to thrive, and may be fatal. It is caused by mother's violation of taboo. (Romero-Daza 2004: 961), the verb (senyehile) is used to describe young girls who become pregnant before marriage.

Sesotho: language and culture of Basotho people.

Thakaneng: female dominated equivalent to the male *khotla*. Court of women's issues, which is headed by the chief's senior wife. Adolescent unmarried girls spend nights there together with an adult lady who supervises and instructs them towards womanhood.

Thokolosi: evil human shaped spirits which transfer witchcraft and travel deploying animals as carriers.

Thothobolo: waste place in proximity of the *seotlo*.

Tsotsi: criminal person.

Voortrekkers: White settlers of Dutch Boer origin who founded the states of Free State, Transvaal and Natalia.

Clans and their totemic animals: Mokoena (crocodile), Motaung (Lion), Motloung (Elephant), Mofokeng (Rabbit), Motobatsi (Cat), Mokhoho (Chicken), Motsoeneng (Monkey), Motlokoa (Nakeli) etc.

Annex: Bibliography

Adair, T. (2007). *Desire for Children and Unmet Need for Contraception Among HIV-Positive Women in Lesotho*. Calverton: Macro International Inc. Retrieved March 1, 2015 from http://dhsprogram.com/pubs/pdf/WP32/WP32.pdf.

Alber, E. (2004). Meidung als Modus des Umgangs mit Konflikten. In: J. M. Eckert (Ed.), *Kultur und soziale Praxis. Anthropologie der Konflikte. Georg Elwerts konflikttheoretische Thesen in der Diskussion*. Bielefeld: transcript-Verlag, 169-185.

Almroth, S., Mohale M. & Latham M. C. (2000). Unnecessary Water Supplementation for Babies: Grandmothers Blame Clinics. *Acta Pædiatrica* 89 (12), 1397-1507.

Ansell, N. & Blerk, Van L. (2004). Children's Migration as a Household/Family Strategy: Coping with AIDS in Lesotho and Malawi. *Journal of Southern African Studies* 30 (30), 673-690.

Apitzsch, U. & Jansen, M. M. (2003). *Migration, Biographie und Geschlechterverhältnisse*. Münster: Westfälisches Dampfboot.

Appadurai, A. (1986). *The Social Life of Things: Commodities in Cultural Perspective.* Cambridge: Cambridge University Press.

ARASA & Human Rights Watch (2008). *A Testing Challenge: The Experience of Lesotho's Universal HIV Counseling and Testing Campaign.* New York and others.

Arendt, H. (1996). *Macht und Gewalt.* München: Piper.

Ashforth, A. (2010). Spiritual Insecurity and AIDS in South Africa. In: H. Dilger & U. Luig (Eds.) *Morality, Hope and Grief. Anthropologies of AIDS in Africa.* New York: Berghahn Books, 43-60.

Ashton, H. (1952). *The Basuto: A Social Study of Traditional and Modern Lesotho*. London: Oxford University Press.

Avishai, O. (2011). Managing the Lactating Body: The Breastfeeding Project in the Age of Anxiety. In: P. Liamputtong (Ed.), *Infant Feeding Practices. A Cross-Cultural Perspective.* New York: Springer Science+Business Media LLC, 23-38.

Bailey, F. G. (1969). *Stratagems and Spoils. A Social Anthropology of Politics.* Oxford: Blackwell.

Beck, K. (2009). The Art of Truck Modding on the Nile (Sudan): An Attempt to Trace Creativity. In: J.-B. Gewald, S. Luning & K. van Walraven (Eds.), *The Speed of Change. Motor Vehicles and People in Africa, 1890-2000.* Leiden: Brill, 151-173.

Beck, U. (1986). *Risikogesellschaft: Auf dem Weg in eine andere Moderne.* Frankfurt am Main: Suhrkamp Taschenbuch-Verlag.

Becker-Schmidt, R. (2003). *Zur doppelten Vergesellschaftung von Frauen.* gender…politik…online, Retrieved March 1, 2015 from http://web.fuberlin.de/gpo/pdf/becker_schmidt/ becker_schmidt_ohne.pdf

Bennett, L., Casey, K. & Austin, P. (1996). Issues for Women as Carers in HIV/AIDS. In: L. Sherr, C. Hankins, L. Bennett (Eds). *AIDS as a Gender Issue.* London: Bristol, PA: Taylor & Francis, 177-190.

Biancuzzo, M. (2005). *Stillberatung: Mutter und Kind professionell unterstützen.* München: Elsevier Urban und Fischer.

Binder-Fritz, C. (1995). Der Wandel der Geburtshilfe bei den Maori in Neuseeland. In: W. Schiefenhövel, D. Sich & C. E. Gottschalk-Batschkus (Eds.), *Gebären. Ethnomedizinische Perspektiven und neue Wege.* Berlin: Verlag für Wissenschaft und Bildung, 93-103.

Binder-Fritz, C. (2003). Gender, Körper und Kultur: Ethnomedizinische Perspektiven auf Gesundheit von Frauen. In: T. Lux (Ed.), *Kulturelle Dimensionen der Medizin. Ethnomedizin – Medizinethnologie – Medical Anthropology.* Berlin: Reimer, 89-123.

Bland, R., Rollins, N., Coovadia, H., Coutsoudis, A. & Newell M. (2007). Infant Feeding Counselling for HIV-infected and Uninfected Women: Appropriateness of Choice and Practice. *Bulletin of the World Health Organization* 85 (4), 289-296, Retrieved March 1, 2015 from http://www.ncbi.nlm.nih.gov/pubmed/17546310.

Bland, R., Little, K., Coovadia, H., Coutsoudis, A., Rollins, N., & Newell, M. (2008). Intervention to Promote Exclusive Breast-Feeding for the First 6 Months of Life in a High HIV Prevalence Area. *AIDS-Official Journal of the International AIDS Society* 22 (7), 883-891.

Bledsoe, C. H. (2002). *Contingent Lives.* Chicago: University of Chicago Press.

Bloemertz, L., Macamo, E., Doevenspeck, M. & Müller-Mahn, D. (Eds.) (2012). *Risk and Africa – Multi-disciplinary Empirical Approaches.* Beiträge zur Afrikaforschung. Berlin (and others): LIT.

Blystad, A. & Moland, K. M. (2009). Technologies of Hope?: Motherhood, HIV and Infant Feeding in Eastern Africa. *Anthropology & Medicine* 16 (2), 105-118.

Bochow, A. (2007). Valentinstag in Kumasi, Ghana: Sexualität und Generationenbeziehungen im Wandel. *Africa Spectrum* 42 (2), 195-218.

Böhm, C. (2003). The Social Life of Fields: Labour Markets and Agrarian Change in Lesotho. *Paideusis – Journal for Interdisciplinary and Cross-Cultural Studies* (3), 1-20.

Booth, K. M. (2004). *Local Women, Global Science: Fighting AIDS in Kenya.* Bloomington: Indiana University Press.

Borck, C. (2003). Zwischen Vermittlungskrise und Biopolitik. Der Aktionsradius der modernen Medizin. In: T. Lux, *Kulturelle Dimensionen der Medizin.* Ethnomedizin - Medizinethnologie – Medical Anthropology, Berlin (Reimer): 124-144.

Bourdieu, P. (2002). Pierre Bourdieu on Marriage Strategies. *Population and Development Review* 28 (3), 549-558.

Bretschneider, P. (1995). *Polygyny: A Cross Cultural Study*. University Uppsala, Diss. 1995. Uppsala.

Brown, L., Thurman, T. R., Kendall, C. & Bloem, J. (2005). *Magnitude of Sexual Violence in Lesotho.* 133rd Annual Meeting & Exposition, December 10-14, 2005, American Public Health Association, Philadelphia, PA. Retrieved from March 1, 2015 https://apha.confex.com/apha/133am/techprogram/paper_114115.htm.

Brown, P. & Levinson, S. C. (1987). *Politeness: Some Universals in Language Usage.* Cambridge: Cambridge University Press.

Browner, C. H. & Press, N. (1997). The Production of Authoritative Knowledge in American Prenatal Care. In: R. E. Davis-Floyd & C.

F. Sargent (Eds.), *Childbirth and Authoritative Knowledge: Cross-cultural Perspectives.* Berkeley: University. of California Press, 113-131.

Bundesamt für Gesundheit (2009). *Factsheet: Quecksilber.* Retrieved March 1, 2015 from http://www.bag.admin.ch/themen/chemikalien/00228/03912/index.html?lang=de.

Caldwell, J. C. (1982). *Theory of Fertility Decline.* London, New York: Academic Press.

Central Intelligence Agency (2010). *The Worldfactbook: Lesotho.* Retrieved March 1, 2015 from https://www.cia.gov/library/publications/the-world-factbook/geos/lt.html.

Chipeta, L. K. (2005). Gendered Separation of Space in Blantyre City, Malawi. In: F. Kalabamu, M. Mapetla & A. Schlyter (Eds.), *Gender, Generation and Urban Living Conditions in Southern Africa.* Roma Lesotho: Institute of Southern African Studies National University of Lesotho, 35-52.

Christiansen, C., Vigh, H. E. & Utas, M. (Eds.) (2006). *Navigating Youth, Generating Adulthood: Social becoming in an African context.* Uppsala: Nordic Africa Institute.

Cobbe, J. (2004). *Lesotho: Will the Enclave Empty?* Retrieved March 1, 2015 from http://www.migrationinformation.org/Profiles/display.cfm?ID=248.

Comaroff, J. & Comaroff, J. (2012), *Theory from the South: Or, how Euro-America is Evolving Toward Africa.* Boulder, Colo., London: Paradigm Publishers.

Comaroff, J. (1980). Healing and the Cultural Order: The Case of the Barolong Boo Ratshidi of Southern Africa. *American Ethnologist* 7 (4), 637-657.

Comaroff, J. (1985). *Body of Power, Spirit of Resistance: The Culture and History of a South African People.* Chicago: University. of Chicago Press.

Comaroff, J. (2010). Beyond Bare Life: AIDS, (Bio) Politics, and the Neoliberal Order. In: H. Dilger & U. Luig (Eds.), *Morality, Hope and*

Grief. Anthropologies of AIDS in Africa. New York: Berghahn Books, 21-42.

Conrad, P. & Schneider, J. (1983). Medicine as an Institution of Social Control: Consequences for Society. In: M. Zuckerman (Ed.), *Biological Bases of Sensation Seeking, Impulsivity, and Anxiety.* Hillsdale, NJ: Erlbaum, 485-515.

Conrad, P. (1975). *Identifying Hyperactive Children: The Medicalization of deviant behavior.* Aldershot: Ashgate.

Conrad, P. (1992). Medicalization and Social Control. *Annual Review of Sociology* (18), 209-232.

Cooper, E. R., Charurat, M., Mofenson, L., Hanson, I. C., Pitt, J., Diaz, C., et al. (2002). Combination Antiretroviral Strategies for the Treatment of Pregnant HIV-1-infected Women and Prevention of Perinatal HIV-1 Transmission. *Journal of Acquired Immune Deficiency Syndromes*, 29(5), 484-494.

Coovadia, H., Rollins, N., Bland, R., Little, K., Coutsoudis, A., Bennish, M., et al. (2007). *Mother-to-Child Transmission of HIV-1 Infection during Exclusive Breastfeeding in the First 6 Months of Life: An Intervention Cohort Study.* The Lancet, 369(9567), 1107-1116, Retrieved March 1, 2015 from http://www.sciencedirect.com/science/article/pii/S0140673607602839.

Coplan, D. B. (2003*).* Land from the Ancestors: Popular Religious Pilgrimage Along the South African-Lesotho Border. *Journal of Southern African Studies* 29 (4), 977-993.

Corno, L. & Walque, D. de (2007). *The Determinants of HIV Infection and Related Sexual Behaviors: Evidence from Lesotho.* Policy Research Working Paper 4421. Washington: The World Bank.

Cosminsky, S. (1986). Traditional Birth Practices and Pregnancy Avoidance in the Americas. In: M. Maglacas, J. Simons & World Health Organization (Eds.), *The Potential of the Traditional Birth Attendant.* 75-89.

Coutsoudis, A., Pillay, K., Kuhn, L., Spooner, E., Tsai, W.-Y., Coovadia, H., et al. (2001). Method of Feeding and Transmission of HIV-1 from Mothers to Children by 15 Months of Age: Prospective Cohort Study from Durban, South Africa. *AIDS-Official Journal of the International AIDS Society* 15 (3), 379-387.

Coutsoudis, A., Pillay, K., Spooner, E., Kuhn, L., Coovadiaa, H. & the South African Vitamin A Study Group (1999). Influence of Infant-Feeding Patterns on Early Mother-to-Child Transmission of HIV-1 in Durban, South Africa: A Prospective Cohort Study. *The Lancet*, 354 (9177), 471-476.

Crush, J., Williams, V. & Peberdy, S. (2005). *Migration in Southern Africa*. Geneva: The Global Commission on International Migration.

Cutting, W. A. M. (1992). Breast Feeding and HIV Infection: Advice Depends on the Circumstances. *British Medical Journal* (305), 788-789.

Davis-Floyd, R. E. & Sargent, C. F. (Eds.) (1997). *Childbirth and Authoritative Knowledge: Cross-Cultural Perspectives.* Berkeley: University of California Press.

Desclaux, A. & Alfieri, C. (2009). Counseling and Choosing Between Infant-Feeding Options: Overall Limits and Local Interpretations by Health Care Providers and Women Living with HIV in Resource-poor Countries (Burkina Faso, Cambodia, Cameroon). In: A. Desclaux, P. Msellati & S. Walentowitz (Eds.), *Women, Mothers and HIV Care in Resource Poor Settings.* 821-829.

Desclaux, A. & Alfieri, C. (2011). Facing Competing Cultures of Breastfeeding. In: P. Liamputtong (Ed.). *Infant Feeding Practices: A Cross-Cultural Perspective.* New York, NY: Springer Science+Business Media LLC. 195-210.

Desclaux, A., & Taverne, B. (Eds.) (2000). *Allaitement et VIH en Afrique de l'Ouest: De l'anthropologie à la Santé publique.* Paris: Karthala.

Desclaux, A., Msellati, P. & Walentowitz, S. (Eds.) (2009). Women, Mothers and HIV Care in Resource Poor Settings. *Special Issue Social Science & Medicine* 69 (6).

Dettwyler, K. A. (1988). More than Nutrition: Breastfeeding in Urban Mali. *Medical Anthropology Quarterly* 2 (2), 172-183.

Dettwyler, K. A. (1995). A Time to Wean: The Hominid Blueprint for the Natural Age of Weaning in Modern Human Populations. In: P. Stuart-Macadam & K. A. Dettwyler (Eds.), *Evolutionary Foundations of Human Behavior. Breastfeeding. Biocultural Perspectives*, New York: Aldine de Gruyter, 39-74.

Dilger, H. & Hadolt, B. (2010). *Medizin im Kontext. Krankheit und Gesundheit in einer vernetzten Welt*. Frankfurt am Peter Lang.

Dilger, H. (2005). *Leben mit Aids: Krankheit, Tod und soziale Beziehungen in Afrika; eine Ethnographie*. Freie Universität, Diss.-Berlin, 2004. Frankfurt am Main: Campus.

Dilger, H. (2010). 'My Relatives are Running Away from Me!': Kinship and Care in the Wake of Structural Adjustment, Privatisation and HIV/AIDS in Tanzania. In: H. Dilger & U. Luig (Eds.), *Morality, Hope and Grief. Anthropologies of AIDS in Africa.*, New York: Berghahn Books, 102-126.

Douglas, M. (1994). *Purity and Danger: An Analysis of the Concepts of Pollution and Taboo*. London: Routledge.

Du Plessis, G. (2003). *HIV/AIDS and Fertility*. In: Department of Social Development. Fertility. Cape Town: Chicago, IL: Distributed worldwide except Africa by Independent Publishers Group: HSRC Publishers, 77-116.

Easterlin, R. A. & Crimmins, E. M. (1985). *The Fertility Revolution*. Chicago: University of Chicago Press.

Eckert, J. M. (2004). Einleitung: Gewalt, Meidung und Verfahren: zur Konflikttheorie Georg Elwerts. In: J. M. Eckert (Ed.), *Kultur und soziale Praxis. Anthropologie der Konflikte. Georg Elwerts konflikttheoretische Thesen in der Diskussion.*, Bielefeld: transcript-Verlag, 7-25.

Einarsdóttir, J. (2005). Restoration of Social Order through the Extinction of Non-human Children. In: R. Jenkins, V. Steffen, & H. Jessen (Eds.), *Managing Uncertainty. Ethnographic Studies of Illness, Risk and the Struggle for Control*. Copenhagen: Museum Tusculanum Press, 31-52.

Elwert, G. (2004). Anthropologische Perspektiven auf Konflikt. In: J. M. Eckert (Ed.), *Kultur und soziale Praxis. Anthropologie der Konflikte. Georg Elwerts konflikttheoretische Thesen in der Diskussion*. Bielefeld: transcript-Verlag, 26-38.

Elwert, G. (Ed.) (1999). *Beihefte/Supplements to Sociologus: Dynamics of Violence: Processes of Escalation and De-escalation in Violent Group Conflicts*. Berlin: Duncker & Humblot.

Erdheim, M. (1984). *Die gesellschaftliche Produktion von Unbewußtheit: Eine Einführung in den ethnopsychoanalytischen Prozeß*. Frankfurt am Main: Suhrkamp.

Erny, P. (1981). *The Child and his Environment in Black Africa: An Essay on Traditional Education*. Nairobi: Oxford University Press.

Evans-Pritchard, E. E. & Gillies, E. (1978). *Hexerei, Orakel und Magie bei den Zande*. Frankfurt Main: Suhrkamp.

Farmer, P. (2005). *Pathologies of Power: Health, Human Rights, and the New War on the Poor*. Berkeley: University of California Press.

Farmer, P. (1996). On Suffering and Structural Violence: A View from Below. *Daedalus* 125 (1), 261-283.

Feierman, S. & Janzen, J. M. (Eds.) (1992). *The Social Basis of Health and Healing in Africa*. Berkeley: University of California Press.

Ferguson, J. (1999). *Expectations of Modernity. Myths and Meanings of urban Life on the Zambian Copperbelt*. Berkeley and others: University of California Press.

Fjeld, E., Siziya, S., Katepa-Bwalya, M., Kankasa, C., Moland K., Tylleskär, T., et al. (2008). 'No Sister, the Breast Alone is not enough for my Baby': A Qualitative Assessment of Potentials and Barriers in the Promotion of Exclusive Breastfeeding in Southern Zambia. *International Breastfeeding Journal* (3), Retrieved March 25, 2015 from http://www.internationalbreastfeedingjournal.com/content/pdf/1746-4358-3-26.pdf.

Föllmer, W. (1983). Besonderheiten der Geburtshilfe in Libyen. In: W. Schiefenhövel & D. Sich (Eds.), *Die Geburt aus ethnomedizinischer Sicht*. IV. Internationale Fachtagung der AG Ethnomedizin über traditionelle Geburtshilfe und Gynäkologie. Braunschweig und Wiesbaden: Vieweg Verlag, 225-228.

Food and Agricultural Organization of the United Nations (2010). *Country Profile: Lesotho: Food Security Indicators*. Retrieved March 1, 2015 from http://www.fao.org/fileadmin/templates/ess/documents/food_security_statistics/country_profiles/eng/Lesotho_E.pdf.

Foster, G. (1998). Today's Children-Challenges to Child Health Promotion in Countries with Severe AIDS Epidemics. *AIDS care* 10 (2), 17-23.

Foster, G., Levine, C. & Williamson, J. (2005). *A Generation at Risk: The Global Impact of HIV/AIDS on Orphans and Vulnerable Children.* Cambridge, New York: Cambridge University Press.

Foucault, M. (1973). *Die Geburt der Klinik: Eine Archäologie des ärztlichen Blicks.* München.

Foucault, M. (1991). *Überwachen und Strafen: Die Geburt des Gefängnisses* (9. Aufl.). Suhrkamp-Taschenbuch Wissenschaft, (184), Frankfurt am Main: Suhrkamp.

Frey, W. H. & Zimmer, Z. (2001). Defining the City. In: R. Paddison (Ed.) *Handbook of Urban Studies*. London: Thousand Oaks, Calif.: Sage, 14-35.

Friebertshäuser, B. (1996). Feldforschende Zugänge zu sozialen Handlungsfeldern: Möglichkeiten und Grenzen ethnographischer Feldforschung. *Neue Praxis* (1), 75-86.

Gausset, Q. (1998). The Changing Meaning of Disease Among the Tonga of Zambia. *Paideusis – Journal for Interdisciplinary and Cross-Cultural Studies* (1), 43-52.

Gausset, Q. (2002). The Cognitive Rationality of Taboos on Production and Reproduction. *Africa* (4), 628-654.

Gausset, Q. & Mogensen, H. (1996). Sida et Pollutions sexuelles chez les Tonga de Zambie. *Cahiers d'Études Africaines* 36 (143), 455-476.

Gay, J. S. (1980). *Basotho Women's Options: A Study of Marital Careers in Rural Lesotho*. Unpublished PhD Thesis. Cambridge.

Geest, S. v. d., Whyte, S. & Hardon, A. (1996). The Anthropology of Pharmaceuticals: A biographical Approach. *Annual Review of Anthropology* (25), 153-178.

Gennep, A.v., Schomburg, K. & Schomburg-Scherff, S. M. (2005). *Übergangsriten.* Frankfurt/Main: Campus-Verlag.

Gill, S. J. (1993). *A Short History of Lesotho: From the late Stone Age Until the 1993 Elections*. Morija: Morija Museum & Archieves.

Girtler, R. (2001). *Methoden der Feldforschung*, Wien: Böhlau.

Goffman, E. (1963). *Stigma: Notes on the Management of Spoiled Identity.* Englewood Cliffs: Prentice-Hall.

Goffman, E. & Weber-Schäfer, P. (2009 [1959]). *Wir alle spielen Theater*. München [u.a.]: Piper.

Gottlieb, D., Shetty, A. K., Mapfungautsi, R. M., Bassett, M. T., Maldonado, Y. & Katzenstein, D. A. (2004). Infant Feeding Practice of HIV-infected and Uninfected Women in Zimbabwe. *AIDS Patient Care and STDs* 18 (1), 45-53.

Government of Lesotho (2000). *National AIDS Strategic Plan 2000/2001-2003/2004.* Maseru, Retrieved March 2, 2015 from http://www.ilo.org/wcmsp5/groups/public/---ed_protect/---protrav/---ilo_aids/documents/legaldocument/wcms_126750.pdf.

Government of Lesotho (2004). *Guidelines to Prevent Mother to Child Transmission of HIV.* Maseru.

Government of Lesotho (2007). *Coordination Framework for the National Response to HIV and AIDS.* Maseru.

Government of Lesotho (2009). *National Guidelines for the Prevention of Mother to Child Transmission of HIV.* Maseru.

Government of Lesotho & National AIDS Commission (2009). *Report of the Mid-Term Review of the National HIV and AIDS Strategic Plan 2006 - 2011.* Maseru. Retrieved March 1, 2015, from http://hivhealthclearinghouse.unesco.org/sites/default/files/resources/iiep_lesotho_review_2009.pdf

Government of Lesotho & World Bank (2009). *Lesotho - HIV Prevention Response and Modes of Transmission Analysis*. Washington, DC: World Bank, Retrieved March 2, 2015 from http://documents.worldbank.org/curated/en/2009/03/10592758/lesotho-hiv-prevention-response-modes-transmission-analysis.

Green, E. (1985). Traditional Healers, Mothers and Childhood Diarrheal Disease in Swaziland: The Interface of Anthropology and Health Education. *Social Science & Medicine* 20 (3), 277-285.

Greifeld, K. (2003). *Ritual und Heilung*. Berlin: Reimer.

Griffiths, A. (1990). *Negotiating Pregnancy: Women's Strategies Concerning Marriage and Compensation Among the Kwena in Botswana.* Edinburgh: Centre of African Studies.

Gronemeyer, R. (2006a). *So stirbt man in Afrika an AIDS: Warum westliche Gesundheitskonzepte im südlichen Afrika scheitern; eine Streitschrift.* Frankfurt am Main: Brandes & Apsel.

Gronemeyer, R. (2006b). Über HIV/AIDS und Modernisierung im südlichen Afrika. In: M. Drescher & S. Kläger (Eds.), *Kommunikation über HIV/Aids. Interdisziplinäre Beiträge zur Prävention im subsaharischen Afrika.* Berlin: LIT, 237-260.

Guz D. & Hobcraft J. (1991). Breastfeeding and Fertility: A Comparative Analysis. Population Studies 45 (1), 91-108.

Häberlein, T. (2007). Das abgewandte Gesicht. *Zeitschrift für Ethnologie.* 132 (2), 287-314.

Halfmann, D. (2011). Recognizing Medicalization and Demedicalization: Discourses, Practices, and Identities. *Health: An Interdisciplinary Journal for the Social Study of Health, Illness and Medicine* (3), 1-22.

Hall, D. & Malahleha, G. (1989). *Health and Family Planning Services in Lesotho: The People's Perspective.* Morija: Morija Printing Works.

Hannerz, U. (1980). *Exploring the City Inquiries toward an Urban Anthropology*. New York and others: Columbia University Press.

Haram, L. (2004). 'Prostitutes' or Modern Women? Negotiating Respectability in Northern Tanzania. In: S. Arnfred, *Re-thinking Sexualities in Africa*. Uppsala, Sweden: Nordiska Afrikainstitutet, 211-229.

Haram, L. & Yamba, B. (2004). Visiting the Issue of Uncertainty in Contemporary African Lives: An Introduction. *African Sociological Review* (8), 1-10.

Hartge, R. (1983). Zur Geburtshilfe und Säuglingsfürsorge im Spiegel der Geschichte Afrikas. In: W. Schiefenhövel & D. Sich (Eds.), *Die Geburt aus ethnomedizinischer Sicht. IV. Internationale Fachtagung der AG Ethnomedizin über traditionelle Geburtshilfe und Gynäkologie.* Braunschweig und Wiesbaden: Vieweg Verlag, 95-108.

Hausmann R., Tyson L. D. & Zahidi, S. (2010). *The Global Gender Gap Report 2010.* Geneva: The World Economic Forum. Retrieved March 1, 2015 from http://www.weforum.org/reports/global-gender-gap-report-2010.

Hazam, N. L. (1983). *The Pursuit of Health in Lesotho: Changing Perceptions of Illness and Healing in an African Country.* Dissertation. Dallas, Texas.

Heap, M. (1989). *Health and Disease in South-eastern Lesotho: A Social Anthropological Perspective of two Villages.* Cape Town: Centre for African Studies University of Cape Town.

Helman, C. G. (2007). *Culture, Health and Illness*. London: Hodder Arnold.

Hirschman, A. O. (1974). *Abwanderung und Widerspruch. Reaktionen auf Leistungsabfall bei Unternehmungen, Organisationen und Staaten.* Tübingen: J.C.B. Mohr.

Hirschman, A. O. (2010). Abwanderung und Widerspruch. In: S. Neckel (Ed.): *Sternstunden der Soziologie. Wegweisende Theoriemodelle des soziologischen Denkens*. Frankfurt am Main and others: Campus, 204-225.

Hobsbawm, E. J. (1962). *Sozialrebellen: archaische Sozialbewegungen im 19. und 20. Jahrhundert.* Neuwied: Luchterhand.

Horstmann, S. (2006). Bearbeitung traditioneller Wissensbestände in Ausbildungskursen für Peer Educators. In: M. Drescher & S. Kläger (Eds.), *Kommunikation über HIV/Aids. Interdisziplinäre Beiträge zur Prävention im subsaharischen Afrika.* Berlin: LIT, 93-116.

Hughes, N. & Stewart, D. (1983). Curanderismo in Taos County, New Mexico – A possible Case of Anthropological Romanticism? *Western Journal of Medicine* 139 (6), 875-884.

Illich, I. (1977). *Die Nemesis der Medizin: Von den Grenzen des Gesundheitswesens.* Reinbek bei Hamburg: Rowohlt.

ILO-International Labour Office (n.d.). Decent Work Country Programme Lesotho 2006 to 2009. n.p. Retrieved October, 19 2010 from http://www.ilo.org/public/english/bureau/program/dwcp/download/lesotho.pdf.

Inhetveen, K. (2006). *Flucht als Politik*. Köln: Köppe.

International Center for AIDS Care and Treatment Programs (2009). *Prevention of Mother-to-Child Transmission: Mafeteng Hospital*. (u.d.), Mafeteng.

International Organisation for Migration (n.d. [2006]). *Briefing Note on HIV and labour migration in Lesotho*. Pretoria. South Africa, Retrieved September, 12 2010 from http://www.iom.int/jahia/webdav/site/myjahiasite/shared/shared/mainsite/events/docs/Briefing_Notes_HIV_Lesotho.pdf.

Jacoby, A. (1994). Felt Versus Enacted Stigma: A Concept Revisited: Evidence from a Study of People with Epilepsy in Remission. *Social Science & Medicine* 38 (2), 269-274.

Janzen, J. (1978). *The Quest for Therapy: Medical Pluralism in Lower Zaire.* Berkeley and others, University of California Press.

Jenkins, R., Steffen, V. & Jessen, H. (Eds.) (2005). *Managing Uncertainty: Ethnographic Studies of Illness, Risk and the Struggle for Control.* Copenhagen: Museum Tusculanum Press.

Jordan, B. (1997). Authoritative Knowledge and its Construction. In: R. E. Davis-Floyd & C. F. Sargent (Eds.), *Childbirth and authoritative Know-ledge: Cross-cultural Perspectives.* Berkeley: University of California Press, 55-79.

Jordan, B. & Davis-Floyd, R. (1993). *Birth in Four Cultures: A Crosscultural Investigation of Childbirth in Yucatan, Holland, Sweden, and the United States.* Prospect Heights, Ill: Waveland Press.

Kalabamu, F., Mapetla, M. & Schlyter, A. (Eds.) (2005). *Gender, Generation and Urban Living Conditions in Southern Africa.* Roma Lesotho: Institute of Southern African Studies National University of Lesotho.

Kaufman, C. E. (2000). *Adolescent Pregnancy and Parenthood in South Africa. Policy Research Division Working Papers.* New York: Population Council.

Kimane, I. & Ntimo-Makara, M. (1998). The Gender Dimension of urban Migration in Lesotho. In: A. Larsson (Ed.), *Changing Gender Relations in Southern Africa. Issues of urban Life.* Roma: Institute of Southern African Studies.

Kipp, W. (2007). AIDS-related Stigma. *World Health and Population* 9 (2), 5-13.

Kisanga, P. (2000). *Protection, Support, and Promotion of Breastfeeding in HIV: Policy Guidelines by IBFAN Africa.* Mbabane Swaziland: IBFAN Africa.

Kleinman, A. (2003). *Patients and Healers in the Context of Culture: An Exploration of the Borderland Between Anthropology, Medicine, and Psychiatry.* 8 (3), Berkeley: University of California Press.

Kneuper, E. (2003). Die "natürliche Geburt": Eine globale Errungenschaft? In: A. Wolf & V. Hörbst (Eds.), *Medizin und Globalisierung. Universelle Ansprüche, lokale Antworten.* Münster: LIT, 107-128.

Krings-Ney, B. & Kotanyi, S. (2009). Introduction of Culturally Sensitive HIV Prevention in the Context of Female Initiation Rites: An Applied Anthropological Approach in Mozambique. *African Journal of AIDS Research* 8 (4), 491-502.

Kroeker, L. (2011). Lesotho's Performance in the Global Gender Gap Index 2010: Conflicts Over Resources and Roles of the Female Breadwinner. In: A. Daniel, K. Fink, L. Kroeker, & J. Schütze (Eds.), *Women's Life Worlds 'In-Between'. Journal of the Bayreuth International Graduate School of African Studies (BIGSAS).* Bayreuth, 80-100.

Kroeker, L. & Beckwith A. (2011). Safe Infant Feeding in Lesotho in the Era of HIV/AIDS. In: B. P. Brenton, J. Mazzeo, A. Rödlach, S. Kedia & D. Himmelgreen (Eds.), *HIV/AIDS and Food Insecurity in Sub-Saharan Africa.* Hoboken, NJ: Wiley-Blackwell, 50-66.

Kroeker, L. (2014). Meidung als Alltagshandlung in langfristigen Abhängigkeitsbeziehungen - Schwangere Frauen mit HIV/AIDS und ihre Kommunikation in asymmetrischen Machtverhältnissen. *Zeitschrift für Ethnologie* 139, 179-198.

Kroeker, L. (forthcoming) Low Fertility and Secret Family Planning in Lesotho, In: A. Bochow & P. Kraeger, *Fertility in Subpopulation*, Berghahn.

Kroeker, L. (forthcoming a) *Ich war wie eine Schlafwandlering, Die Situation von HIV-Infizierten in Bamako (Mali) im sozialen und kulturellen Umfeld aus Sicht der Betroffenen*. Magisterarbeit, J.W.Goethe Universität Frankfurt/M.

Kücholl, V. (1985). *Ethnomedical Evaluation in Lesotho 1984-1985: Final report.* Thaba-Tseka: Paray Hospital.

Kukla, R. (2006). Ethics and Ideology in Breastfeeding Campaigns. *Hypatia* 21 (1), 157-180.

Kuntner, L. (1983). Die Gebärhaltung der Frau. In: W. Schiefenhövel & D. Sich (Eds.), *Die Geburt aus ethnomedizinischer Sicht.* IV. Internationale Fachtagung der AG Ethnomedizin über traditionelle Geburtshilfe und Gynäkologie. Braunschweig und Wiesbaden: Vieweg Verlag, 81-92.

Kuntner, L. (1985). *Die Gebärhaltung der Frau: Schwangerschaft u. Geburt aus geschichtlicher, völkerkundlicher und medizinischer Sicht.* München: Marseille.

Kuntner, L. (1995). Geburtshilfe ausserhalb des Krankenhauses in traditionellen Gesellschaften. In: W. Schiefenhövel, D. Sich & C. E. Gottschalk-Batschkus (Eds.), *Gebären. Ethnomedizinische Perspektiven und neue Wege.* Berlin: Verlag für Wissenschaft und Bildung, 127-138.

Kuntner, L. (2004). Zum Umgang mit der Nachgeburt: Planzentabestattung im Kulturvergleich. *Curare* 27 (3), 279-293.

Kuper, H. (1950). Kinship among the Swazi. In: A. R. Radcliffe-Brown & C. D. Forde (Eds.), *African Systems of Kinship and Marriage*. London/New York: Oxford University Press, 87-110.

Labouvie, E. (1999). *Beistand in Kindsnöten: Hebammen und weibliche Kultur auf dem Land (1550-1910).* Universität Saarbrücken, Habil.1997. Frankfurt am Main: Campus-Verlag.

Larsson, A., Mapetla, M. & Schlyter, A. (Eds.) (1998). *Changing Gender Relations in Southern Africa: Issues of Urban Life.* Roma: Institute of Southern African Studies.

Latour, B. (1986). The Powers of Association In: J. Law (Ed.), *Power, Action and Belief.* London: Routledge & Paul, 264-280.

Lazarus, E. (1997). What do Women Want?: Issues of Choice, Control, and Class in American Pregnancy and Childbirth. In: R. E. Davis-Floyd & C. F. Sargent (Eds.), *Childbirth and Authoritative Knowledge: Cross-cultural Perspectives.* Berkeley: University of California Press, 132-158.

Ledermann, S. A. (1992). Estimating Infant Mortality from Human Immunodeficiency Virus and other Causes in Breast-Feeding and Bottle-Feeding Populations. *Acta Pædiatrica* 98 (2), 290-296.

Leshabari S., Blystad A., de Paoli M. & Moland K. (2007a). HIV and Infant Feeding Counselling: Challenges Faced by Nurse-Counsellors in Northern Tanzania. *Human Resources for Health* 18 (5).

Leshabari S. C., Blystad A. & Moland, K. M. (2007b). Difficult Choice: Infant Feeding Decisions Among HIV-positive Mothers in Northern Tanzania. *SAHARA Journal* (4), 544-555.

Liamputtong, P. (2011). Infant Feeding Beliefs and Practices Across Cultures: An Introduction. In: P. Liamputtong. (Ed.) (2011). *Infant Feeding Practices: A Cross-cultural Perspective.* New York, NY: Springer Science+Business Media LLC, 1-20.

Lipp, W. (1975). Selbststigmatisierung. In: M. Brusten & J. Hohmeier (Eds.), *Stigmatisierung I. Zur Produktion gesellschaftlicher Randgruppen.* Darmstadt: Luchterhand Verlag GmbH, 5-53.

Loimeier, R., Neubert, D. & Weißköppel, C. (2005). Einleitung: Globalisierung im lokalen Kontext - Perspektiven und Konzepte von Handeln in Afrika. In: R. Loimeier, D. Neubert & C. Weißköppel (Eds.): *Globalisierung im lokalen Kontext – Perspektiven und Konzepte von Handeln in Afrika.* Münster: LIT, 1-30.

Long, D., Hunter, C. & Geest, v. d. S. (2008). When the Field is Ward or a Clinic: Hospital Ethnography. *Anthropology & Medicine* 15 (2), 71-78.

Lucas, D. (1992). Fertility and Family Planning in Southern and Central Africa. *Studies in Family Planning* 23 (3), 145-158.

Lucius-Hoene, G. & Deppermann, A. (2002). *Rekonstruktion narrativer Identität: Ein Arbeitsbuch zur Analyse narrativer Interviews.* Lehrtexte Soziologie. Opladen: Leske + Budrich.

Luhmann, N. (1990). Familiarity, Confidence, Trust: Problems and Alternatives. In: D. Gambetta (Ed.), *Trust. Making and Breaking Cooperative Relations.* Oxford: Blackwell Publishers, 94-107.

Macamo, E. (unpublished, 2009). *The Taming of Fate: Approaching Risk from a Social Action Perspective*. Habil. University of Bayreuth.

Mafeteng Government Hospital (1993). *Mafeteng Government Hospital: Annual Report 1993*, (unpublished document). Mafeteng.

Mafeteng Government Hospital (2008). *ARV Defaulters Follow-up Report done from 18th-22nd February 2008*, (unpublished document). Mafeteng.

Maher, V. (1992). *The Anthropology of Breast-Feeding: Natural Law or Social Construct. Cross-cultural Perspectives on Women.* Oxford: Berg.

Mapetla, M. M. T. (2005). Perspectives on Living Conditions of Women Factory Workers in Ha Tetsane, Lesotho. In: F. Kalabamu, M. Mapetla & A. Schlyter (Eds.), *Gender, Generation and Urban Living Conditions in Southern Africa.* Roma Lesotho: Institute of Southern African Studies National University of Lesotho. 131-152.

Mapetla, N. & Moultrie T. A. (2011). *Fertility and Women's Labour Force Participation in Lesotho.* 6th African Population Conference: African Population: Past, Present, and Future, Ouagadougou 5-9 Dec. 2011. Retrieved March 1, 2015 from http://uaps2011.princeton.edu/papers/110714.

Maqutu, W. C. M. (2005). *Contemporary Family Law: The Lesotho Position.* Roma Lesotho: National University of Lesotho Pub. House.

Matete-Lieb, T. (1997). Frauen und Räume: Geschlechtsspezifische Auswirkungen von Tradition und Gesetz in Lesotho. *Frauen in der einen Welt – Zeitschrift für interkulturelle Frauenalltagsforschung* (2), 64-76.

Mauss, M. (1968). *Die Gabe: Form und Funktion des Austauschs in archaischen Gesellschaften.* Frankfurt am Main: Suhrkamp.

Ministry of Health and Social Welfare (2004). *HIV Testing and Counselling 2004.* Training guide, Maseru.

Ministry of Health and Social Welfare & ICF Macro. (2010). *Lesotho Demographic and Health Survey 2009.* Maseru.

Ministry of Health and Social Welfare, & National AIDS Commission (2009). *National HIV and AIDS Estimates for Lesotho 2009.* Maseru.

Ministry of Health and Social Welfare, B. o. S. a. O. M. (2005). *Lesotho Demographic and Health Survey 2004.* Maseru.

Mogensen, H. (2010). New Hopes and New Dilemmas: Disclosure and Recognition in the Time of Antiretroviral Treatment. In: H. Dilger & U. Luig (Eds.), *Morality, Hope and Grief. Anthropologies of AIDS in Africa*. New York: Berghahn Books. 61-79.

Moland, K. M. (2004). Mother's Milk: An Ambiguous Blessing in the Era of AIDS: The Case of the Chagga in Kilimanjaro. *African Sociological Review* 8 (1), 83-99.

Morgan, D. L. (1997). *Focus Groups as Qualitative Research.* Thousand Oaks, Calif.: Sage Publ.

Morija (1998) *English-Sotho Sotho-English Pocket Dictionary*. Morija Sesuto Book Depot: Morija-Lesotho.

Motsoeli, N. (2009). *Rape Victims Suffer in Silence.* Lesotho Times, October 8, 2009. Retrieved March 1, 2015 from http://www.lestimes.com/?p=2357.

Mturi, A. J. & Moerane, W. (2001). Premarital Childbearing among Adolescents in Lesotho. *Journal of Southern African Studies* 27 (2), 259-275.

Muzvidziwa, V. N. (2003). *Gender and Urban Housing in Mafeteng District: Life Experiences of Basotho Women Tenants.* Roma, Lesotho: Institute of Southern African Studies, National University of Lesotho.

Mvududu, S. C. (2002). *Lobola: Its Implications for Women's Reproductive Rights in Botswana, Lesotho, Malawi, Mozambique, Swaziland, Zambia, and Zimbabwe.* Harare, Zimbabwe: Weaver.

Ng'andwe, T. (2007). Diet of Breast Milk Alone Reduces HIV Transmission. *SciDevNet* 30 (3). Retrieved March 1, 2015 from http://www.scidev.net/en/news/diet-of-breast-milk-alone-reduces-hiv-transmission.html.

Ngubane, H. (1976). Some Notions of 'Purity' and 'Impurity' Among the Zulu. *Africa* 46 (3), 274-284.

Ngubane, H. (1992). Clinical Practice and Organization of Indigenous Healers in South Africa. In: S. Feierman & J. M. Janzen (Eds.), *The Social Basis of Health and Healing in Africa.* Berkeley: University of California Press, 366-375.

Nguyen, V. K. (2005). Antiretroviral Globalism, Biopolitics, and Therapeutic Citizenship. In: A.-h. Ong & S. J. Collier (Eds.), *Global Assemblages. Technology, Politics, and Ethics as Anthropological Problems.* Malden, MA: Blackwell Publishing, 124-144.

Nguyen, V. K. & Peschard, K. (2003). Anthropology, Inequality, and Disease: A Review. *Annual Review of Anthropology* (32), 447-474.

Nguyen, V. K. (2010). *The Republic of Therapy: Triage and Sovereignty in West Africa's Time of AIDS. Body, Commodity, Text.* Durham, NC: Duke University Press.

Nolen, S., Dürr, K., Peschel, U. & Ströle, W. (2007). *28 Stories über Aids in Afrika.* München: Piper.

Ntimo-Makara, M. & Makara- Khatleli, N. (2005). Gender and Administrative Conflicts over Land in Peri-urban Areas in Maseru, Lesotho. In: F. Kalabamu, M. Mapela & A. Schlyter (Ed.), *Gender, Generation and Urban Living Conditions in Southern Africa.* Roma Lesotho: Institute of Southern African Studies National University of Lesotho, 195-217.

Nyanguru, A. C. (2005). Elderly Women as Caregivers to Relatives Affected by HIV/AIDS in Urban Lesotho. In: F. Kalabamu, M. Mapetla & A. Schlyter (Eds.), *Gender, Generation and urban Living Conditions in southern Africa.* Roma Lesotho: Institute of Southern African Studies National University of Lesotho, 219-236.

Nzioka, C. (2003). *A Baseline Study on the Magnitude of Abortion Among Women of Child-bearing Age in Lesotho.* Maseru.

Ochs, E. & Capps, L. (2001). *Living Narrative: Creating Lives in Everyday Storytelling.* Cambridge, Mass.: Harvard University Press.

Parsons, T. (1964). *The Social System.* New York: Free Press of Glencoe.

Paslack, R. (1999). Technikfolgenabschätzung in der Medizin. In: S. Bröchler, G. Simonis & K. Sundermann (Eds.), *Handbuch Technikfolgenabschätzung*, Rainer Bohn Verlag: Berlin, 837-856.

Peltzer, K. (2007). Barriers to Prevention of HIV Transmission from Mother to Child (PMTCT) in a Resource Poor Setting in the Eastern Cape, South Africa. *African Journal of Reproductive Health* 11(1), 57-66.

Peltzer, K., Chao, L.-W. & Dana, P. (2009a). Family Planning among HIV-positive and negative: Prevention of Mother to Child Transmission (PMTCT) Clients in a Resource Poor Setting in South Africa. *AIDS and Bahavior* (13), 973-979.

Peltzer, K., Phaswana-Mafuya, N. & Treger, L. (2009b). Use of Traditional and Complementary Health Practices in Prenatal, Delivery and Postnatal Care in the Context of HIV-Transmission from Mother to Child (PMTCT) in the Eastern Cape, South Africa. *African Journal of Traditional, Complementary and Alternative Medicines* 6 (2), 155-162.

Peltzer, K., Ladzani, R., Mlambo, M., Majaja, M., Phaweni, K., Matseke, G., Shikwane, E. & Majaja, M. (2010). *Implementing a Rural Programme of Prevention of Mother-to-Child Transmission of HIV Nkangala South Africa: A Baseline Evaluation.* Pretoria. Retrieved March 1, 2015 from http://www.hsrc.ac.za/en/research-outputs/view/5195.

Phaswana-Mafuya, N. (2008). Obstacles in Executing Prevention Plans for HIV Birth Infections. *Human Sciences Research Council Review* 6 (3).

Piwoz, E. G. (2005). Women's Voices, Women's Choices: The Challenge of Nutrition and HIV/AIDS. *JN – The Journal of Nutrition* (135), 933-937.

Preston-Whyte, E. & Zondi, M. (1989) To Control their Own Reproduction: The Agenda of Black Teenage Mothers in Durban. *Agenda* 4, 47-68.

Quandt, S. (1995). Sociocultural Aspects of the Lactation Process. In: P. Stuart-Macadam & K. A. Dettwyler (Eds.), *Evolutionary Founda-*

tions of Human Behavior. Breastfeeding. Biocultural Perspectives. New York: Aldine de Gruyter. 127-144.

Rieck, C. (1993). *Spieltheorie. Einführung für Wirtschafts- und Sozialwissenschaftler*. Wiesbaden: Gabler Verlag.

Riemann, G. (2006). Erzählanalyse. In: R. Bohnsack, W. Marotzki & M. Meuser (Eds.) *Hauptbegriffe qualitativer Sozialforschung.* Opladen: Budrich. 45-48.

v. Rijn, K. (2006). The Politics of Uncertainty: The AIDS Debate, Thabo Mbeki and the South African Government Response. *Social History of Medicine* 19 (3), 521-538.

Riordan, J. & Auerbach, K. G. (1998). *Breastfeeding and Human Lactation.* Boston: Jones and Barlett.

Romero-Daza, N. & Himmelgreen, D. (2004). The Sotho. In: C. R. Ember (Ed.), *Encyclopedia of Medical Anthropology. Health and Illness in the World's Cultures.* New York, NY: Springer, 957-964.

Romero-Daza, N., Himmelgreen D. A., Noble, C. A. & Turkon, D. (2009). Dealing with the Global Food Crisis in Local Settings: Nonintensive Agriculture in Lesotho. Southern Africa. *NAPA Bulletin* (32), 23-41.

Rompel, M. (2003). *"It Will Really Knock on to Everybody's Door ...": Die sozialen Folgen der AIDS-Epidemie in Namibia: Eine Untersuchung in Katutura und Ovamboland.* Dissertation in Social- and Cultural Sciences. Giessen.

Rompel, M. (2006). Prevention is Like Telling People: Ey, Stop Loving: Ansätze und Problemfelder massenmedial vermittelter Aids-Prävention im südlichen Afrika. In: M. Drescher & S. Kläger (Eds.), *Kommunikation über HIV/Aids. Interdisziplinäre Beiträge zur Prävention im subsaharischen Afrika.* Berlin: LIT, 219-235.

Rosenberg, S., Weisfelder, R. F. & Frisbie-Fulton, M. (2004). *Historical Dictionary of Lesotho.* Lanham, Md: Scarecrow Press.

Rottenburg, R. (1996). When Organization Travels. On Intercultural Translation. In: B. Czarniawska-Joerges, G. Sevón & W. d. Gruyter (Eds.), *Translating Organizational Change.* Berlin/New York, 191-240.

Rottenburg, R. (2002). *Weit hergeholte Fakten: Eine Parabel der Entwicklungshilfe.* Stuttgart: Lucius & Lucius.

Rottenburg, R. (2009). *Far-fetched Facts. A Parable of Development Aid.* Cambridge: MIT Press.

Sachse, R., Fasbender, J. & Sachse, M. (2011). Die Bearbeitung von Vermeidung in der klärungsorientierten Psychotherapie. In: R. Sachse, J. Fasbender, J. Breil & M. Sachse (Eds.), P*erspektiven klärungsorientierter Psychotherapie II.* Lengerich: Pabst, 156-183.

Sargent, C. F. (1982). *Factors Influencing Women's Choices of Obstetrical Care in a Northern District in the People's Republik of Benin.* University East Lansing (Mich.), Diss., 1979: University East Lansing.

Sargent, C. F. (1989). Maternity, Medicine, and Power: Reproductive Decisions in Urban Benin. *Comparative Studies of Health Systems and medical Care,* 22. Berkeley, Calif.: University of California Press.

Sargent, C. F. & Bascope, G. (1997). Ways of Knowing About Birth in Three Cultures. In: R. E. Davis-Floyd & C. F. Sargent (Eds.), *Childbirth and Authoritative Knowledge: Cross-cultural Perspectives.* Berkeley: University of California Press. 183-208.

Schiefenhövel, W. (1983). Geburten bei den Eipo. In: W. Schiefenhövel & D. Sich (Eds.), *Die Geburt aus ethnomedizinischer Sicht. IV. Internationale Fachtagung der AG Ethnomedizin über traditionelle Geburtshilfe und Gynäkologie.* Braunschweig und Wiesbaden: Vieweg Verlag. 41-56.

Schiefenhövel, W. (2005). Die Vertikale als optimale Gebärhaltung. *Curare* (28), 67-74.

Scott, J. C. (1985). *Weapons of the Weak: Everyday Forms of Peasant Resistance.* New Haven: Yale University Press.

Scott, J. C. (1990). *Domination and the Arts of Resistance: Hidden Transcripts.* New Haven: Yale University Press.

Sechefo, J. M. (n.d. (Reprint 1900)). *Customs and Superstitions in Lesotho.* Roma, Lesotho.

Sich, D. (1983). Geburtshilfliche Pathologie im Schnittpunkt des traditionellen und modernen gebutshilflichen Systems in Korea. In: W. Schiefenhövel & D. Sich (Eds.), *Die Geburt aus ethnomedizinischer Sicht. IV. Internationale Fachtagung der AG Ethnomedizin über traditionelle Geburtshilfe und Gynäkologie.* Braunschweig und Wiesbaden: Vieweg Verlag. 21-40.

Silase, M. (n.d. [2001]). *Way Ahead with Social Studies: Textbook for Primary Education in Lesotho, Std.6,* Morija.

Silberschmidt, M. (2004). Masculinities, Sexuality and Socio-Economic Change in Rural and Urban East Africa. In: S. Arnfred (ed.), *Rethinking Sexualities in Africa.* Uppsala, Sweden: Nordiska Afrikainstitutet, 233-248.

Silberschmidt, M. & Rasch, V. (2001). Adolescent Girls, Illegal Abortions and 'Sugar-Daddies' in Dar es Salaam: Vulnerable Victims and Active Social Agents. *Social Science and Medicine* 52, 1815-1826.

Silverman, D. (1997). *Discourses of Counselling: HIV Counselling as Social Interaction.* London: Sage.

Simbayi, L. C., Kalichman, S., Strebel, A., Cloete, A., Henda, N. & Mqeketo, A. (2007). Internalized Stigma, Discrimination, and Depression among Men and Women Living with HIV/AIDS in Cape Town, South Africa. In: *Social Science & Medicine* (64), 1823-1831.

Singh, S., Darroch, J. E., Ashford, L. S. & Vlassoff, M. (2009). *Adding it up: The Costs and Benefits of Investing in Family Planning and Maternal and Newborn Health.* New York: Guttmacher Institute and United Nations Population Fund.

Spittler, G. (2001). Teilnehmende Beobachtung als Dichte Teilnahme. *Zeitschrift für Ethnologie* (126), 1-25.

Steffen, V. (2005). Challenging Control: Antabuse Medication in Denmark. In: R. Jenkins, V. Steffen, & H. Jessen (Eds.), *Managing Uncertainty. Ethnographic Studies of Illness, Risk and the Struggle for Control.* Copenhagen: Museum Tusculanum Press, 173-196.

Stuart-Macadam, P. & Dettwyler, K. A. (1995). *Breastfeeding: Biocultural Perspectives. Evolutionary Foundations of Human Behavior.* New York: Aldine de Gruyter.

Tavengwa, N. V., Piwoz E. G., Iliff, P. J., Moulton, L. H., Zunguza, C. D., Nathoo, K. J., Hargrove, J. W., ZVITAMBO Study Group &

Humphrey, J. H. (2007). Adoption of Safer Infant Feeding and Postpartum Sexual Practices and their Relationship to Maternal HIV Status and Risk Acquiring HIV in Zimbabwe. *Tropical Medicine and International Health* 12 (1), 97-106.

Teijlingen, E. R. v. (2000). *Midwifery and the Medicalization of Childbirth: Comparative Perspectives.* Huntington, NY: Nova Science Publishers.

Thairu, L., Pelto, G., Rollins, N., Bland, R. & Ntshangase, N. (2005). Sociocultural Influences on Infant Feeding Decisions Among HIV-infected Women in Rural Kwa-Zulu Natal, South Africa. *Maternal and Child Nutrition* (1), 2-10.

Thornton, A. C., Romanelli, F. & Collins, J. D. (2004). *Reproduction Decision Making for Couples affected by HIV: A Review of the Literature, Review – Reproduction Decision Making.* 2 (12), Retrieved October 20, 2010 from https://iasusa.org/sites/default/files/tam/12-2-61.pdf.

Timaeus, I. M. & Moultrie, T. A. (2008). On Postponement and Birth Intervals. *Population and Development Review*, 34 (3), 483-510.

Tomlinson, R. J. & Madjarov, A. (2002). Global Voices on HIV/AIDS. Pasteurised human Breastmilk should be considered. *BMJ* 324 (7344), 1034-5.

Tonwe-Gold B., Ekouevi D. K., Viho I., Amani-Bosse, C. & Toure, S. (2007). Antiretroviral Treatment and Prevention of Peripartum and Postnatal HIV Transmission in West Africa: Evaluation of a Two-tiered Approach. *Public Library of Science* 4 (8), 1362-1373.

Trevathan, W. R. (1997). An Evolutionary Perspective on Authoritative Knowledge About Birth. In: R. E. Davis-Floyd & C. F. Sargent (Eds.), *Childbirth and Authoritative Knowledge: Cross-cultural Perspectives*. Berkeley: University of California Press. 80-88.

Tuoane, M., Diamond, I. & Madise, N. (2003). Use of Family Planning in Lesotho. The Importance of Quality of Care and Access. *African Population Studies* 18 (2), 105-132.

Tuoane, M., Madise, N. J. & Diamond, I. (2004). Provision of Family Planning Services in Lesotho. *International Family Planning Perspectives* 30 (2), 77-86.

Turner, V. (2005). *Das Ritual: Struktur und Anti-Struktur*. Frankfurt am Main: Campus-Verlag.

UNAIDS (2010). *UNAIDS Report on the Global AIDS Epidemic 2010*. Joint United Nations Programme on HIV/AIDS.

Unesco (2005). *Literacy for Life. EFA Global Monitoring Report: Vol. 2006.* Paris.

Ungruhe, C. (2011). Migration, Marriage and Modernity: Motives, Impacts and Negotiations of Rural-Urban Circulation Amongst Young Women in Northern Ghana. In: A. Daniel, K. Fink, L. Kroeker & J. Schütze (Eds.), *Women's Life Worlds 'In-Between'. Journal of the Bayreuth International Graduate School of African Studies (BIGSAS)*. Bayreuth, 58-79.

United Nations - INSTRAW. (n.d.). *Remittances in Lesotho. Retrieved March 1, 2015* from http://www.un-instraw.org/index.php?option=com_content&id=331&lang=en&task=view&Itemid=449.

United Nations Children's Fund (UNICEF) (2007). *UNICEF Humanitarian Action Report 2007.* Geneva/New York.

United Nations Children's Fund (UNICEF) (n.d.). *The Baby-Friendly Hospital Initiative.* Retrieved March 1, 2015 from http://www.unicef.org/programme/breastfeeding/baby.htm.

UNINSTRAW & UNDP (2010). *Migration, Remittances and Gender-responsive local Development: The case of Lesotho*. Retrieved March 2, 2015 from http://www.queensu.ca/samp/sampresources/samppublications/sampreports/SAMP_Report1.pdf.

United Nations Programme on HIV/AIDS. (n.d.). *AIDSinfo Country Fact Sheets: Lesotho.* Retrieved March 1, 2015 from http://www.unaids.org.

United Nations-INSTRAW/UNDP (2010). *Migration, Remittances and Gender-Responsive Local Development: The Case of Lesotho.* Santo Domingo, New York, Maseru.

USAID (2006). *ISSUE BRIEF –- Adding Family Planning to PMTCT Sites Increases PMTCT Benefit.* Washington, DC.

Utas, M. (2005). West-African Warscapes: Victimcy, Girlfriending, Soldiering: tactic Agency in a Young Woman's Social Navigation of the Liberian War Zone. *Anthropological Quarterly* 78 (2), 403-430.

Vidal, L. (2000). Penser le Risque de Transmission: Transmission de la Mère à l'enfant et Allaitement. In: A. Desclaux & B. Taverne (Eds.), *Allaitement et VIH en Afrique de l'Ouest. De l'anthropologie à la Santé publique*. Paris: Karthala. 1-22.

Vigh, H. (2006). *Navigating Terrains of War: Youth and Soldiering in Guinea Bissau.* New York: Berghahn Books.

Vigh, H. (2009). Motion Squared: A Second Look at the Concept of Social Navigation. *Anthropological Theory* 9 (4), 419-438.

Wahlberg, A. (2009). Serious Disease as Kinds of Living. In: S. Bauer & A. Wahlberg (Eds.) *Contested Categories*. Farnham, England: Burlington, VT: Ashgate, 89-111.

Walker, C. (1990). Gender and the Development of the Migrant Labour System c. 1850-1930. In: C. Walker (Ed.) *Women and Gender in Southern Africa to 1945.* London: David Philip Publishers. 168-196.

Warren, C., Phafoli, S., Majara, B. & Tsukulu, T. (2008). *Extending Prevention of Mother-to-Child Transmission through Postpartum Family Planning in Lesotho.* Retrieved March 1, 2015 from https://www.k4health.org/sites/default/files/Extending%20 prevention%20of%20mother%20to%20child%20tranmssion.pdf

Whyte, S. R. (1997). *Questioning Misfortune: The Pragmatics of Uncertainty in Eastern Uganda.* Cambridge: Cambridge University Press.

Whyte, S. R. (2002). Materia Medica: Ideen und Substanzen in verflochtenen Welten. In: B. Hauser-Schäublin (Ed.). *Ethnologie der Globalisierung. Perspektiven kultureller Verflechtungen.* Berlin: Reimer, 31-46.

Whyte, S. R. (2005). *Going Home?: Belonging and Burial in the Era of AIDS.* Africa, 75(2), 154-172.

Whyte, S. R., Whyte, M. A. & Kyaddond, D. (2010). Health Workers Entangled: Confidentiality and Certification. In: H. Dilger & U. Luig (Eds.), *Morality, Hope and Grief. Anthropologies of AIDS in Africa.* New York: Berghahn Books, 80-101.

Whyte, S. R., Geest, S. v. d. & Hardon, A. (2002). *Social Lives of Medicines.* Cambridge: Cambridge University. Press.

Williams, C. (2006). Dilemmas in Fetal Medicine: Premature Application of Technology or Responding to Women's Choice? *Sociology of Health and Illness* 28 (1), 1-20.

Wolf, A. (2006). Das, was kommt, schlägt nicht die Trommel: Botschaften von Aids-Aufklärungsplakaten der postkolonialen Wendezeit in Malawi. In: M. Drescher & S. Kläger (Eds.), *Kommunikation über HIV/Aids. Interdisziplinäre Beiträge zur Prävention im subsaharischen Afrika.* Berlin: LIT, 117-154.

Wolf, A. (2010). Orphans' Ties: Belonging and Relatedness in Child-headed Households in Malawi. In: H. Dilger & U. Luig (Eds.) *Morality, Hope and Grief. Anthropologies of AIDS in Africa*, New York: Berghahn Books, 292-311.

Wolf, A. & Dilger, H. (2003). Universalismus versus lokale Besonderheiten. Medizin, Globalisierung und AIDS. In: T. Lux (Ed.), *Kulturelle Dimensionen der Medizin. Ethnomedizin - Medizinethnologie – Medical Anthropology*, Berlin (Reimer), 252-276.

Wolf, A. & Hörbst, V. (Eds.) (2003). *Medizin und Globalisierung. Universelle Ansprüche, lokale Antworten.* Münster (LIT).

Women Thrive Worldwide (2010). *How Women in Lesotho got the Right to own Property.* Retrieved March 1, 2015 from http://www.womenthrive.org/index.php?option=com_content&task=view&id=392&Itemid=121.

World Health Organization (2001). *Antenatal Care for HIV-infected Women:* Geneva.

World Health Organization (2003). *Nutrient Requirements forPeople Living with HIV/AIDS: Report of a Technical Consultation.*

World Health Organization, & United Nations Children's Fund (UNICEF). *Innocenti Declaration: On the Protection, Promotion and Support of Breastfeeding.* Meeting of Policy Makers "Breastfeeding in the 1990s: A Global Initiative", Florence, Italy, on 30 July - 1 August 1990.

World Health Organization, UNAIDS, UNFPA & Unicef (2010). *Guidelines on HIV and Infant Feeding. 2010. Principles and Recommendations for Infant Feeding in the Context of HIV and a Summary of Evidence*. World Health Organization: Geneva.

Yovsi, R. D. (2003). *Ethnotheories about Breastfeeding and Mother – Infant –Interaction: The Case of Sedentary Nso Farmers and Nomadic Fulani Pastorals with their Infants 3 – 6 months of Age in Mbven Sub Division of the Northwest Province of Cameroon*. Universität Osnabrück, Diss. 2002, Münster: LIT.

Zola, I. (1972). Medicine as an Institution of Social Control. *The Sociological Review* (20), 487-504.

Annex: List of Study Participants

No referring to table in Chapter 9	Alias	Key characteristics
1	Nnoe	aged 27, married with one child, secondary education; previously employed in the textile factory but currently unemployed; lives with husband, was tested HIV+ while pregnant with her first child; sees PMTCT as a chance to have a second child; baby delivered in hospital, exclusive breastfeeding.
2	Peli (Chapter 5.4)	aged 25, married with one child, primary education; unemployed and financially dependent on her husband who is working abroad and only comes home on weekends; she tested HIV+ earlier but denied the result to be true and refused to take treatment; she decided on traditional medication for herself but biomedical treatment for her baby. Baby delivered in hospital, mixed feeding.
3	Tharo (Chapter 9.2)	aged 26, married with two children, primary education; lives on her own, husband works abroad and only comes home on weekends; tested HIV+ earlier but denied the result to be true and refused treatment, delivered in a home delivery with her neighbour. Tharo passed away a few weeks after the baby is born.
4	Nne (Prologue and 5.1.6)	aged 23, single, no children, secondary education, employed as a maid; staying at her grandmother's but frequently changing residence to stay with her other grandmother who is a traditional healer; wanted to get married to the father of her child but negotiations failed; chose to exclusively breastfeed but cannot comply with her choice, since she had not disclosed her HIV status.

No referring to table in Chapter 9	Alias	Key characteristics
5	Hlano	aged 32, married with two children, secondary education; employed in the textile factory and living with her husband in town while the children are with relatives; decided on feeding with formula milk from the factory but mixed it with other nutriments. The baby turned out HIV+.
6	Tselela (Chapter 7.6)	aged 32, married with two children, primary education; unemployed and dependent on the husband's remittances; baby delivered in a home delivery and mixed fed.
7	Supa	aged 20, married with one HIV+ child, primary education, unemployed; lives in a house with her mother and 6 younger siblings, only source of income is from the sale of her mother's vegetables, husband sells handicrafts in another town, very poor living conditions; first child was mixed fed (malnutrition?) and opted for exclusive breastfeeding this time but unsure if it can be sustained due to malnutrition of the mother.
8	Robeli (Chapter 5.1.5)	aged 24, married, primary education, primagravida, unemployed and dependent on husband's remittances, living with husband who denied that HIV existed and refused to get tested or to allocate money for her check-ups and delivery. Robeli left the marriage for her parental home.
9	Robong	aged 22, primagravida, wanted to get married but negotiations failed, secondary education, living on her own while her mother is in labour migration; tried to inform her mother indirectly about her infection and asked a counsellor to step in to mediate.

No referring to table in Chapter 9	Alias	Key characteristics
10	Leshome (Chapter 7.5)	aged 36, with boyfriend in separate household, primagravida, secondary education, works in the textile factory and self-employed, peer educator for HIV awareness and hosts a support group for PLHIV; decided on a caesarean section and formula feeding.
11	LeMong	aged 36, widowed with two children from her marriage, now pregnant by her boyfriend, boyfriend in separate household, secondary education, working in a shop; opted for formula milk and delivered in the hospital. Her husband's death from AIDS urges her to adhere solely to PMTCT and her HAART treatment, whereas in the past she used traditional medication complementarily.
12	LeMeli	aged 27, married one child, secondary education, working in the textile factory; the husband is sick due to AIDS and in need of care; baby delivered in hospital; exclusive breastfeeding.
13	LeTharo (Chapter 6.5.1)	aged 29, married, but husband passes away due to a criminal attack while she is pregnant; tertiary education, LeTharo is a pastor and assumes witchcraft to be the reason for her unfortunate events during pregnancy and delivery, delivery by caesarean section after complications appeared during labour at home; opted for formula milk due to her breast milk being bewitched.
14	LeNne (Chapter 6.5)	aged 31, married with two children, primary education, unemployed but trained as peer educator for HIV awareness; staying with her sister in town to be closer to the hospital but decides then to deliver at the traditional clinic since she feared maltreatment from the nurses and had delivered twice at home before.

No referring to table in Chapter 9	Alias	Key characteristics
15	LeHlano	aged 24, married, primary education, working in a shop; delivery by caesarean section due to a STD; opted for short exclusive breastfeeding until she returned to work and exclusive formula feeding thereafter; believes that her first child passed away due to an undetected infection with AIDS.
16	LeTselela	aged 22, hoped to get married but negotiations failed, secondary education, works in the textile factory, lives on her own; delivered in the traditional clinic and decided on formula feeding. Her mother stays at her place after the delivery and looks after the baby as well as after another grandson. LeTselela brings formula milk from the factory which is used for both babies and LeTselela supplements with breast milk.
17	LeSupa	aged 22, student in secondary education, marriage negotiations failed, lives with her parents and her siblings. She fell pregnant aged 17 (crude birth) and again aged 22 before finishing school. Her father named the child "Thuto", meaning 'lecture'.
18	LeRobeli	aged 23, married, primagravida, works in a shop; tested HIV- in her 3rd month and HIV+ in her 6th month of gestation; discordant couple; staying in the waiting mother shelters after a rupture of membranes without labour pains. The child was stillborn days later. The medical records lack information on the progress of her delivery.
19	LeRobong (Chapter 4.7 and 9.4)	aged 23, married with one child, secondary education; stayed at in-laws' when working in the textile factory but moved to a single household to further education; husband is working abroad; she delivers in the hospital and feeds formula milk. The baby passes away aged three months presumably of a witchcraft disease ("pulsing fontanelles").

No referring to table in Chapter 9	Alias	Key characteristics
20	MaMapeli (Chapter 7.4)	aged 25, primary education, gets married while pregnant, lost two babies presumably due to HIV which was not detected at that time; stays with her mother who discusses PMTCT with MaMapeli's in-laws; MaMapeli stays with her mother for several months after delivery to secure exclusive breastfeeding.
21	MaMong	aged 23, gets married while pregnant, tertiary education; as part of a church community she offered biblical health counselling to fellow students including some HIV awareness; she opted for a caesarean section and exclusive formula feeding, after she returned from her maternal homestead she moved with her husband to his work place in the rural mountains where milk formula may be in short supply.
22	MaMeli (Chapter 3.2 and 4.9)	aged 19, gets married while pregnant, secondary education; she overheard her in-laws talking with her mother about HIV and thinks they may know about her status while she did not manage to disclose to her mother. Her mother advises her on traditional medication which she takes in combination with PMTCT; her mother leaves to be trained as a traditional healer, leaving MaMeli by herself after having delivered in hospital. The baby passes away in childbed, perhaps due to a neonatal sepsis. For the mourning she returns to her in-laws.
23	MaTharo	aged 25, with a boyfriend in separate households, primary education, working in the factory; father passed away of AIDS, mother and sister are also receiving treatment. MaTharo's first baby passed away and she reckons now that it may have died of undetected AIDS, her mother assumes the baby's sickness was due to traditional medication to induce an abortion. Now, she opted for exclusive formula milk until the factory ran out of stock.

No referring to table in Chapter 9	Alias	Key characteristics
24	MaNne	aged 26, married, working as a maid, primary education, lost her first baby aged four months and her in-laws believe it was due to missed rites while she believes the baby died of undetected AIDS; staying at her employer's house without her husband. The first baby was delivered at home and the second is now delivered in hospital.
25	MaHlano	aged 32, married with two children, but separates during pregnancy, tertiary education, works as a pharmacist, separates due to domestic violence (third child to mend relationship?), delivered by caesarean section, opted for formula feeding.
26	MaTselela	aged 34, widowed and married again, primary education, self-employed, pregnant with her fifth child, lost one due to AIDS, considers PMTCT as an opportunity; delivered in hospital; baby is mixed fed.
27	MaSupa	aged 33, widowed with boyfriend in separate households, tertiary education, works as an accountant; lives in her own house with two children; marriage preparations fail during pregnancy; delivered by caesarean section and opted for short-term exclusive breastfeeding and formula feeding thereafter; baby passed away shortly after the delivery for unknown reasons.
28	MaRobeli (Chapter 6.4.2 and 9.5)	aged 25, married, secondary education, unemployed; stays with mother-in-law, while husband works abroad; miscarried a baby and her mother-in-law argued she did not perform rites properly and was bewitched, MaRobeli assumes that she was already HIV+ but not yet tested; stays in waiting mother shelters due to constant conflicts with her mother-in-law; delivered twins in hospital and one passed away. Opted for exclusive breastfeeding, but difficulties to sustain it.

No referring to table in Chapter 9	Alias	Key characteristics
29	MaRobong (Chapter 4.8)	aged 22, married, secondary education, research assistant; discordant couple and conflicts since she wanted to leave the marriage after her HIV+ test result; family elders decide that she must stay in the marriage even though she does not see a future in marriage after their HIV tests; both her family and her family-in-law use traditional medication and she fulfils all rites and takes HIV therapy as prescribed. The baby is delivered by caesarean section, she opts for exclusive breastfeeding.
30	MaMararo	aged 22, with boyfriend, secondary education, working as a traditional healer; expects to get married soon; delivers in hospital and attends hospital counselling with her mother who is also a traditional healer.